Movement Disorders
SOURCEBOOK

Second Edition

Health Reference Series

Second Edition

Movement Disorders
SOURCEBOOK

Basic Consumer Health Information about the Symptoms and Causes of Movement Disorders, Including Parkinson Disease, Amyotrophic Lateral Sclerosis, Cerebral Palsy, Muscular Dystrophy, Multiple Sclerosis, Myasthenia, Myoclonus, Spina Bifida, Dystonia, Essential Tremor, Choreatic Disorders, Huntington Disease, Tourette Syndrome, and Other Disorders That Cause Slowed, Absent, or Excessive Movements

Along with Information about Surgical and Nonsurgical Interventions, Physical Therapies, Strategies for Independent Living, a Glossary of Related Terms, and a Directory of Resources for Additional Help and Information

Edited by
Amy L. Sutton

Omnigraphics

P.O. Box 31-1640, Detroit, MI 48231

Bibliographic Note

Because this page cannot legibly accommodate all the copyright notices, the Bibliographic Note portion of the Preface constitutes an extension of the copyright notice.

Edited by Amy L. Sutton

Health Reference Series

Karen Bellenir, *Managing Editor*
David A. Cooke, M.D., *Medical Consultant*
Elizabeth Collins, *Research and Permissions Coordinator*
Cherry Edwards, *Permissions Assistant*
EdIndex, Services for Publishers, *Indexers*

* * *

Omnigraphics, Inc.

Matthew P. Barbour, *Senior Vice President*
Kevin M. Hayes, *Operations Manager*

* * *

Peter E. Ruffner, *Publisher*

Copyright © 2009 Omnigraphics, Inc.

ISBN 978-0-7808-1034-1

Library of Congress Cataloging-in-Publication Data

Movement disorders sourcebook : basic consumer health information about the symptoms and causes of movement disorders ... / edited by Amy L. Sutton. -- 2nd ed.
   p. cm.
 Summary: "Provides basic consumer health information about diagnosis, treatment, and management of Parkinson disease and other hypokinetic and hyperkinetic movement disorders, along with advice for family members and caregivers"--Provided by publisher.
 Includes bibliographical references and index.
 ISBN 978-0-7808-1034-1 (hardcover : alk. paper) 1. Movement disorders--Popular works. I. Sutton, Amy L.
 RC376.5.M693 2009
 616.8'3--dc22

                                                        2008054682

∞

This book is printed on acid-free paper meeting the ANSI Z39.48 Standard. The infinity symbol that appears above indicates that the paper in this book meets that standard.

Printed in the United States

Table of Contents

Visit www.healthreferenceseries.com to view *A Contents Guide to the Health Reference Series*, a listing of more than 14,000 topics and the volumes in which they are covered.

Part III: Other Hypokinetic Movement Disorders: Slowed or Absent Movements

Part IV: Hyperkinetic Movement Disorders: Excessive or Unwanted Movements

Part V: Diagnosis and Treatment of Movement Disorders

Part VI: Living with Movement Disorders

Part VII: Additional Help and Information

Preface

About This Book

Nearly 40 million Americans—about one in seven people—experience the slowed, stiff, jerky, or excessive motions that characterize the neurological conditions known as movement disorders. For many, movement disorders cause chronic pain, weakness, and disability and make employment and independent living difficult or impossible. Although most movement disorders cannot be cured, patients who get timely diagnoses and educate themselves about medications, surgeries, and therapies may find relief of painful symptoms and face fewer limitations.

Movement Disorders Sourcebook, Second Edition provides information about the common types and symptoms of movement disorders in children and adults. The *Sourcebook* details the causes and treatments of Parkinson disease and provides information on other hypokinetic movement disorders, such as amyotrophic lateral sclerosis, cerebral palsy, muscular dystrophy, multiple sclerosis, myasthenia, myoclonus, spina bifida, and spinal cord injury. Basic facts about hyperkinetic movement disorders, including dystonia, essential tremor, choreatic disorders, Huntington disease, movement disorders during sleep, and Tourette syndrome, are provided. In addition, the book offers information about surgical and nonsurgical treatments, physical therapies, strategies for independent living, and tips for spouses, caregivers, and parents of people with movement disorders. The volume concludes with a glossary of related terms and a directory of resources.

xi

How to Use This Book

This book is divided into parts and chapters. Parts focus on broad areas of interest. Chapters are devoted to single topics within a part.

Part I: Introduction to Movement Disorders provides general information about how the brain, bones, muscles, and joints contribute to the body's movement. This part also offers an overview of some of the most common types of movement disorders and their related symptoms, including ataxia, spasticity, stiffness, cramps, twitching, and tremor.

Part II: Parkinson Disease offers detailed facts on the causes, symptoms, and progression of this well-known movement disorder and its related syndromes. Information on PD therapies and treatments, such as deep brain stimulation, as well as strategies for coping with pain, nutrition, relationships, and employment concerns are also discussed.

Part III: Other Hypokinetic Movement Disorders: Slowed or Absent Movements identifies the symptoms and treatments for hypokinetic movement disorders, including amyotrophic lateral sclerosis, cerebellar or spinocerebellar degeneration, cerebral palsy, muscular dystrophy, multiple sclerosis, myasthenia, myoclonus, spina bifida, and spinal cord injury.

Part IV: Hyperkinetic Movement Disorders: Excessive or Unwanted Movements explains the basics of hyperkinetic disorders, such as dystonia, tremor disorders, chorea, Huntington disease, restless legs syndrome and periodic limb movement disorders, neuroacanthocytosis and neurodegeneration, spastic paraplegia, and Tourette syndrome.

Part V: Diagnosis and Treatment of Movement Disorders highlights specific tests and procedures used to diagnose movement disorders and offers patients advice on assembling a trusted health care team. Current therapies used to treat the symptoms of movement disorders—including botulinum toxin injections, surgical options, medications, and physical therapy—are also discussed, as is the future potential of stem cell therapy for reducing the pain and disability associated with movement disorders.

Part VI: Living with Movement Disorders identifies the everyday concerns of people with movement disorders and their caregivers. Tips on choosing health care facilities, assembling legal documents, dressing, driving, working independently, coping with chronic illness, and supporting and parenting a loved one with a movement disorder are all included in this part.

Part VII: Additional Help and Information includes a glossary of important terms and a directory of organizations for patients with movement disorders and their families.

Bibliographic Note

This volume contains documents and excerpts from publications issued by the following U.S. government agencies: National Cancer Institute (NCI); National Eye Institute (NEI); National Human Genome Research Institute; National Institute of Neurological Disorders and Stroke (NINDS); National Institute on Deafness and Other Communication Disorders (NIDCD); National Institute on Drug Abuse (NIDA); National Institutes of Health (NIH); National Library of Medicine; Social Security Administration (SSA); U.S. Department of Health and Human Services (HHS); and the U.S. Food and Drug Administration (FDA).

In addition, this volume contains copyrighted documents from the following organizations and individuals: A.D.A.M., Inc.; American Academy of Neurology; American Association of Neurological Surgeons; American Psychological Association; Pamela A. Cazzolli, R.N.; Center on Aging, University of Hawaii at Manoa; Children's Hospital of Pittsburgh Spasticity and Movement Disorder Clinic; Cleveland Clinic Foundation; Dystonia Medical Research Foundation; Dystonia Society; Family Caregiver Alliance; International Radiosurgery Association; Lippincott Williams and Wilkins; Muscular Dystrophy Association of the United States; Myasthenia Gravis Foundation of America; NAMI: The Nation's Voice on Mental Illness; National Ataxia Foundation; National Multiple Sclerosis Society; National Parkinson Foundation; The Nemours Foundation; Northwest Hospital Gamma Knife Center; Parkinson's Disease Foundation; Rehabilitation Institute of Chicago; Rush University Medical Center; Society for Progressive Supranuclear Palsy; Spastic Paraplegic Foundation; and the St. Louis Children's Hospital Center for Cerebral Palsy Spasticity.

Full citation information is provided on the first page of each chapter or section. Every effort has been made to secure all necessary rights to reprint the copyrighted material. If any omissions have been made, please contact Omnigraphics to make corrections for future editions.

Acknowledgements

Thanks go to the many organizations, agencies, and individuals who have contributed materials for this *Sourcebook* and to medical consultant Dr. David Cooke and document engineer Bruce Bellenir. Special thanks go to managing editor Karen Bellenir and research and permissions coordinator Liz Collins for their help and support.

About the Health Reference Series

The *Health Reference Series* is designed to provide basic medical information for patients, families, caregivers, and the general public. Each volume takes a particular topic and provides comprehensive coverage. This is especially important for people who may be dealing with a newly diagnosed disease or a chronic disorder in themselves or in a family member. People looking for preventive guidance, information about disease warning signs, medical statistics, and risk factors for health problems will also find answers to their questions in the *Health Reference Series*. The *Series*, however, is not intended to serve as a tool for diagnosing illness, in prescribing treatments, or as a substitute for the physician/patient relationship. All people concerned about medical symptoms or the possibility of disease are encouraged to seek professional care from an appropriate health care provider.

A Note about Spelling and Style

Health Reference Series editors use *Stedman's Medical Dictionary* as an authority for questions related to the spelling of medical terms and the *Chicago Manual of Style* for questions related to grammatical structures, punctuation, and other editorial concerns. Consistent adherence is not always possible, however, because the individual volumes within the *Series* include many documents from a wide variety of different producers and copyright holders, and the editor's primary goal is to present material from each source as accurately as is possible following the terms specified by each document's producer. This sometimes means that information in different chapters or sections may follow other guidelines and alternate spelling authorities. For example, occasionally a copyright holder may require that eponymous terms be shown in possessive forms (Crohn's disease *vs.* Crohn disease) or that British spelling norms be retained (leukaemia *vs.* leukemia).

Locating Information within the Health Reference Series

The *Health Reference Series* contains a wealth of information about a wide variety of medical topics. Ensuring easy access to all the fact sheets, research reports, in-depth discussions, and other material contained within the individual books of the *Series* remains one of our highest priorities. As the *Series* continues to grow in size and scope, however, locating the precise information needed by a reader may become more challenging.

A Contents Guide to the Health Reference Series was developed to direct readers to the specific volumes that address their concerns. It presents an extensive list of diseases, treatments, and other topics of general interest compiled from the Tables of Contents and major index headings. To access *A Contents Guide to the Health Reference Series*, visit www.healthreferenceseries.com.

Medical Consultant

Medical consultation services are provided to the *Health Reference Series* editors by David A. Cooke, M.D. Dr. Cooke is a graduate of Brandeis University, and he received his M.D. degree from the University of Michigan. He completed residency training at the University of Wisconsin Hospital and Clinics. He is board-certified in Internal Medicine. Dr. Cooke currently works as part of the University of Michigan Health System and practices in Ann Arbor, MI. In his free time, he enjoys writing, science fiction, and spending time with his family.

Our Advisory Board

We would like to thank the following board members for providing guidance to the development of this *Series*:

- Dr. Lynda Baker,
  Associate Professor of Library and Information Science,
  Wayne State University, Detroit, MI

- Nancy Bulgarelli,
  William Beaumont Hospital Library, Royal Oak, MI

- Karen Imarisio,
  Bloomfield Township Public Library, Bloomfield Township, MI

- Karen Morgan,
  Mardigian Library, University of Michigan-Dearborn,
  Dearborn, MI

- Rosemary Orlando,
  St. Clair Shores Public Library, St. Clair Shores, MI

Health Reference Series *Update Policy*

The inaugural book in the *Health Reference Series* was the first edition of *Cancer Sourcebook* published in 1989. Since then, the *Series* has been enthusiastically received by librarians and in the medical community. In order to maintain the standard of providing high-quality health information for the layperson the editorial staff at Omnigraphics felt it was necessary to implement a policy of updating volumes when warranted.

Medical researchers have been making tremendous strides, and it is the purpose of the *Health Reference Series* to stay current with the most recent advances. Each decision to update a volume is made on an individual basis. Some of the considerations include how much new information is available and the feedback we receive from people who use the books. If there is a topic you would like to see added to the update list, or an area of medical concern you feel has not been adequately addressed, please write to:

Editor
Health Reference Series
Omnigraphics, Inc.
P.O. Box 31-1640
Detroit, MI 48231
E-mail: editorial@omnigraphics.com

Part One

Introduction to Movement Disorders

Chapter 1

Anatomy of the Brain: How the Brain Controls the Body's Movements

The brain consists of several large regions, each responsible for some of the activities vital for living. These include the brainstem, cerebellum, limbic system, diencephalon, and cerebral cortex.

The brainstem is the part of the brain that connects the brain and the spinal cord. It controls many basic functions, such as heart rate, breathing, eating, and sleeping. The brainstem accomplishes this by directing the spinal cord, other parts of the brain, and the body to do what is necessary to maintain these basic functions.

The cerebellum, which represents only one eighth of the total weight of the human brain, coordinates the brain's instructions for skilled repetitive movements and for maintaining balance and posture. It is a prominent structure located above the brainstem.

On top of the brainstem and buried under the cortex, there is a set of more evolutionarily primitive brain structures called the limbic system (e.g., amygdala and hippocampus. The limbic system structures are involved in many of our emotions and motivations, particularly those that are related to survival, such as fear, anger, and sexual behavior. The limbic system is also involved in feelings of pleasure that are related to our survival, such as those experienced from eating and sex. The large limbic system structure, the hippocampus, is also involved in memory. One of the reasons that drugs of abuse can exert

"Brain's Response to Drugs: Teacher's Guide," from the National Institute on Drug Abuse (NIDA, www.nida.nih.gov), part of the National Institutes of Health, May 2005.

such powerful control over our behavior is that they act directly on the more evolutionarily primitive brainstem and limbic system structures, which can override the cortex in controlling our behavior. In effect, they eliminate the most human part of our brain from its role in controlling our behavior.

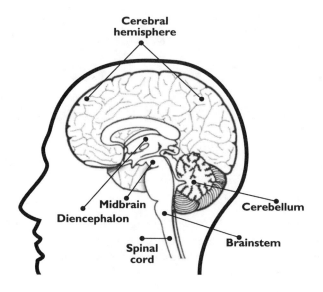

Figure 1.1. *This drawing of a brain cut in half demonstrates some of the major regions of the brain.*

The diencephalon, which is also located beneath the cerebral hemispheres, contains the thalamus and hypothalamus. The thalamus is involved in sensory perception and regulation of motor functions (i.e., movement). It connects areas of the cerebral cortex that are involved in sensory perception and movement with other parts of the brain and spinal cord that also have a role in sensation and movement. The hypothalamus is a very small but important component of the diencephalon. It plays a major role in regulating feeding hormones, the pituitary gland, body temperature, the adrenal glands, and many other vital activities.

The cerebral cortex, which is divided into right and left hemispheres, encompasses about two thirds of the human brain mass and lies over and around most of the remaining structures of the brain. It is the most highly developed part of the human brain and is responsible for thinking, perceiving, and producing and understanding

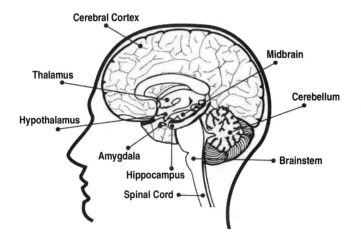

Figure 1.2. This drawing of a brain cut in half demonstrates some of the brain's internal structures. The amygdala and hippocampus are actually located deep within the brain, but are shown as an overlay in the approximate areas that they are located.

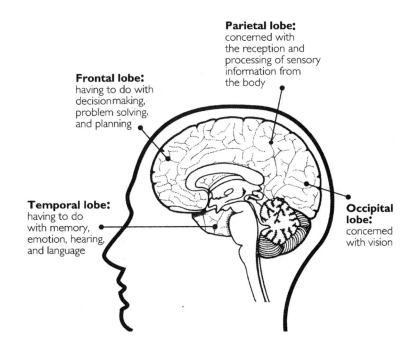

Figure 1.3. This drawing of a brain cut in half demonstrates the lobes of the cerebral cortex and their functions.

language. It is also the most recent structure in the history of brain evolution. The cerebral cortex can be divided into areas that each has a specific function. For example, there are specific areas involved in vision, hearing, touch, movement, and smell. Other areas are critical for thinking and reasoning. Although many functions, such as touch, are found in both the right and left cerebral hemispheres, some functions are found in only one cerebral hemisphere. For example, in most people, language abilities are found in the left hemisphere.

Nerve Cells and Neurotransmission

The brain is made up of billions of nerve cells, also known as neurons. Typically, a neuron contains three important parts: a central cell body that directs all activities of the neuron; dendrites, short fibers that receive messages from other neurons and relay them to the cell body; and an axon, a long single fiber that transmits messages from the cell body to the dendrites of other neurons or to body tissues, such as muscles. Although most neurons contain all of the three parts, there is a wide range of diversity in the shapes and sizes of neurons as well as their axons and dendrites.

The transfer of a message from the axon of one nerve cell to the dendrites of another is known as neurotransmission. Although axons and dendrites are located extremely close to each other, the transmission of a message from an axon to a dendrite does not occur through direct contact. Instead, communication between nerve cells occurs mainly through the release of chemical substances into the space between the axon and dendrites. This space is known as the synapse. When neurons communicate, a message, traveling as an electrical impulse, moves down an axon and toward the synapse. There it triggers the release of molecules called neurotransmitters from the axon into the synapse. The neurotransmitters then diffuse across the synapse and bind to special molecules, called receptors, that are located within the cell membranes of the dendrites of the adjacent nerve cell. This, in turn, stimulates or inhibits an electrical response in the receiving neuron's dendrites. Thus, the neurotransmitters act as chemical messengers, carrying information from one neuron to another.

There are many different types of neurotransmitters, each of which has a precise role to play in the functioning of the brain. Generally, each neurotransmitter can only bind to a very specific matching receptor. Therefore, when a neurotransmitter couples to a receptor, it is like fitting a key into a lock. This coupling then starts a whole cascade of events at both the surface of the dendrite of the receiving nerve cell and inside the cell. In this manner, the message carried by the neurotransmitter is received and processed by the receiving nerve cell. Once this has occurred, the neurotransmitter is inactivated in one of two ways. It is either broken down by an enzyme or reabsorbed back into the nerve cell that released it. The reabsorption (also known as reuptake) is accomplished by what are known as transporter molecules. Transporter molecules reside in the cell membranes of the axons that release the neurotransmitters. They pick up specific neurotransmitters from the synapse and carry them back across the cell membrane and into the axon. The neurotransmitters are then available for reuse at a later time.

As noted above, messages that are received by dendrites are relayed to the cell body and then to the axon. The axons then transmit the messages, which are in the form of electrical impulses, to other neurons or body tissues. The axons of many neurons are covered in a fatty substance known as myelin. Myelin has several functions. One of its most important is to increase the rate at which nerve impulses travel along the axon. The rate of conduction of a nerve impulse along a heavily myelinated axon can be as fast as 120 meters/second. In contrast, a nerve impulse can travel no faster than about 2 meters/second along an axon without myelin. The thickness of the myelin covering on an axon is closely linked to the function of that axon. For example, axons that travel a long distance, such as those that extend from the spinal cord to the foot, generally contain a thick myelin covering to facilitate faster transmission of the nerve impulse. The axons that transmit messages from the brain or spinal cord to muscles and other body tissues are what make up the nerves of the human body. Most of these axons contain a thick covering of myelin, which accounts for the whitish appearance of nerves.

Chapter 2

Bones, Muscles, and Joints: What They Do and How They Move

Every time you walk, settle into a chair, or hug your child, you're using your bones, muscles, and joints. Without these important body parts, we wouldn't be able to stand, walk, run, or even sit.

Bones and What They Do

From our head to our toes, our bones provide support for our bodies and help form our shape. The skull protects the brain and forms the shape of our face. The spinal cord, a pathway for messages between the brain and the body, is protected by the backbone, or spinal column.

The ribs form a cage that shelters the heart, lungs, liver, and spleen, and the pelvis helps protect the bladder, intestines, and in women, the reproductive organs.

Although they're very light, bones are strong enough to support our entire weight.

The human skeleton has 206 bones, which begin to develop before birth. When the skeleton first forms, it is made of flexible cartilage, but within a few weeks it begins the process of ossification. Ossification is when the cartilage is replaced by hard deposits of calcium phosphate and stretchy collagen, the two main components of bone. It takes about 20 years for this process to be completed.

"Bones, Muscles, and Joints," March 2007, reprinted with permission from www.kidshealth.org. Copyright © 2007 The Nemours Foundation. This information was provided by KidsHealth, one of the largest resources online for medically reviewed health information written for parents, kids, and teens. For more articles like this one, visit www.KidsHealth.org, or www.TeensHealth.org.

The bones of kids and young teens are smaller than those of adults and contain "growing zones" called growth plates. These plates consist of columns of multiplying cartilage cells that grow in length, and then change into hard, mineralized bone. These growth plates are easy to spot on an X-ray. Because girls mature at an earlier age than boys, their growth plates change into hard bone at an earlier age.

Bone building continues throughout life, as a body constantly renews and reshapes the bones' living tissue. Bone contains three types of cells: osteoblasts, which make new bone and help repair damage; osteocytes, which carry nutrients and waste products to and from blood vessels in the bone; and osteoclasts, which break down bone and help to sculpt and shape it.

Osteoclasts are very active in kids and teens, working on bone as it is remodeled during growth. They also play an important role in the repair of fractures.

Bones are made up of calcium, phosphorus, sodium, and other minerals, as well as the protein collagen. Calcium is needed to make bones hard, which allows them to support body weight. Bones also store calcium and release some into the bloodstream when it's needed by other parts of the body. The amounts of certain vitamins and minerals that you eat, especially vitamin D and calcium, directly affect how much calcium is stored in the bones.

The soft bone marrow inside many of the bones is where most of the blood cells are made. The bone marrow contains stem cells, which produce the body's red blood cells and platelets. Red blood cells carry oxygen to the body's tissues, and platelets help with blood clotting when someone has a cut or wound.

Bones are made up of two types of bone:

1. **Compact bone** is the solid, hard, outside part of the bone. It looks like ivory and is extremely strong. Holes and channels run through it, carrying blood vessels and nerves from the periosteum, the bone's membrane covering, to its inner parts.

2. **Cancellous bone**, which looks like a sponge, is inside the compact bone. It is made up of a mesh-like network of tiny pieces of bone called trabeculae. The spaces in this network are filled with red marrow, found mainly at the ends of bones, and yellow marrow, which is mostly fat.

Bones are fastened to other bones by long, fibrous straps called ligaments. Cartilage, a flexible, rubbery substance in our joints, supports bones and protects them where they rub against each other.

10

Muscles and What They Do

Bones don't work alone—they need help from the muscles and joints. Muscles pull on the joints, allowing us to move. They also help your body perform other functions so you can grow and remain strong, such as chewing food and then moving it through the digestive system.

The human body has more than 650 muscles, which make up half of a person's body weight. They are connected to bones by tough, cord-like tissues called tendons, which allow the muscles to pull on bones. If you wiggle your fingers, you can see the tendons on the back of your hand move as they do their work.

Humans have three different kinds of muscle:

1. **Skeletal muscle** is attached to bone, mostly in the legs, arms, abdomen, chest, neck, and face. Skeletal muscles are called striated because they are made up of fibers that have horizontal stripes when viewed under a microscope. These muscles hold the skeleton together, give the body shape, and help it with everyday movements (known as voluntary muscles because you can control their movement). They can contract (shorten or tighten) quickly and powerfully, but they tire easily and have to rest between workouts.

2. **Smooth, or involuntary, muscle** is also made of fibers, but this type of muscle looks smooth, not striated. Generally, we can't consciously control our smooth muscles; rather, they're controlled by the nervous system automatically (which is why they're also called involuntary). Examples of smooth muscles are the walls of the stomach and intestines, which help break up food and move it through the digestive system. Smooth muscle is also found in the walls of blood vessels, where it squeezes the stream of blood flowing through the vessels to help maintain blood pressure. Smooth muscles take longer to contract than skeletal muscles do, but they can stay contracted for a long time because they don't tire easily.

3. **Cardiac muscle** is found in the heart. The walls of the heart's chambers are composed almost entirely of muscle fibers. Cardiac muscle is also an involuntary type of muscle. Its rhythmic, powerful contractions force blood out of the heart as it beats.

Even when you sit perfectly still, muscles throughout your body are constantly moving. Muscles enable your heart to beat, your chest to

11

rise and fall as you breathe, and your blood vessels to help regulate the pressure and flow of blood through your body. When we smile and talk, muscles are helping us communicate, and when we exercise, they help us stay physically fit and healthy.

The movements your muscles make are coordinated and controlled by the brain and nervous system. The involuntary muscles are controlled by structures deep within the brain and the upper part of the spinal cord called the brain stem. The voluntary muscles are regulated by the parts of the brain known as the cerebral motor cortex and the cerebellum.

When you decide to move, the motor cortex sends an electrical signal through the spinal cord and peripheral nerves to the muscles, causing them to contract. The motor cortex on the right side of the brain controls the muscles on the left side of the body and vice versa.

The cerebellum coordinates the muscle movements ordered by the motor cortex. Sensors in the muscles and joints send messages back through peripheral nerves to tell the cerebellum and other parts of the brain where and how the arm or leg is moving and what position it's in. This feedback results in smooth, coordinated motion. If you want to lift your arm, your brain sends a message to the muscles in your arm and you move it. When you run, the messages to the brain are more involved, because many muscles have to work in rhythm.

Muscles move body parts by contracting and then relaxing. Your muscles can pull bones, but they can't push them back to the original position. So they work in pairs of flexors and extensors. The flexor contracts to bend a limb at a joint. Then, when you've completed the movement, the flexor relaxes and the extensor contracts to extend or straighten the limb at the same joint. For example, the biceps muscle, in the front of the upper arm, is a flexor, and the triceps, at the back of the upper arm, is an extensor. When you bend at your elbow, the biceps contracts. Then the biceps relaxes and the triceps contracts to straighten the elbow.

Joints and What They Do

Joints occur where two bones meet. They make the skeleton flexible—without them, movement would be impossible.

Joints allow our bodies to move in many ways. Some joints open and close like a hinge (such as knees and elbows), whereas others allow for more complicated movement—a shoulder or hip joint, for example, allows for backward, forward, sideways, and rotating movement.

Joints are classified by their range of movement. Immovable, or fibrous, joints don't move. The dome of the skull, for example, is made of bony plates, which must be immovable to protect the brain. Between the edges of these plates are links, or joints, of fibrous tissue. Fibrous joints also hold the teeth in the jawbone.

Partially movable, or cartilaginous, joints move a little. They are linked by cartilage, as in the spine. Each of the vertebrae in the spine moves in relation to the one above and below it, and together these movements give the spine its flexibility.

Freely movable, or synovial, joints move in many directions. The main joints of the body—found at the hip, shoulders, elbows, knees, wrists, and ankles—are freely movable. They are filled with synovial fluid, which acts as a lubricant to help the joints move easily.

Three kinds of freely movable joints play a big part in voluntary movement:

1. **Hinge joints** allow movement in one direction, as seen in the knees and elbows.

2. **Pivot joints** allow a rotating or twisting motion, like that of the head moving from side to side.

3. **Ball-and-socket joints** allow the greatest freedom of movement. The hips and shoulders have this type of joint, in which the round end of a long bone fits into the hollow of another bone.

Problems with the Bones, Muscles, and Joints

As strong as bones are, they can break. Muscles can weaken, and joints (as well as tendons, ligaments, and cartilage) can be damaged by injury or disease.

Problems that can affect the bones, muscles, and joints include:

Arthritis: Arthritis is the inflammation of a joint, and people who have it experience swelling, warmth, pain, and often have trouble moving. Although we often think of arthritis as a condition that affects only older people, arthritis can also occur in children and teens. Health problems that involve arthritis in kids and teens include juvenile rheumatoid arthritis (JRA), lupus, Lyme disease, and septic arthritis (a bacterial infection of a joint).

Fracture: A fracture occurs when a bone breaks; it may crack, snap, or shatter. After a fracture, new bone cells fill the gap and repair the break. Applying a strong plaster cast, which keeps the bone in the correct position until it heals, is the usual treatment. If the fracture is complicated, metal pins and plates can be placed to better stabilize it while the bone heals.

Muscular dystrophy: Muscular dystrophy is an inherited group of diseases that affect the muscles, causing them to weaken and break down over time. The most common form in childhood is called Duchenne muscular dystrophy, and it most often affects boys.

Osgood-Schlatter disease (OSD): Osgood-Schlatter disease is an inflammation (pain and swelling) of the bone, cartilage, and/or tendon at the top of the shinbone, where the tendon from the kneecap attaches. OSD usually strikes active teens around the beginning of their growth spurts, the approximately 2-year period during which they grow most rapidly.

Osteomyelitis: Osteomyelitis is a bone infection often caused by *Staphylococcus aureus* bacteria, though other types of bacteria can cause it, too. In kids and teens, osteomyelitis usually affects the long bones of the arms and legs. Osteomyelitis often develops after an injury or trauma.

Osteoporosis: In osteoporosis, bone tissue becomes brittle, thin, and spongy. Bones break easily, and the spine sometimes begins to crumble and collapse. Although the condition usually affects older people, kids and teens with eating disorders can get the condition, as can girls with female athlete triad—a combination of three conditions that some girls who exercise or play sports may be at risk for: disordered eating, amenorrhea (loss of a girl's period), and osteoporosis. Participation in sports where a thin appearance is valued can put a girl at risk for female athlete triad.

Repetitive stress injuries (RSIs): RSIs are a group of injuries that happen when too much stress is placed on a part of the body, resulting in inflammation (pain and swelling), muscle strain, or tissue damage. This stress generally occurs from repeating the same movements over and over again. RSIs are becoming more common in kids and teens because they spend more time than ever using computers. Playing sports like tennis that involve repetitive motions can also lead to RSIs. Kids and teens who spend a lot of time playing musical instruments or video games are also at risk for RSIs.

Scoliosis: Every person's spine curves a little bit; a certain amount of curvature is necessary for people to move and walk properly. But 3–5 people out of 1,000 have scoliosis, which causes the spine to curve too much. It can be hereditary, so someone who has scoliosis often has family members who have it.

Strains and sprains: Strains occur when muscles or tendons are overstretched. Sprains are an overstretching or a partial tearing of the ligaments. Strains usually happen when a person takes part in a strenuous activity when the muscles haven't properly warmed up or the muscle is not used to the activity (such as a new sport or playing a familiar sport after a long break). Sprains, on the other hand, are usually the result of an injury, such as twisting an ankle or knee. A common sprain injury is a torn Achilles tendon, which connects the calf muscles to the heel. This tendon can snap, but it usually can be repaired by surgery. Both strains and sprains are common in kids and teens because they're active and still growing.

Tendinitis: This common sports injury usually happens after overexercising a muscle. The tendon and tendon sheath become inflamed, which can be painful. Resting the muscles and taking anti-inflammatory medication can bring relief.

Chapter 3

Types of Movement Disorders

Ataxia

A degenerative disorder affecting the brain, brainstem, or spinal cord. This can result in clumsiness, inaccuracy, instability, imbalance, tremor, or a lack of coordination while performing voluntary movements. Movements are not smooth and may appear disjointed or jerky. Patients may fall down frequently due to an unsteady gait. Ataxia can also affect speech and movement of the eyes.

If a metabolic disorder can be identified as the underlying cause, specific treatment may be available in select cases. The cornerstone of treatment for ataxia of parkinsonism (or parkinsonism of any cause) is the use of oral L-DOPA. Other medications used to treat ataxia associated with parkinsonism (or parkinsonism of any cause) include anticholinergics, dopamine agonists, amantadine, selegiline, and entacapone. In children with ataxia, generally only anticholinergics are prescribed.

Dystonia

A neurological muscle disorder characterized by involuntary muscle spasms. Dystonia results from abnormal functioning of the basal ganglia, a deep part of the brain which helps control coordination of movement. These regions of the brain control the speed and fluidity of movement and prevent unwanted movements. Patients with dystonia may experience uncontrollable twisting, repetitive movements, or abnormal postures and positions. These can affect any part of the body, including the arms, legs, trunk, eyelids and vocal cords. General dystonia involves the entire body. Focal dystonias involve only one body location, most commonly the neck (spasmodic torticollis), eyelids (blepharospasm), lower face (Meige syndrome), or hand (writer's cramp or limb dystonia). Depending on what part of the body is affected, the condition can be very disabling.

There is a three-tiered approach to treating dystonia: botulinum toxin (Botox) injections, medication, and surgery. These may be used alone or in combination. Botox injections help block the communication between the nerve and the muscle and may lessen abnormal movements and postures. Surgery is considered when other treatments have proven ineffective. The goal of surgery is to interrupt the pathways responsible for the abnormal movements at various levels of the nervous system. Some operations purposely damage small regions of the thalamus (thalamotomy), globus pallidus (pallidotomy), or other deep centers in the brain. Deep brain stimulation (DBS) has been tried recently with some success. Other surgeries include cutting nerves leading to the nerve roots deep in the neck close to the spinal cord (anterior cervical rhizotomy) or removing the nerves at the point they enter the contracting muscles (selective peripheral denervation).

Essential Tremor

An uncontrolled shaking or trembling, usually of one or both hands or arms, that worsens when basic movements are attempted. Essential tremor affects about 5 million people in the United States, with a higher incidence in people age 60 and older. It is caused by abnormalities in areas of the brain that control movement and is not tied to an underlying disease (e.g., Parkinson's disease). About 50 percent of patients have a family history of the condition. This condition usually does not result in serious complications, but it can certainly interfere with daily activities and cause distress.

In some cases, physical therapy or changes in lifestyle may improve symptoms. If the condition affects a patient's ability to perform daily tasks and has a negative impact on quality of life, medication or surgery are considered. About 50 to 75 percent of patients taking medications have a reduction of their tremor. Beta-blockers, antiseizure medications, benzodiazepines, and carbonic anhydrase inhibitors often are prescribed. Beta-blockers are usually prescribed for younger patients because they may cause memory loss and confusion in older patients. Botox injections help block the communication between the nerve and the muscle and may lessen tremor.

If the tremor is so severe that is causes a disability, surgery may be recommended. Thalamotomy purposely destroys a portion of the area deep within the brain that receives sensory messages (thalamus). About 75 percent of patients undergoing this procedure find relief on one side of their body. Surgery on both sides of the thalamus is rarely done due to the high risk of speech loss. DBS is another surgical option in severe cases of essential tremor that have not responded to medication. A hair-thin wire is implanted in the thalamus and connected to a neurostimulator implanted under the collarbone. The neurostimulator sends electrical impulses along the wire to the thalamus, interrupting signals that cause tremor.

Huntington's Disease

A progressive, degenerative, and fatal disease caused by the deterioration of certain nerve cells in the brain. Onset most often occurs between ages 35 and 50, with the condition progressing without remission over 10 to 25 years. Huntington's disease affects an estimated one in every 10,000 people in the United States. A juvenile form of the disease affects patients age 20 and younger, accounting for about 16 percent of all cases. Symptoms include jerking; uncontrollable movements of the limbs, trunk, and face; progressive loss of mental abilities; and the development of psychiatric problems. The condition is hereditary—a child with one affected parent has a 50 percent chance of developing Huntington's disease.

There is no cure for Huntington's disease, so treatment focuses on reducing symptoms, preventing complications, and helping patients and family members cope with daily challenges. Doctors may prescribe antipsychotics, antidepressants, tranquilizers, mood stabilizers, or Botox injections. These are prescribed in the lowest effective dosage, as all of these medications may have side effects. Huntington's disease usually runs its full terminal course in 10 to 30 years. Researchers have observed that the earlier in life the symptoms occur, the faster the disease often progresses.

Multiple System Atrophy (MSA)

A progressive, neurodegenerative disease affecting movement, blood pressure, and other body functions. Because symptoms, onset, and severity of MSA vary from person to person, differing ranges of symptoms were designated initially as three different diseases: Shy-Drager syndrome, striatonigral degeneration, and olivopontocerebellar atrophy. All of these are now classified under MSA. Symptoms include stiffness or rigidity; freezing or slowed movements; instability; loss of balance; loss of coordination; a significant fall in blood pressure when standing, causing dizziness, lightheadedness, fainting, or blurred vision (orthostatic hypotension); male impotence; urinary difficulties; constipation; and speech and swallowing difficulties.

Medication may be prescribed to treat some of the symptoms associated with this disease. Levodopa and dopamine agonists used to treat Parkinson's disease may be effective in treating slowness and rigidity in some patients. Orthostatic hypotension can be improved by prescribing drugs that raise blood pressure. As this disease progresses, the benefits of medication lessen. In cases that have progressed and are more severe, a feeding tube may be needed when the patient cannot swallow food on his or her own.

Myoclonus

A twitching or intermittent spasm of a muscle or group of muscles. Myoclonus is classified into several major types and many subcategories. The most common type is cortical myoclonus, arising from an area of the brain known as the sensorimotor cortex. Jerky movements usually have a regular rhythm and may be limited to one muscle or muscle group (focal) or several different muscle groups (multifocal). They may occur without an obvious cause or be a result of many diseases. Some of the diseases associated with myoclonus are celiac disease, Angelman syndrome, Huntington's disease, Rett syndrome, Creutzfeldt-Jakob disease, and Alzheimer's disease. Subcortical myoclonus usually affects many muscle groups (generalized) and may be the result of abnormally low levels of oxygen in the brain (hypoxia) or a metabolic process, such as kidney or liver failure. Spinal myoclonus is usually caused by a focal spinal lesion, such as multiple sclerosis, syringomyelia, trauma, ischemic myelopathy, or an infection such as herpes zoster, Lyme disease, *E. coli,* or HIV [human immunodeficiency syndrome]. The jerking often lasts longer and is more variable than in cortical or subcortical myoclonus and continues during sleep. The most common type of peripheral myoclonus is hemifacial spasm, which may occur for no underlying reason or may be caused by compression of the facial nerve. Movements persist during sleep and may last for only a few days or for as long as a few months. The exact type of myoclonus is delineated further by the parts of the body affected and by the underlying causes.

Myoclonus is treated through prescribing medications that may help reduce symptoms. In some cases, effective results are achieved by combining multiple drugs. Some of the medications prescribed are barbiturates, phenytoin, primidone, sodium valproate, or the tranquilizer clonazepam. All of these medications have potential side effects, so it is very important for patients to work closely with their doctor on medication management.

Parkinson's Disease

A progressive disorder that is caused by degeneration of nerve cells in the part of the brain called the substantia nigra, which controls movement. These nerve cells die or become impaired, losing the ability to produce an important chemical called dopamine. Parkinson's produces many common symptoms, including: tremor; muscle rigidity or stiffness of the limbs; gradual loss of spontaneous movement, often leading to decreased mental skill or reaction time, voice changes, or decreased facial expression; gradual loss of automatic movement, often leading to decreased blinking, decreased frequency of swallowing, and drooling; a stooped, flexed posture, with bending at the elbows, knees, and hips; an unsteady walk or balance; and depression or dementia. It is estimated that 60,000 new cases of Parkinson's disease are diagnosed each year, adding to the estimated 1 to 1.5 million Americans who currently have the disease. While the condition usually develops after the age of 55, the disease may affect people in their 30s and 40s.

Most Parkinson's patients are treated with medications to relieve the symptoms of the disease. Some common medications used are dopamine precursors, dopamine agonists, and anticholinergics. Surgery is considered when medications have proven ineffective. DBS of the subthalamic nucleus or globus pallidus can be effective in treating all of the primary motor features of Parkinson's and sometimes allows for significant decreases in medication doses. Thalamotomy can help stop tremor by placing a small lesion in a specific nucleus of the thalamus.

Progressive Supranuclear Palsy (PSP)

A rare brain disorder that causes serious and permanent neurological problems. People with PSP experience a gradual loss of specific brain cells, causing slowing of movement and reduced control of walking, balance, swallowing, speech, and eye movement. Often, there are personality and cognitive changes, causing emotional outbursts and a decrease in intellectual abilities. This disease more commonly affects people ages 40 to 60 and usually runs its full terminal course in 6 to 10 years. It is sometimes misdiagnosed as Parkinson's disease due to the similarity in symptoms. While the cause of PSP is unknown, researchers know that a brain protein called tau accumulates in abnormal clumps in certain brain cells in people with PSP, causing the cells to die. There appears to be a genetic predisposition.

Unfortunately, there is no effective medication to treat PSP, but research is ongoing. Medications that may have a slight benefit are levodopa, amantadine, and amitriptyline. Botox injections may be used to treat the blepharospasm (involuntary eyelid closure) that occurs in some people with PSP.

Rett Syndrome (RTT)

A progressive neurological disorder that causes debilitating symptoms including reduced muscle tone, autistic-like behavior, repetitive hand movements, irregular breathing, decreased ability to express feelings, developmental delays in brain and head growth, gait abnormalities, and seizures. Loss of muscle tone is usually the first symptom. About one in every 10,000 to 15,000 baby girls are diagnosed with RTT, but the prevalence may be much higher due to undiagnosed cases. RTT can affect boys, but they account for only a very small percentage of cases. RTT is caused by mutations in the gene MECP2, located on the X chromosome. Children with RTT appear to develop normally until 6 to 18 months of age, at which point symptoms start to appear. RTT leaves its victims profoundly disabled, requiring maximum assistance with all aspects of daily living.

Unfortunately, there is no cure for RTT. Treatment for the disorder focuses on the management of symptoms and requires a supportive, multidisciplinary approach. The disorder progresses through four major stages, each with characteristic symptoms and medical implications. Medication may be needed for breathing irregularities and motor difficulties. Antiepileptic drugs may be used to control seizures. Occupational therapy, education, and supportive services are geared towards helping individuals with RTT cope with daily challenges and maintain a quality of life. Although it is severely debilitating, individuals with RTT have lived to middle age, but rarely beyond age 40 to 50.

Secondary Parkinsonism

A disorder with symptoms similar to Parkinson's disease, but caused by medication side effects, different neurodegenerative disorders, illness, or brain damage. As in Parkinson's disease, many common symptoms may develop, including tremor; muscle rigidity or stiffness of the limbs; gradual loss of spontaneous movement, often leading to decreased mental skill or reaction time, voice changes, or decreased facial expression; gradual loss of automatic movement, often leading to decreased blinking, decreased frequency of swallowing, and drooling; a stooped, flexed posture with bending at the elbows, knees and hips; an unsteady walk or balance; and depression or dementia. Unlike Parkinson's disease, the risk of developing secondary parkinsonism may be minimized by careful medication management, particularly limiting the usage of specific types of antipsychotic medications.

Many of the medications used to treat this condition have potential side effects, so it is very important to work closely with your doctor on medication management. Unfortunately, secondary parkinsonism does not seem to respond as effectively to medical therapy as Parkinson's disease.

Spasticity

Increased muscle contractions causing stiffness or tightness of the muscles that may interfere with movement, speech, and walking. Spasticity is usually caused by damage to the portion of the brain or spinal cord that controls voluntary movement. It may result from spinal cord injury, multiple sclerosis, cerebral palsy, stroke, brain damage caused by a lack of oxygen, severe head injury, and metabolic diseases such as Lou Gehrig's disease.

Treatment may include medications such as baclofen, diazepam, tizanidine, or clonazepam. Physical therapy with specific muscle exercises may be prescribed, in an effort to help reduce the severity of symptoms. Surgery may be recommended for tendon release or to cut the nerve-muscle pathway. The prognosis depends on the severity of the spasticity and the underlying disorder(s).

Tardive Dyskinesia

A muscle disorder that results from prolonged exposure to some types of antipsychotic and neuroleptic medications. TD is characterized by repetitive, involuntary, purposeless movements such as grimacing, lip smacking, eye blinking, or rapid leg and arm movements. The condition can be quite embarrassing because it cannot be controlled. TD may be mild and reversible in many cases. The percentage of patients who develop severe or irreversible TD is quite low in proportion to those receiving long-term antipsychotic therapy. Older adults are more susceptible to persistent and irreversible TD than younger people. New classes of antipsychotic medications have decreased the prevalence of TD considerably.

While there is no treatment for TD, the risk of developing TD may be minimized by prescribing newer classes of antipsychotics to treat psychosis, restricting the long-term use of neuroleptics to well-defined indications, and prescribing these medications in the lowest effective dosage. It is also important that patients taking these medications are frequently monitored for symptoms.

Tourette Syndrome

A hereditary, neurological disorder characterized by repeated involuntary movements and uncontrollable vocal sounds called tics. This disorder evidences itself most often between the ages of 6 and 15, but may occur as early as age 2, or as late as age 20. The first symptoms are often involuntary movements (tics), most commonly of the face, followed by the arms, legs or trunk. These tics are frequent, repetitive, and quick. Verbal tics (vocalizations) usually occur with the movements; later they may replace one or more movement tics. Vocalizations include grunting, throat clearing, shouting, and barking. Verbal tics may also be expressed as coprolalia (the involuntary use of obscene words or socially unacceptable words and phrases) or copropraxia (obscene gestures). It is estimated that in 70 percent of cases, the tics disappear in a person's early 20s.

The major problem faced by people with TS is socialization and acceptance by peers because the condition can be quite embarrassing. Often, tic symptoms do not cause serious enough impairment to require medication. However, there are many types of medications prescribed for those whose symptoms interfere with functioning. Because all of these medications have potentially serious side effects, they should be prescribed in the lowest effective dosage.

Wilson's Disease

A genetic disorder that causes excessive copper accumulation in the liver or brain. Although copper accumulation begins at birth, symptoms begin appearing between the ages of 6 and 40, but most commonly in late adolescence. Wilson's disease affects an estimated one in 30,000 people worldwide. It is an autosomal recessive disease, occurring equally in males and females. In order to inherit it, both parents must carry a gene that is passed along to the child. Consequences include liver disease and psychiatric and neurological problems. Physical signs include jaundice, abdominal swelling, vomiting of blood, abdominal pain, tremor, and difficulty in walking, talking or swallowing. Psychiatric signs include homicidal or suicidal behavior, depression, and aggression. If undetected and untreated, the disorder is always fatal.

Early diagnosis is crucial since liver damage may occur before the onset of symptoms. Family members of those with a confirmed diagnosis of Wilson's disease require testing and screening for the disease even if they have no symptoms. Screening tests should include the evaluation of serum ceruloplasmin levels and urinary copper output. Treatment of Wilson's disease generally involves removing excess copper from the body and preventing it from reaccumulating. Most cases are treated with the medications zinc acetate, trientine, and penicillamine. Penicillamine and trientine increase urinary excretion of copper, but both can cause serious side effects. Zinc acetate blocks the absorption of copper, increases copper excretion in the stool, and causes no serious side effects; thus, it is often considered the treatment of choice. Treatment is lifelong and also involves avoiding copper-rich foods in one's diet.

Chapter 4

Common Symptoms of Movement Disorders

Chapter Contents

27

Section 4.1

Ataxia

What is ataxia?

Ataxia is a symptom, not a specific disease. Ataxia means clumsiness, or loss of coordination. Ataxia may affect the fingers and hands, the arms or legs, the body, speech, or eye movements. This loss of coordination may be caused by a number of different medical or neurological conditions; for this reason, it is important that a person with ataxia seek medical attention to determine the underlying cause of the symptom and to get the appropriate treatment.

What causes ataxia?

Most often, ataxia is caused by loss of function in the part of the brain which serves as the "coordination center," which is the cerebellum. The cerebellum is located toward the back and lower part of the head. The right side of the cerebellum controls coordination on the left. The central part of the cerebellum is involved in coordinating the very complex movements of gait, or walking. Other parts of the cerebellum help to coordinate eye movements, speech, and swallowing.

Ataxia may also be caused by dysfunction of the pathways leading into and out of the cerebellum. Information comes into the cerebellum from the spinal cord and other parts of the brain, and signals from the cerebellum go out to the spinal cord and to the brain. Although the cerebellum does not directly control strength ("motor function") or feeling (" sensory function"), the motor and sensory pathways must work properly to provide the correct input into the cerebellum. Thus, a person with impaired strength or sensation may notice clumsiness or poor coordination, and the doctor may say that person has ataxia.

How does a physician diagnose ataxia?

Remember, ataxia is a symptom, not a diagnosis. If you have clumsiness or loss of coordination in an arm or both legs or slurred speech, the physician may say that you have an ataxic arm, or ataxic gait, or ataxic speech. Then the physician will first ask many questions about your ataxia, how it came on, whether it is getting worse, whether there are any other symptoms, and so on.

A very important part of the evaluation is the neurological examination. The physician can usually determine whether the ataxia is caused by trouble in the cerebellum, its associated pathways, or other parts of the nervous system by this neurological examination. A careful neurologic and general physical examination can also determine whether other parts of the nervous system are impaired and whether a medical illness may be causing the ataxia.

Blood tests and x-rays including an MRI [magnetic resonance imaging test] may be very helpful in the diagnosing specific medical or neurological conditions that can cause ataxia, or in "ruling out" suspected cases. Genetic testing is available for various types of ataxia.

Here is a list of some medical and neurological conditions that can cause ataxia to appear suddenly:

- Head trauma
- Stroke
- Brain hemorrhage
- Brain tumor
- Congenital abnormality (the back part of the brain was formed in an unusual way)
- Postinfectious (after a severe viral infection)
- Exposure to certain drugs or toxins (e.g., alcohol, seizure medicine)
- Following cardiac or respiratory arrest

Here is a list of some medical and neurological conditions that can cause ataxia to appear gradually:

- Hypothyroidism
- Deficiencies of certain vitamins (e.g., vitamin E, vitamin B12)
- Exposure to certain drugs or toxins (e.g., heavy metals, seizure medicine, chronic alcohol exposure, certain cancer drugs) related to certain kinds of cancer (e.g., ovarian, lung cancer)

- Congenital abnormality (the back part of the brain was formed in an unusual way)

- Multiple sclerosis

- Syphilis (locomotor ataxia)

- Hereditary disorders

- Idiopathic (unknown cause) cerebellar degeneration disorders

You can see that the list of conditions that the physicians must think about as causes of ataxia is rather long; proper diagnosis may require a number of examinations, x-rays, MRIs, and tests.

How is ataxia treated?

There is no medicine which specifically treats the symptoms of ataxia. If ataxia is due to a stroke, a low vitamin level, or exposure to a toxic drug or chemical, then treatment would include treatment of the stroke, vitamin therapy, or avoiding the toxic drug or chemical. There is no reason to think that taking vitamins or thyroid medication will help ataxia that is not caused by vitamin or thyroid deficiency.

The treatment of incoordination or ataxia then mostly involves the use of adaptive devices to allow the ataxia individual to maintain as much independence as possible. Such devices may include a cane, crutches, walker, or wheelchair for those with impaired gait; devices to assist with writing, feeding, and self-care if hand and arm coordination is impaired; and communication devices for those with impaired speech. Many people with hereditary or sporadic forms of ataxia have other symptoms in addition to ataxia. Medication or other therapies such as physical therapy or speech therapy might be appropriate for some of these symptoms, which could include tremor, stiffness, depression, spasticity, and sleep disorders, among others.

How can the National Ataxia Foundation help?

The National Ataxia Foundation is interested in all forms of hereditary ataxias and sporadic ataxia. While treatment and prognosis of ataxia due to other causes such as stroke or tumor depends primarily on the treatment of the underlying cause, for the hereditary and sporadic ataxias, little is understood of the underlying cause and no definite treatment is available.

The National Ataxia Foundation [NAF] is committed to education about ataxia, service to individuals afflicted with the various forms of ataxia, and promoting research to find the causes, better treatments, or a cure for ataxia. NAF can help by providing information for you, your family, and your physician about ataxia.

Section 4.2

Spasticity

"Spasticity," Christina Marciniak, M.D.
© 2008 Rehabilitation Institute of Chicago (www.lifecenter.ric.org).
All rights reserved. Reprinted with permission.

What is spasticity?

Spasticity is a term used to describe abnormal involuntary tightening of muscles that either occurs spontaneously or when the body is stimulated in certain ways (for example, when a joint is moved). Spasticity may be seen in association with rapid repetitive muscle spasms, called clonus. These muscles spasms are often found at the ankle.

What causes spasticity?

Spasticity is a nerve and muscle condition that occurs after an injury to the brain or the spinal cord. Nerve cells below the level of the injury become disconnected from the brain. These nerves are then in a "turned on" state, constantly sending a chemical signal to the muscle, causing it to tighten. Spasticity is often not seen immediately after an injury, but may become gradually worse weeks to months following the event. Conditions that commonly lead to spasticity include strokes, cerebral palsy, spinal cord injuries, traumatic brain injuries, and multiple sclerosis.

What makes spasticity worse?

- Rapidly moving a joint
- Sensory stimulation (such as pressure or touch)

- Medical problems such as pain or skin breakdown
- Infections of the bladder or kidney
- Constipation
- Restrictive or tight clothing
- Certain body positions, e.g., sitting, lying in bed, walking, or other activities
- Fatigue
- Certain times of the day or night

All these factors should be considered and checked if someone experiences a sudden increase in their spasticity.

What are the consequences of spasticity?

Spasticity may be mild and cause only slight muscle stiffness. As it becomes more severe, the stiffness may lead to muscle, tendon, and joint shortening, called contracture. The tightening may also be painful. Involuntary tightening can be reduced with medicines; however, a fixed contracture, which occurs when the muscle and the other structures become permanently short, will not be helped by the anti-spasticity medicine. This can only be treated by stretching, splinting, serial casting (progressive casts that gradually stretch out the muscle), or surgery.

Spasticity and contractures may impact a person's ability to do the daily activities such as dressing, eating, toileting, and grooming. Severe tightness in the armpit, groin, or hand can cause problems for hygiene and can lead to skin breakdown. In the upper body or leg, spasticity can affect sitting, transfers, and walking. Sometimes spasticity is helpful. For example, some people are able to trigger a spasm to help roll over, or leg tightness can help someone stand when his or her leg muscles are weak. These aspects of spasticity need to be considered when spasticity is treated.

What treatments are available to treat spasticity?

Spasticity does not always need to be treated. It is best to consult with a medical professional who is familiar with spasticity and its treatment. There are different types of treatments available.

- Stretching is an important part of any program to help prevent contracture development.

- Splinting can be used in addition to stretching to help maintain joint position.

- Medications that relax the muscles may also be tried. These can be given orally, injected into muscles, or into the space around the spine that contains the spinal fluid. Some patients with severe spasticity may need to be on multiple medicines, or may need to use oral medicines in combination with muscle or nerve injections, called chemodenervation.

With severe spasticity, a treatment team may be needed to assess the best methods of intervention. This team can include rehabilitation professionals and physicians including a physical therapist, occupational therapist, speech therapist, rehabilitation engineer, nurse, and physiatrist (rehabilitation doctor). A neurosurgeon or an orthopedic surgeon may be involved, particularly if surgery is anticipated. Some centers have spasticity clinics where patients may be seen by these multiple professionals for an assessment.

References

- www.WeMove.org

- *Muscle and Nerve,* Supplement 6/1997: Spasticity: Etiology, Evaluation, Management, and the Role of Botulinum Toxin Type A.

Section 4.3

Stiffness, Cramps, and Twitching

Neuromuscular diseases can cause a variety of symptoms other than muscle weakness. Some people may feel their muscles are stiff or don't respond quickly; others might complain of cramps or twitches; while still others get tired quickly during exercise.

Not all of these symptoms are painful, but some can be inconvenient or annoying. Learning the medical names and nature of these symptoms can lead to better discourse between you and your doctor, and sometimes better management of symptoms.

Cramps

A true cramp is a specific condition in which muscles undergo painful involuntary contractions (muscle shortening). The classic muscle cramp is neural in origin, meaning the contractions are caused by abnormal nerve activity rather than abnormal muscle activity. This type of contraction problem usually has a sudden onset and may be ended by stretching the muscle passively.

True cramps can occur in anyone, particularly after exercise or at night. Neuromuscular diseases in which classic cramps are common are amyotrophic lateral sclerosis (ALS) and spinal muscular atrophy (SMA).

A second kind of cramp, which doesn't involve abnormal nerve activity, occurs when a muscle is temporarily locked in a contracted state. This is technically called a contracture, but isn't to be confused with the more common use of "contracture" to indicate fixed joints.

This sensation can be painful and is often described as a cramp. People with paramyotonia congenita, some forms of myotonia, rippling muscle syndrome or metabolic myopathies due to glycolytic defects (McArdle disease, Cori or Forbes disease, Tarui disease, phosphoglycerate kinase deficiency, and lactate dehydrogenase deficiency) may experience muscle pain during exercise due to nonneural muscle cramps.

Fasciculation

"Fasciculation" is basically a fancy term for a twitch. Like classic cramps, fasciculations are caused by abnormal nerve activity, but they tend to involve only a small portion of the affected muscle and aren't generally painful.

While one is occurring, you may observe a small muscle "jump" under the skin. Fasciculations are common in ALS, spinal bulbar muscular atrophy, X-linked SMA, and SMA type 1 (in the tongue and mouth).

Neurologist Valerie Cwik of the University of Arizona Health Sciences Center in Tucson says that everyone gets fasciculations now and then, particularly around the eye, in the small muscle of the back of the hand between the thumb and index finger, and in the feet.

Fasciculations are made worse by stress, lack of sleep, and caffeine. They may also be seen in people with overactive thyroids, and there's a syndrome of benign (harmless) cramps and fasciculations. While some people with cramps and fasciculations develop ALS, in others the problem remains restricted to these symptoms.

Myotonia

Myotonia occurs when contracted muscles relax too slowly due to electrical problems in the muscle or nerve cells. A person with myotonia may have difficulty releasing his grip after holding an object—the sensation is sometimes described as stiffness. Myotonia can be sensitive to exercise, temperature, or diet, and occurs in paramyotonia congenita (PC), myotonia congenita (MC), hyperkalemic periodic paralysis (PP), and myotonic dystrophy (MMD).

Myalgia

Myalgia, or muscle pain, can be caused by mechanical stress without muscle injury (as in classic or nonneural muscle cramps), or by injury. Muscle injury can occur in anyone who "overdoes it" during exercise, including those with types of muscular dystrophy that render muscle cells more fragile.

Muscle injury can also occur in response to problems with the immune system, as in polymyositis and dermatomyositis, or in response to a lack of energy and buildup of toxic metabolites, as in carnitine palmityl transferase deficiency.

Fatigue

Fatigue can mean a subjective feeling of tiredness or an objective measurement of a decline in muscle force with use, but is always distinguished from weakness. Fatigue is associated with myasthenia gravis, ALS, SMA, myotonic disorders, metabolic disorders (McArdle and Tarui diseases), and mitochondrial disease. It can be a feature of many of the muscular dystrophies as muscles weaken and greater energy is expended to move them.

Hypotonia

Hypotonia means "lack of muscle tone," or absence of the normal degree of tension in the muscle at rest. The condition is seen most often in infants and children with neuromuscular problems, who may appear "floppy" because of the lack of muscle tone.

Hypotonia can occur in many muscle disorders, including acid maltase deficiency, mitochondrial disorders, congenital myopathies (central core disease, nemaline myopathy and myotubular myopathy), congenital myotonic dystrophy, congenital muscular dystrophies, neonatal and infantile myasthenia gravis, SMA type 1 and "benign" congenital hypotonia.

These muscle symptoms have many different primary causes. Although not all can be treated, some respond to gentle stretching, heat or cold, while others may respond to drug treatments. Your MDA [Muscular Dystrophy Association] clinic director will help you identify and possibly treat these symptoms.

Section 4.4

Tremor

From "Tremor Information Page," by the National Institute of
Neurological Disorders and Stroke (NINDS, www.ninds.nih.gov),
part of the National Institutes of Health, December 11, 2007.

What is tremor?

Tremor is an unintentional, somewhat rhythmic, muscle movement involving to-and-fro movements of one or more parts of the body. Most tremors occur in the hands, although they can also affect the arms, head, face, vocal cords, trunk, and legs. Sometimes tremor is a symptom of another neurological disorder, but the most common form occurs in otherwise healthy people. Some forms of tremor are inherited and run in families, while others have no known cause. Excessive alcohol consumption or alcohol withdrawal can kill certain nerve cells, resulting in tremor, especially in the hand. Other causes include an overactive thyroid and the use of certain drugs. Tremor may occur at any age but is most common in middle-aged and older persons.

Essential tremor (sometimes called benign essential tremor) is the most common of the more than 20 types of tremor. The hands are most often affected but the head, voice, tongue, legs, and trunk may also be involved. Head tremor may be seen as a "yes-yes" or "no-no" motion. Onset is most common after age 40, although symptoms can appear at any age. Parkinsonian tremor is caused by damage to structures within the brain that control movement. The tremor is classically seen as a "pill-rolling" action of the hands but may also affect the chin, lips, legs, and trunk. Dystonic tremor occurs in individuals of all ages who are affected by dystonia, a movement disorder in which sustained involuntary muscle contractions cause twisting motions or painful postures or positions.

Is there any treatment?

There is no cure for most tremors. The appropriate treatment depends on accurate diagnosis of the cause. Drug treatment for parkinsonian tremor involves levodopa or dopamine-like drugs such as pergolide mesylate, bromocriptine mesylate, and ropinirole. Essential tremor may be treated with propranolol or other beta blockers (such as nadolol) and primidone, an anticonvulsant drug. Dystonic tremor may respond to clonazepam, anticholinergic drugs, and intramuscular injections of botulinum toxin. Eliminating tremor "triggers" such as caffeine and other stimulants from the diet is often recommended. Physical therapy may help to reduce tremor and improve coordination and muscle control for some patients. Surgical intervention, such as thalamotomy and deep brain stimulation, are usually performed only when the tremor is severe and does not respond to drugs.

What is the prognosis?

Although tremor is not life-threatening, it can be embarrassing to some people and make it harder to perform daily tasks.

Part Two

Parkinson Disease

Chapter 5

Understanding Parkinson Disease (PD) and Its Symptoms

What Is Parkinson Disease?

Parkinson disease belongs to a group of conditions called movement disorders. The four main symptoms are tremor, or trembling in hands, arms, legs, jaw, or head; rigidity, or stiffness of the limbs and trunk; bradykinesia, or slowness of movement; and postural instability, or impaired balance. These symptoms usually begin gradually and worsen with time. As they become more pronounced, patients may have difficulty walking, talking, or completing other simple tasks. Not everyone with one or more of these symptoms has PD, as the symptoms sometimes appear in other diseases as well.

PD is both chronic, meaning it persists over a long period of time, and progressive, meaning its symptoms grow worse over time. It is not contagious. Although some PD cases appear to be hereditary, and a few can be traced to specific genetic mutations, most cases are sporadic—that is, the disease does not seem to run in families. Many researchers now believe that PD results from a combination of genetic susceptibility and exposure to one or more environmental factors that trigger the disease.

PD is the most common form of parkinsonism, the name for a group of disorders with similar features and symptoms. PD is also called primary parkinsonism or idiopathic PD. The term idiopathic means

Excerpted from "Parkinson's Disease: Hope Through Research," by the National Institute of Neurological Disorders and Stroke (NINDS, www.ninds.nih .gov), part of the National Institutes of Health, April 10, 2008.

41

a disorder for which no cause has yet been found. While most forms of parkinsonism are idiopathic, there are some cases where the cause is known or suspected or where the symptoms result from another disorder. For example, parkinsonism may result from changes in the brain's blood vessels.

What Causes the Disease?

Parkinson disease occurs when nerve cells, or neurons, in an area of the brain known as the substantia nigra die or become impaired. Normally, these neurons produce an important brain chemical known as dopamine. Dopamine is a chemical messenger responsible for transmitting signals between the substantia nigra and the next "relay station" of the brain, the corpus striatum, to produce smooth, purposeful movement. Loss of dopamine results in abnormal nerve firing patterns within the brain that cause impaired movement. Studies have shown that most Parkinson patients have lost 60 to 80 percent or more of the dopamine-producing cells in the substantia nigra by the time symptoms appear. Recent studies have shown that people with PD also have loss of the nerve endings that produce the neurotransmitter norepinephrine. Norepinephrine, which is closely related to dopamine, is the main chemical messenger of the sympathetic nervous system, the part of the nervous system that controls many automatic functions of the body, such as pulse and blood pressure. The loss of norepinephrine might help explain several of the non-motor features seen in PD, including fatigue and abnormalities of blood pressure regulation.

Many brain cells of people with PD contain Lewy bodies—unusual deposits or clumps of the protein alpha-synuclein, along with other proteins. Researchers do not yet know why Lewy bodies form or what role they play in development of the disease. The clumps may prevent the cell from functioning normally, or they may actually be helpful, perhaps by keeping harmful proteins "locked up" so that the cells can function.

Scientists have identified several genetic mutations associated with PD, and many more genes have been tentatively linked to the disorder. Studying the genes responsible for inherited cases of PD can help researchers understand both inherited and sporadic cases. The same genes and proteins that are altered in inherited cases may also be altered in sporadic cases by environmental toxins or other factors. Researchers also hope that discovering genes will help identify new ways of treating PD.

Although the importance of genetics in PD is increasingly recognized, most researchers believe environmental exposures increase a person's risk of developing the disease. Even in familial cases, exposure to toxins or other environmental factors may influence when symptoms of the disease appear or how the disease progresses. There are a number of toxins, such as 1-methyl-4-phenyl-1,2,3,6-tetrahydropyridine, or MPTP (found in some kinds of synthetic heroin), that can cause parkinsonian symptoms in humans. Other, still-unidentified environmental factors also may cause PD in genetically susceptible individuals.

Viruses are another possible environmental trigger for PD. People who developed encephalopathy after a 1918 influenza epidemic were later stricken with severe, progressive Parkinson-like symptoms. A group of Taiwanese women developed similar symptoms after contracting herpes virus infections. In these women, the symptoms, which later disappeared, were linked to a temporary inflammation of the substantia nigra.

Several lines of research suggest that mitochondria may play a role in the development of PD. Mitochondria are the energy-producing components of the cell and are major sources of free radicals—molecules that damage membranes, proteins, DNA, and other parts of the cell. This damage is often referred to as oxidative stress. Oxidative stress-related changes, including free radical damage to DNA, proteins, and fats, have been detected in brains of PD patients.

Other research suggests that the cell's protein disposal system may fail in people with PD, causing proteins to build up to harmful levels and trigger cell death. Additional studies have found evidence that clumps of protein that develop inside brain cells of people with PD may contribute to the death of neurons, and that inflammation or overstimulation of cells (because of toxins or other factors) may play a role in the disease. However, the precise role of the protein deposits remains unknown. Some researchers even speculate that the protein buildup is part of an unsuccessful attempt to protect the cell. While mitochondrial dysfunction, oxidative stress, inflammation, and many other cellular processes may contribute to PD, the actual cause of the dopamine cell death is still undetermined.

Who Gets Parkinson Disease?

About 50,000 Americans are diagnosed with PD each year, but getting an accurate count of the number of cases may be impossible because many people in the early stages of the disease assume their symptoms are the result of normal aging and do not seek help from a physician. Also, diagnosis is sometimes difficult and uncertain because other conditions may produce symptoms of PD and there is no definitive test for the disease. People with PD may sometimes be told by their doctors that they have other disorders, and people with PD-like diseases may be incorrectly diagnosed as having PD.

PD strikes about 50 percent more men than women, but the reasons for this discrepancy are unclear. While it occurs in people throughout the world, a number of studies have found a higher incidence in developed countries, possibly because of increased exposure to pesticides or other toxins in those countries. Other studies have found an increased risk in people who live in rural areas and in those who work in certain professions, although the studies to date are not conclusive and the reasons for the apparent risks are not clear.

One clear risk factor for PD is age. The average age of onset is 60 years, and the incidence rises significantly with increasing age. However, about 5 to 10 percent of people with PD have "early-onset" disease that begins before the age of 50. Early-onset forms of the disease are often inherited, though not always, and some have been linked to specific gene mutations. People with one or more close relatives who have PD have an increased risk of developing the disease themselves, but the total risk is still just 2 to 5 percent unless the family has a known gene mutation for the disease. An estimated 15 to 25 percent of people with PD have a known relative with the disease.

In very rare cases, parkinsonian symptoms may appear in people before the age of 20. This condition is called juvenile parkinsonism. It is most commonly seen in Japan but has been found in other countries as well. It usually begins with dystonia and bradykinesia, and the symptoms often improve with levodopa medication. Juvenile parkinsonism often runs in families and is sometimes linked to a mutated parkin gene.

What are the Symptoms of the Disease?

Early symptoms of PD are subtle and occur gradually. Affected people may feel mild tremors or have difficulty getting out of a chair. They may notice that they speak too softly or that their handwriting is slow and looks cramped or small. They may lose track of a word or thought, or they may feel tired, irritable, or depressed for no apparent reason. This very early period may last a long time before the more classic and obvious symptoms appear.

Friends or family members may be the first to notice changes in someone with early PD. They may see that the person's face lacks expression and animation (known as "masked face") or that the person does not move an arm or leg normally. They also may notice that the person seems stiff, unsteady, or unusually slow.

As the disease progresses, the shaking or tremor that affects the majority of Parkinson patients may begin to interfere with daily activities. Patients may not be able to hold utensils steady or they may find that the shaking makes reading a newspaper difficult. Tremor is usually the symptom that causes people to seek medical help.

People with PD often develop a so-called parkinsonian gait that includes a tendency to lean forward, small quick steps as if hurrying forward (called festination), and reduced swinging of the arms. They also may have trouble initiating movement (start hesitation), and they may stop suddenly as they walk (freezing).

PD does not affect everyone the same way, and the rate of progression differs among patients. Tremor is the major symptom for some patients, while for others, tremor is nonexistent or very minor.

PD symptoms often begin on one side of the body. However, as it progresses, the disease eventually affects both sides. Even after the disease involves both sides of the body, the symptoms are often less severe on one side than on the other. The four primary symptoms of PD are:

- **Tremor:** The tremor associated with PD has a characteristic appearance. Typically, the tremor takes the form of a rhythmic back-and-forth motion at a rate of 4-6 beats per second. It may involve the thumb and forefinger and appear as a "pill rolling" tremor. Tremor often begins in a hand, although sometimes a foot or the jaw is affected first. It is most obvious when the hand is at rest or when a person is under stress. For example, the shaking may become more pronounced a few seconds after the hands are rested on a table. Tremor usually disappears during sleep or improves with intentional movement.

- **Rigidity:** Rigidity, or a resistance to movement, affects most people with PD. A major principle of body movement is that all muscles have an opposing muscle. Movement is possible not just because one muscle becomes more active, but because the opposing muscle relaxes. In PD, rigidity comes about when, in response to signals from the brain, the delicate balance of opposing muscles is disturbed. The muscles remain constantly tensed and contracted so that the person aches or feels stiff or weak. The rigidity becomes obvious when another person tries to move the patient's arm, which will move only in ratchet-like or short, jerky movements known as "cogwheel" rigidity.

45

- **Bradykinesia:** Bradykinesia, or the slowing down and loss of spontaneous and automatic movement, is particularly frustrating because it may make simple tasks somewhat difficult. The person cannot rapidly perform routine movements. Activities once performed quickly and easily—dressing—may take several hours.

- **Postural instability:** Postural instability, or impaired balance, causes patients to fall easily. Affected people also may develop a stooped posture in which the head is bowed and the shoulders are drooped.

A number of other symptoms may accompany PD. Some are minor; others are not. Many can be treated with medication or physical therapy. No one can predict which symptoms will affect an individual patient, and the intensity of the symptoms varies from person to person.

- **Depression:** This is a common problem and may appear early in the course of the disease, even before other symptoms are noticed. Fortunately, depression usually can be successfully treated with antidepressant medications.

- **Emotional changes:** Some people with PD become fearful and insecure. Perhaps they fear they cannot cope with new situations. They may not want to travel, go to parties, or socialize with friends. Some lose their motivation and become dependent on family members. Others may become irritable or uncharacteristically pessimistic.

- **Difficulty with swallowing and chewing:** Muscles used in swallowing may work less efficiently in later stages of the disease. In these cases, food and saliva may collect in the mouth and back of the throat, which can result in choking or drooling. These problems also may make it difficult to get adequate nutrition. Speech-language therapists, occupational therapists, and dietitians can often help with these problems.

- **Speech changes:** About half of all PD patients have problems with speech. They may speak too softly or in a monotone, hesitate before speaking, slur or repeat their words, or speak too fast. A speech therapist may be able to help patients reduce some of these problems.

- **Urinary problems or constipation:** In some patients, bladder and bowel problems can occur due to the improper functioning of the autonomic nervous system, which is responsible for regulating smooth muscle activity. Some people may become incontinent, while others have trouble urinating. In others, constipation may occur because the intestinal tract operates more slowly. Constipation can also be caused by inactivity, eating a poor diet, or drinking too little fluid. The medications used to treat PD also can contribute to constipation. It can be a persistent problem and, in rare cases, can be serious enough to require hospitalization.

- **Skin problems:** In PD, it is common for the skin on the face to become very oily, particularly on the forehead and at the sides of the nose. The scalp may become oily too, resulting in dandruff. In other cases, the skin can become very dry. These problems are also the result of an improperly functioning autonomic nervous system. Standard treatments for skin problems can help. Excessive sweating, another common symptom, is usually controllable with medications used for PD.

- **Sleep problems:** Sleep problems common in PD include difficulty staying asleep at night, restless sleep, nightmares and emotional dreams, and drowsiness or sudden sleep onset during the day. Patients with PD should never take over-the-counter sleep aids without consulting their physicians.

- **Dementia or other cognitive problems:** Some, but not all, people with PD may develop memory problems and slow thinking. In some of these cases, cognitive problems become more severe, leading to a condition called Parkinson dementia late in the course of the disease. This dementia may affect memory, social judgment, language, reasoning, or other mental skills. There is currently no way to halt PD dementia, but studies have shown that a drug called rivastigmine may slightly reduce the symptoms. The drug donepezil also can reduce behavioral symptoms in some people with PD-related dementia.

- **Orthostatic hypotension:** Orthostatic hypotension is a sudden drop in blood pressure when a person stands up from a lying-down position. This may cause dizziness, lightheadedness, and, in extreme cases, loss of balance or fainting. Studies have suggested that, in PD, this problem results from a loss of nerve endings in the sympathetic nervous system that controls heart rate, blood pressure, and other automatic functions in the body. The medications used to treat PD also may contribute to this symptom.

- **Muscle cramps and dystonia:** The rigidity and lack of normal movement associated with PD often causes muscle cramps, especially in the legs and toes. Massage, stretching, and applying heat may help with these cramps. PD also can be associated with dystonia—sustained muscle contractions that cause forced or twisted positions. Dystonia in PD is often caused by fluctuations in the body's level of dopamine. It can usually be relieved or reduced by adjusting the person's medications.

- **Pain:** Many people with PD develop aching muscles and joints because of the rigidity and abnormal postures often associated with the disease. Treatment with levodopa and other dopaminergic drugs often alleviates these pains to some extent. Certain exercises also may help. People with PD also may develop pain due to compression of nerve roots or dystonia-related muscle spasms. In rare cases, people with PD may develop unexplained burning, stabbing sensations. This type of pain, called "central pain," originates in the brain. Dopaminergic drugs, opiates, antidepressants, and other types of drugs may all be used to treat this type of pain.

- **Fatigue and loss of energy:** The unusual demands of living with PD often lead to problems with fatigue, especially late in the day. Fatigue may be associated with depression or sleep disorders, but it also may result from muscle stress or from overdoing activity when the person feels well. Fatigue also may result from akinesia—trouble initiating or carrying out movement. Exercise, good sleep habits, staying mentally active, and not forcing too many activities in a short time may help to alleviate fatigue.

- **Sexual dysfunction:** PD often causes erectile dysfunction because of its effects on nerve signals from the brain or because of poor blood circulation. PD-related depression or use of antidepressant medication also may cause decreased sex drive and other problems. These problems are often treatable.

What Other Diseases Resemble Parkinson?

A number of disorders can cause symptoms similar to those of PD. People with symptoms that resemble PD but that result from other causes are sometimes said to have parkinsonism. Some of these disorders are listed below.

- **Postencephalitic parkinsonism:** Just after the first World War, a viral disease, encephalitis lethargica, attacked almost 5 million people throughout the world, and then suddenly disappeared in the 1920s. Known as sleeping sickness in the United States, this disease killed one third of its victims and led to postencephalitic parkinsonism in many others. This resulted in a particularly severe form of movement disorder that appeared sometimes years after the initial illness. (In 1973, neurologist Oliver Sacks published *Awakenings*, an account of his work in the late 1960s with surviving postencephalitic patients in a New York hospital. Using the then-experimental drug levodopa, Dr. Sacks was able to temporarily "awaken" these patients from their statue-like state). In rare cases, other viral infections, including western equine encephalomyelitis, eastern equine encephalomyelitis, and Japanese B encephalitis, have caused parkinsonian symptoms.

- **Drug-induced parkinsonism:** A reversible form of parkinsonism sometimes results from use of certain drugs, such as chlorpromazine and haloperidol, which are prescribed for patients with psychiatric disorders. Some drugs used for stomach disorders (metoclopramide), high blood pressure (reserpine), and epilepsy (valproate) may also produce parkinsonian symptoms. Stopping the medication or lowering the dosage of these medications usually causes the symptoms to go away.

- **Toxin-induced parkinsonism:** Some toxins—such as manganese dust, carbon disulfide, and carbon monoxide—can cause parkinsonism. The chemical MPTP also causes a permanent form of parkinsonism that closely resembles PD. Investigators discovered this reaction in the 1980s when heroin addicts in California who had taken an illicit street drug contaminated with MPTP began to develop severe parkinsonism. This discovery, which showed that a toxic substance could damage the brain and produce parkinsonian symptoms, caused a dramatic breakthrough in Parkinson research: for the first time, scientists were able to simulate PD in animals and conduct studies to increase understanding of the disease.

- **Arteriosclerotic parkinsonism:** Sometimes known as pseudoparkinsonism, vascular parkinsonism, or atherosclerotic parkinsonism, arteriosclerotic parkinsonism involves damage to the brain due to multiple small strokes. Tremor is rare in this type of parkinsonism, while dementia—the loss of mental skills and abilities—is common. Antiparkinsonian drugs are of little help to patients with this form of parkinsonism.

- **Parkinsonism-dementia complex of Guam:** This disease occurs among the Chamorro populations of Guam and the Mariana Islands and may be accompanied by a motor neuron disease resembling amyotrophic lateral sclerosis (Lou Gehrig disease). The course of the disease is rapid, with death typically occurring within 5 years.

- **Posttraumatic parkinsonism:** Also known as posttraumatic encephalopathy or "punch-drunk syndrome," parkinsonian symptoms can sometimes develop after a severe head injury or frequent head trauma that results from boxing or other activities. This type of trauma also can cause a form of dementia called dementia pugilistica.

- **Essential tremor:** Essential tremor, sometimes called benign essential tremor or familial tremor, is a common condition that tends to run in families and progresses slowly over time. The tremor is usually equal in both hands and increases when the hands are moving. The tremor may involve the head but usually spares the legs. Patients with essential tremor have no other parkinsonian features. Essential tremor is not the same as PD, and usually does not lead to it, although in some cases the two conditions may overlap in one person. Essential tremor does not respond to levodopa or most other PD drugs, but it can be treated with other medications.

- **Normal pressure hydrocephalus:** Normal pressure hydrocephalus (NPH) is an abnormal increase of cerebrospinal fluid (CSF) in the brain's ventricles, or cavities. It occurs if the normal flow of CSF throughout the brain and spinal cord is blocked in some way. This causes the ventricles to enlarge, putting pressure on the brain. Symptoms include problems with walking, impaired bladder control leading to urinary frequency or incontinence, and progressive mental impairment and dementia. The person also may have a general slowing of movements or may complain that his or her feet feel "stuck." These symptoms may sometimes be mistaken for PD. Brain scans, intracranial pressure monitoring, and other tests can help to distinguish NPH from PD and other disorders. NPH can sometimes be treated by surgically implanting a CSF shunt that drains excess cerebrospinal fluid into the abdomen, where it is absorbed.

- **Progressive supranuclear palsy:** Progressive supranuclear palsy (PSP), sometimes called Steele-Richardson-Olszewski syndrome, is a rare, progressive brain disorder that causes problems with control of gait and balance. People often tend to fall early in the course of PSP. One of the most obvious signs of the disease is an inability to move the eyes properly. Some patients describe this effect as a blurring. PSP patients often show alterations of mood and behavior, including depression and apathy as well as mild dementia. The symptoms of PSP are caused by a gradual deterioration of brain cells in the brainstem. It is often misdiagnosed because some of its symptoms are very much like those of PD, Alzheimer disease, and other brain disorders. PSP symptoms usually do not respond to medication.

- **Corticobasal degeneration:** Corticobasal degeneration results from atrophy of multiple areas of the brain, including the cerebral cortex and the basal ganglia. Initial symptoms may first appear on one side of the body, but eventually affect both sides. Symptoms are similar to those found in PD, including rigidity, impaired balance and coordination, and dystonia. Other symptoms may include cognitive and visual-spatial impairments, apraxia (loss of the ability to make familiar, purposeful movements), hesitant and halting speech, myoclonus (muscular jerks), and dysphagia (difficulty swallowing). Unlike PD, corticobasal degeneration usually does not respond to medication.

- **Multiple system atrophy:** Multiple system atrophy (MSA) refers to a set of slowly progressive disorders that affect the central and autonomic nervous systems. MSA may have symptoms that resemble PD. It also may take a form that primarily produces poor coordination and slurred speech, or it may have a mixture of these symptoms. Other symptoms may include breathing and swallowing difficulties, male impotence, constipation, and urinary difficulties. The disorder previously called Shy-Drager syndrome refers to MSA with prominent orthostatic hypotension—a fall in blood pressure every time the person stands up. MSA with parkinsonian symptoms is sometimes referred to as striatonigral degeneration, while MSA with poor coordination and slurred speech is sometimes called olivopontocerebellar atrophy.

- **Dementia with Lewy bodies:** Dementia with Lewy bodies is a neurodegenerative disorder associated with abnormal protein deposits (Lewy bodies) found in certain areas of the brain. Symptoms can range from traditional parkinsonian symptoms, such as bradykinesia, rigidity, tremor, and shuffling gait, to symptoms similar to those of Alzheimer disease. These symptoms may fluctuate, or wax and wane dramatically. Visual hallucinations may be one of the first symptoms, and patients may suffer from other psychiatric disturbances such as delusions and depression. Cognitive problems also occur early in the course of the disease. Levodopa and other antiparkinsonian medications can help with the motor symptoms of dementia with Lewy bodies, but they may make hallucinations and delusions worse.

- **Parkinsonism accompanying other conditions:** Parkinsonian symptoms may also appear in patients with other, clearly distinct neurological disorders such as Wilson disease, Huntington disease, Alzheimer disease, spinocerebellar ataxias, and Creutzfeldt-Jakob disease. Each of these disorders has specific features that help to distinguish them from PD. MSA, corticobasal degeneration, and progressive supranuclear palsy are sometimes referred to as "Parkinson-plus" diseases because they have the symptoms of PD plus additional features.

How Is Parkinson Disease Diagnosed?

There are currently no blood or laboratory tests that have been proven to help in diagnosing sporadic PD. Therefore the diagnosis is based on medical history and a neurological examination. The disease can be difficult to diagnose accurately. Early signs and symptoms of PD may sometimes be dismissed as the effects of normal aging. The physician may need to observe the person for some time until it is apparent that the symptoms are consistently present. Doctors may sometimes request brain scans or laboratory tests in order to rule out other diseases. However, CT and MRI brain scans of people with PD usually appear normal. Since many other diseases have similar features but require different treatments, making a precise diagnosis as soon as possible is essential so that patients can receive the proper treatment.

What Is the Prognosis?

PD is not by itself a fatal disease, but it does get worse with time. The average life expectancy of a PD patient is generally the same as for people who do not have the disease. However, in the late stages of the disease, PD may cause complications such as choking, pneumonia, and falls that can lead to death. Fortunately, there are many treatment options available for people with PD.

The progression of symptoms in PD may take 20 years or more. In some people, however, the disease progresses more quickly. There is no way to predict what course the disease will take for an individual person. One commonly used system for describing how the symptoms of PD progress is called the Hoehn and Yahr scale.

Table 5.1. Hoehn and Yahr Staging of Parkinson Disease

Stage one	Symptoms on one side of the body only.
Stage two	Symptoms on both sides of the body. No impairment of balance.
Stage three	Balance impairment. Mild to moderate disease. Physically independent.
Stage four	Severe disability, but still able to walk or stand unassisted.
Stage five	Wheelchair-bound or bedridden unless assisted.

Another commonly used scale is the Unified Parkinson Disease Rating Scale (UPDRS). This much more complicated scale has multiple ratings that measure mental functioning, behavior, and mood; activities of daily living; and motor function. Both the Hoehn and Yahr scale and the UPDRS are used to measure how individuals are faring and how much treatments are helping them.

With appropriate treatment, most people with PD can live productive lives for many years after diagnosis.

How Is the Disease Treated?

At present, there is no cure for PD. But medications or surgery can sometimes provide dramatic relief from the symptoms.

Drug Treatments

Medications for PD fall into three categories. The first category includes drugs that work directly or indirectly to increase the level of dopamine in the brain. The most common drugs for PD are dopamine precursors—substances such as levodopa that cross the blood-brain barrier and are then changed into dopamine. Other drugs mimic dopamine or prevent or slow its breakdown.

The second category of PD drugs affects other neurotransmitters in the body in order to ease some of the symptoms of the disease. For example, anticholinergic drugs interfere with production or uptake of the neurotransmitter acetylcholine. These drugs help to reduce tremors and muscle stiffness, which can result from having more acetylcholine than dopamine.

The third category of drugs prescribed for PD includes medications that help control the non-motor symptoms of the disease, that is, the symptoms that don't affect movement. For example, people with PD-related depression may be prescribed antidepressants.

The cornerstone of therapy for PD is the drug levodopa (also called L-dopa). Levodopa (from the full name L-3,4-dihydroxyphenylalanine) is a simple chemical found naturally in plants and animals. Levodopa is the generic name used for this chemical when it is formulated for drug use in patients. Nerve cells can use levodopa to make dopamine and replenish the brain's dwindling supply. People cannot simply take dopamine pills because dopamine does not easily pass through the blood-brain barrier, a lining of cells inside blood vessels that regulates the transport of oxygen, glucose, and other substances into the brain. Usually, patients are given levodopa combined with another substance called carbidopa. When added to levodopa, carbidopa delays the conversion of levodopa into dopamine until it reaches the brain, preventing or diminishing some of the side effects that often accompany levodopa therapy. Carbidopa also reduces the amount of levodopa needed.

Levodopa is very successful at reducing the tremors and other symptoms of PD during the early stages of the disease. It allows the majority of people with PD to extend the period of time in which they can lead relatively normal, productive lives.

Although levodopa helps most people with PD, not all symptoms respond equally to the drug. Levodopa usually helps most with bradykinesia and rigidity. Problems with balance and other non-motor symptoms may not be alleviated at all.

People who have taken other medications before starting levodopa therapy may have to cut back or eliminate these drugs in order to feel the full benefit of levodopa. People often see dramatic improvement in their symptoms after starting levodopa therapy. However, they may need to increase the dose gradually for maximum benefit. A high-protein diet can interfere with the absorption of levodopa, so some physicians recommend that patients taking the drug restrict their protein consumption during the early parts of the day or avoid taking their medications with protein-rich meals.

Levodopa is often so effective that some people may temporarily forget they have PD during the early stages of the disease. But levodopa is not a cure. Although it can reduce the symptoms of PD, it does not replace lost nerve cells and it does not stop the progression of the disease.

Levodopa can have a variety of side effects. The most common initial side effects include nausea, vomiting, low blood pressure, and restlessness. The drug also can cause drowsiness or sudden sleep onset, which can make driving and other activities dangerous. Long-term use of levodopa sometimes causes hallucinations and psychosis. The nausea and vomiting caused by levodopa are greatly reduced by combining levodopa and carbidopa, which enhances the effectiveness of a lower dose.

Dyskinesias, or involuntary movements such as twitching, twisting, and writhing, commonly develop in people who take large doses of levodopa over an extended period. These movements may be either mild or severe and either very rapid or very slow. The dose of levodopa is often reduced in order to lessen these drug-induced movements. However, the PD symptoms often reappear even with lower doses of medication. Doctors and patients must work together closely to find a tolerable balance between the drug's benefits and side effects. If dyskinesias are severe, surgical treatment may be considered. Because dyskinesias tend to occur with long-term use of levodopa, doctors often start younger PD patients on other dopamine-increasing drugs and switch to levodopa only when those drugs become ineffective.

Other troubling and distressing problems may occur with long-term levodopa use. Patients may begin to notice more pronounced symptoms before their first dose of medication in the morning, and they may develop muscle spasms or other problems when each dose begins to wear off. The period of effectiveness after each dose may begin to shorten, called the wearing-off effect. Another potential problem is referred to as the on-off effect—sudden, unpredictable changes in movement, from normal to parkinsonian movement and back again. These effects probably indicate that the patient's response to the drug is changing or that the disease is progressing.

One approach to alleviating these side effects is to take levodopa more often and in smaller amounts. People with PD should never stop taking levodopa without their physician's knowledge or consent because rapidly withdrawing the drug can have potentially serious side effects, such as immobility or difficulty breathing.

Fortunately, physicians have other treatment choices for some symptoms and stages of PD. These therapies include the following:

- **Dopamine agonists:** These drugs, which include bromocriptine, apomorphine, pramipexole, and ropinirole, mimic the role of dopamine in the brain. They can be given alone or in conjunction with levodopa. They may be used in the early stages of the disease, or later on in order to lengthen the duration of response to levodopa in patients who experience wearing off or on-off effects. They are generally less effective than levodopa in controlling rigidity and bradykinesia. Many of the potential side effects are similar to those associated with the use of levodopa, including drowsiness, sudden sleep onset, hallucinations, confusion, dyskinesias, edema (swelling due to excess fluid in body tissues), nightmares, and vomiting. In rare cases, they can cause compulsive behavior, such as an uncontrollable desire to gamble, hypersexuality, or compulsive shopping. Bromocriptine can also cause fibrosis, or a buildup of fibrous tissue, in the heart valves or the chest cavity. Fibrosis usually goes away once the drugs are stopped.

- **MAO-B inhibitors:** These drugs inhibit the enzyme monoamine oxidase B, or MAO-B, which breaks down dopamine in the brain. MAO-B inhibitors cause dopamine to accumulate in surviving nerve cells and reduce the symptoms of PD. Selegiline, also called deprenyl, is an MAO-B inhibitor that is commonly used to treat PD. Studies supported by the NINDS have shown that selegiline can delay the need for levodopa therapy by up to a year or more. When selegiline is given with levodopa, it appears to enhance and prolong the response to levodopa and thus may reduce wearing-off fluctuations. Selegiline is usually well-tolerated, although side effects may include nausea, orthostatic hypotension, or insomnia. It should not be taken with the antidepressant fluoxetine or the sedative meperidine, because combining selegiline with these drugs can be harmful. An NINDS-sponsored study of selegiline in the late 1980s suggested that it might help to slow the loss of nerve cells in PD. However, follow-up studies cast doubt on this finding. Another MAO-B inhibitor, rasagiline, was approved by the FDA [U.S. Food and Drug Administration] in May 2006 for use in treating PD.

- **COMT inhibitors:** COMT stands for catechol-O-methyltransferase, another enzyme that helps to break down dopamine. Two COMT inhibitors are approved to treat PD in the United States: entacapone and tolcapone. These drugs prolong the effects of levodopa by preventing the breakdown of dopamine. COMT inhibitors can decrease the duration of "off" periods, and they usually make it possible to reduce the person's dose of levodopa. The most common side effect is diarrhea. The drugs may also cause nausea, sleep disturbances, dizziness, urine discoloration, abdominal pain, low blood pressure, or hallucinations. In a few rare cases, tolcapone has caused severe liver disease. Because of this, patients taking tolcapone need regular monitoring of their liver function.

- **Amantadine:** An antiviral drug, amantadine, can help reduce symptoms of PD and levodopa-induced dyskinesia. It is often used alone in the early stages of the disease. It also may be used with an anticholinergic drug or levodopa. After several months, amantadine's effectiveness wears off in up to half of the patients taking it. Amantadine's side effects may include insomnia, mottled skin, edema, agitation, or hallucinations. Researchers are not certain how amantadine works in PD, but it may increase the effects of dopamine.

- **Anticholinergics:** These drugs, which include trihexyphenidyl, benztropine, and ethopropazine, decrease the activity of the neurotransmitter acetylcholine and help to reduce tremors and muscle rigidity. Only about half the patients who receive anticholinergics are helped by it, usually for a brief period and with only a 30 percent improvement. Side effects may include dry mouth, constipation, urinary retention, hallucinations, memory loss, blurred vision, and confusion.

When recommending a course of treatment, a doctor will assess how much the symptoms disrupt the patient's life and then tailor therapy to the person's particular condition. Since no two patients will react the same way to a given drug, it may take time and patience to get the dose just right. Even then, symptoms may not be completely alleviated.

Medications for Non-Motor Symptoms

Doctors may prescribe a variety of medications to treat the non-motor symptoms of PD, such as depression and anxiety. For example, depression can be treated with standard antidepressant drugs such as amitriptyline or fluoxetine (however, as stated earlier, fluoxetine should not be combined with MAO-B inhibitors). Anxiety can sometimes be treated with drugs called benzodiazepines. Orthostatic hypotension may be helped by increasing salt intake, reducing antihypertension drugs, or prescribing medications such as fludrocortisone.

Hallucinations, delusions, and other psychotic symptoms are often caused by the drugs prescribed for PD. Therefore reducing or stopping PD medications may alleviate psychosis. If such measures are not effective, doctors sometimes prescribe drugs called atypical antipsychotics, which include clozapine and quetiapine. Clozapine also may help to control dyskinesias. However, clozapine also can cause a serious blood disorder called agranulocytosis, so people who take it must have their blood monitored frequently.

Surgery

Treating PD with surgery was once a common practice. But after the discovery of levodopa, surgery was restricted to only a few cases. Studies in the past few decades have led to great improvements in surgical techniques, and surgery is again being used in people with advanced PD for whom drug therapy is no longer sufficient.

Pallidotomy and thalamotomy: The earliest types of surgery for PD involved selectively destroying specific parts of the brain that contribute to the symptoms of the disease. Investigators have now greatly refined the use of these procedures. The most common of these procedures is called pallidotomy. In this procedure, a surgeon selectively destroys a portion of the brain called the globus pallidus. Pallidotomy can improve symptoms of tremor, rigidity, and bradykinesia, possibly by interrupting the connections between the globus pallidus and the striatum or thalamus. Some studies have also found that pallidotomy can improve gait and balance and reduce the amount of levodopa patients require, thus reducing drug-induced dyskinesias and dystonia. A related procedure, called thalamotomy, involves surgically destroying part of the brain's thalamus. Thalamotomy is useful primarily to reduce tremor.

Because these procedures cause permanent destruction of brain tissue, they have largely been replaced by deep brain stimulation for treatment of PD.

Deep brain stimulation: Deep brain stimulation, or DBS, uses an electrode surgically implanted into part of the brain. The electrodes are connected by a wire under the skin to a small electrical device called a pulse generator that is implanted in the chest beneath the collarbone. The pulse generator and electrodes painlessly stimulate the brain in a way that helps to stop many of the symptoms of PD. DBS has now been approved by the U.S. Food and Drug Administration, and it is widely used as a treatment for PD.

DBS can be used on one or both sides of the brain. If it is used on just one side, it will affect symptoms on the opposite side of the body. DBS is primarily used to stimulate one of three brain regions: the subthalamic nucleus, the globus pallidus, or the thalamus. However, the subthalamic nucleus, a tiny area located beneath the thalamus, is the most common target. Stimulation of either the globus pallidus or the subthalamic nucleus can reduce tremor, bradykinesia, and rigidity. Stimulation of the thalamus is useful primarily for reducing tremor.

DBS usually reduces the need for levodopa and related drugs, which in turn decreases dyskinesias. It also helps to relieve on-off fluctuation of symptoms. People who initially responded well to treatment with levodopa tend to respond well to DBS. While the benefits of DBS can be substantial, it usually does not help with speech problems, "freezing," posture, balance, anxiety, depression, or dementia.

One advantage of DBS compared to pallidotomy and thalamotomy is that the electrical current can be turned off using a handheld device. The pulse generator also can be externally programmed.

Patients must return to the medical center frequently for several months after DBS surgery in order to have the stimulation adjusted by trained doctors or other medical professionals. The pulse generator must be programmed very carefully to give the best results. Doctors also must supervise reductions in patients' medications. After a few months, the number of medical visits usually decreases significantly, though patients may occasionally need to return to the center to have their stimulator checked. Also, the battery for the pulse generator must be surgically replaced every 3 to 5 years, though externally rechargeable batteries may eventually become available. Long-term results of DBS are still being determined. DBS does not stop PD from progressing, and some problems may gradually return. However, studies up to several years after surgery have shown that many people's symptoms remain significantly better than they were before DBS.

DBS is not a good solution for everyone. It is generally used only in people with advanced, levodopa-responsive PD who have developed dyskinesias or other disabling "off" symptoms despite drug therapy. It is not normally used in people with memory problems, hallucinations, a poor response to levodopa, severe depression, or poor health. DBS generally does not help people with "atypical" parkinsonian syndromes such as multiple system atrophy, progressive supranuclear palsy, or posttraumatic parkinsonism. Younger people generally do better than older people after DBS, but healthy older people can undergo DBS and they may benefit a great deal.

As with any brain surgery, DBS has potential complications, including stroke or brain hemorrhage. These complications are rare, however. There is also a risk of infection, which may require antibiotics or even replacement of parts of the DBS system. The stimulator may sometimes cause speech problems, balance problems, or even dyskinesias. However, those problems are often reversible if the stimulation is modified.

Researchers are continuing to study DBS and to develop ways of improving it. They are conducting clinical studies to determine the best part of the brain to receive stimulation and to determine the long-term effects of this therapy. They also are working to improve the technology used in DBS.

Complementary and Supportive Therapies

A wide variety of complementary and supportive therapies may be used for PD. Among these therapies are standard physical, occupational, and speech therapy techniques, which can help with such problems as gait and voice disorders, tremors and rigidity, and cognitive decline. Other types of supportive therapies include the following:

Diet: At this time there are no specific vitamins, minerals, or other nutrients that have any proven therapeutic value in PD. Some early reports have suggested that dietary supplements might be protective in PD. In addition, a phase II clinical trial of a supplement called co-enzyme Q10 suggested that large doses of this substance might slow disease progression in patients with early-stage PD. The NINDS and other components of the National Institutes of Health are funding research to determine if caffeine, antioxidants, and other dietary factors may be beneficial for preventing or treating PD. While there is currently no proof that any specific dietary factor is beneficial, a normal, healthy diet can promote overall well-being for PD patients just as it would for anyone else. Eating a fiber-rich diet and drinking plenty of fluids also can help alleviate constipation. A high protein diet, however, may limit levodopa's effectiveness.

Exercise: Exercise can help people with PD improve their mobility and flexibility. Some doctors prescribe physical therapy or muscle-strengthening exercises to tone muscles and to put underused and rigid muscles through a full range of motion. Exercises will not stop disease progression, but they may improve body strength so that the person is less disabled. Exercises also improve balance, helping people minimize gait problems, and can strengthen certain muscles so that people can speak and swallow better. Exercise can also improve the emotional well-being of people with PD, and it may improve the brain's dopamine synthesis or increase levels of beneficial compounds called neurotrophic factors in the brain. Although structured exercise programs help many patients, more general physical activity, such as walking, gardening, swimming, calisthenics, and using exercise machines, also is beneficial. People with PD should always check with their doctors before beginning a new exercise program.

Other complementary therapies that are used by some individuals with PD include massage therapy, yoga, tai chi, hypnosis, acupuncture, and the Alexander technique, which optimizes posture and muscle activity. There have been limited studies suggesting mild benefits with some of these therapies, but they do not slow PD and there is no convincing evidence that they are beneficial.

How Can People Cope with Parkinson Disease?

While PD usually progresses slowly, eventually the most basic daily routines may be affected—from socializing with friends and enjoying normal relationships with family members to earning a living and taking care of a home. These changes can be difficult to accept. Support groups can help people cope with the disease emotionally. These groups can also provide valuable information, advice, and experience to help people with PD, their families, and their caregivers deal with a wide range of issues, including locating doctors familiar with the disease and coping with physical limitations. Individual or family counseling also may help people find ways to cope with PD.

People with PD also can benefit from being proactive and finding out as much as possible about the disease in order to alleviate fear of the unknown and to take a positive role in maintaining their health. Many people with PD continue to work either full- or part-time, although eventually they may need to adjust their schedule and working environment to cope with the disease.

Chapter 6

Parkinson Plus Syndromes (PPS)

The term "parkinsonism" refers to a group of diseases that are all linked to an insufficiency of dopamine in the basal ganglia—the part of the brain that controls movement. Symptoms include tremor, bradykinesia (extreme slowness of movement), flexed posture, postural instability, and rigidity. A diagnosis of parkinsonism requires the presence of at least two of these symptoms, one of which must be tremor or bradykinesia.

By far the most common form of parkinsonism is idiopathic, or classic, Parkinson's disease (PD), but for a significant minority of diagnoses—about 15 percent of the total—one of the Parkinson's plus syndromes (PPS) may be present.

These syndromes, also known as atypical parkinsonism, include corticobasal degeneration, Lewy body dementia, multiple system atrophy, and progressive supranuclear palsy. Each of these syndromes has its own distinctive set of symptoms that can help doctors diagnose them. Although there is currently no cure for Parkinson's plus syndromes, researchers are making advances to better understand and manage them.

- **Corticobasal degeneration:** The main symptoms of corticobasal degeneration (CBD) are apraxia (inability to perform coordinated movements or use familiar objects), pronounced asymmetry, stiffness that is more severe than classic Parkinson's, and myoclonus (twitching or jerking) usually in the hand.

"Understanding Parkinson's Plus Syndromes and Atypical Parkinsonism," © 2008 Parkinson's Disease Foundation (www.pdf.org). Reprinted with permission.

- **Lewy body dementia:** Lewy body dementia (LBD) is one of the most common types of progressive dementia. Its central feature is progressive cognitive decline, combined with pronounced fluctuations in alertness and attention, complex visual hallucinations and motor symptoms, such as rigidity and the loss of spontaneous movement.

- **Multiple system atrophy:** Multiple system atrophy (MSA) is characterized by symptoms of autonomic nervous system failure (such as lightheadedness or fainting spells, constipation, erectile failure in men, and urinary retention), combined with tremor and rigidity, slurred speech, or loss of muscle coordination.

- **Progressive supranuclear palsy:** The cardinal symptoms of progressive supranuclear palsy (PSP) include frequent falls, an inability to aim the eyes properly, especially in a downward gaze, and emotional and personality changes.

Diagnosis: Is It PD or PPS?

Initial signs indicating that the diagnosis may be PPS and not PD include early and severe dementia, falling, and difficulty with voluntary eye movements. Tremor is often not a presenting symptom. Stepwise deterioration (a series of episodes that result in a sudden decline in functioning followed by periods of time where the individual's condition remains relatively stable, but resulting in an overall worsening of that condition) might also point toward a PPS diagnosis.

Another measure used to differentiate PPS and PD is the individual's response to medications typically used to treat Parkinson's. When given these medications (primarily levodopa), individuals with PPS generally have only a slight response or no response at all. In some cases, there may be an initially strong response to the medication, but this response will not be long lasting. For this reason, a doctor may conduct a trial of levodopa at doses higher than those normally used to treat Parkinson's. If this approach is used, it is important that the individual with PPS and his/her care partner have easy access to the doctor during this time. If these high doses do not significantly help the symptoms, the doctor may gradually lower the dose and possibly discontinue the medication altogether.

Treatment Approaches for PPS

For some people with PPS, a low dose of levodopa helps with mobility and reduces rigidity and stiffness. At this time, people with PPS are not considered to be candidates for any of the surgical treatment techniques available for PD including deep brain stimulation (DBS). Because there are currently no medications that effectively treat PPS, the prognosis for these syndromes is not as positive as for medication-responsive PD.

A common problem for people who live with PPS is swallowing or choking. In such cases, the doctor will usually order a swallow study, which involves a series of x-rays that allow the doctor to see how a liquid such as barium passes from the mouth to the throat and down the esophagus. Depending on the results, the doctor may direct adjustments in diet, such as the pureeing of food and/or the thickening of liquids. At some point, gastrostomy (a surgical procedure that involves the placement of a tube through the skin of the abdomen into the stomach for feeding purposes) may be considered.

Cognitive problems may also arise for some individuals with PPS. If a person is experiencing hallucinations, these may be alleviated somewhat with the use of quetiapine or clozapine. For dementia, a comprehensive neuropsychological evaluation once a year can accurately measure the decline of cognitive abilities and suggest coping strategies. There are techniques that can reduce frustration and encourage the maximum amount of independence for the person with PPS. These include limiting the number of choices offered and cueing. For additional information, please see the PDF Fact Sheet, "Coping with Dementia: Advice for Caregivers," at www.pdf.org. A growing number of clinical trials are studying PPS.

For more information on these trials and to find one in your community, please visit www.PDtrials.org.

Complementary Treatment Approaches for PPS

Although there are currently no effective treatments for Parkinson's plus syndromes, some relief may be found in complementary approaches, including exercise and physical, occupational, and speech therapy. For all PPS conditions (as for classic Parkinson's disease), a regular daily exercise program is vital for maintaining muscle tone, strength, and flexibility. A physical therapist trained in neurological conditions and PD can design an appropriate program as well as suggest a walker (one with wheels and brakes) that meets the special needs of a person who lives with one of the PPS conditions. An occupational therapist can be brought in to assess the individual's abilities and home environment and make recommendations that will allow for greater independence while at the same time assuring safety.

A speech therapist can be asked to develop a program to improve voice articulation and volume.

In summary, Parkinson's plus syndromes can be very difficult to diagnose and are difficult to treat. Because the cardinal symptoms of the individual disorders may take a long time to become visible or may never appear at all, a doctor may not be able to say exactly what is causing the parkinsonism. In addition, because these syndromes are complex and rare, complete diagnostic clarity may only come after the patient has been followed for several years by a movement disorder specialist (MDS)—that is, a neurologist who has completed additional, specialized training in movement disorders. For more information or to locate a MDS in your area, please contact PDF's Parkinson's Information Service helpline at 800-457-6676.

Chapter 7

The Genetics of PD

What Do We Know about Heredity and Parkinson Disease?

Parkinson disease (PD) is a neurological condition that typically causes tremor and/or stiffness in movement. The condition affects about 1 to 2 percent of people over the age of 60 years and the chance of developing PD increases as we age. Most people affected with PD are not aware of any relatives with the condition but in a number of families, there is a family history. When three or more people are affected in a family, especially if they are diagnosed at an early age (under 50 years) we suspect that there may be a gene making this family more likely to develop the condition.

Genetics: The Basics

Our genetic material is stored in the center of every cell in our bodies (skin cells, hair cells, blood cells). This genetic material comes in individual units called genes. We all have thousands of genes. Genes carry the information the body needs to make proteins, which are the substances in the body that actually carry out all the functions we need to live and grow. Our genes affect many things about us: our height, eye color, why we respond to some medications better than others, and our likelihood of developing certain conditions. We have

"Learning about Parkinson's Disease," from the National Human Genome Research Institute (NHGRI, www.genome.gov), May 27, 2008.

two copies of every gene: we inherit one copy, one member of each pair, from our mother and the other from our father. We then pass only one copy of a gene from each pair of genes to the next generation. Whether we pass on the gene we got from our father or the one from our mother is purely by chance, like flipping a coin heads or tails.

We all have genes that don't work properly. In most cases the other copy of the gene makes up for the one that does not work properly and we are healthy. A problem only arises if we meet someone else who has a nonworking copy of the same gene and we have a child who inherits two nonworking copies of that gene. This is called recessive inheritance.

Sometimes if one of our genes is not working properly the other copy of the gene cannot make up for it and that causes a condition or an increased risk of developing a condition. Each time we have a child we randomly pass on one copy of each gene. If the child inherits the copy that doesn't work properly, they too may develop the condition. This is called dominant inheritance.

What Genes Are Linked to Parkinson Disease?

In 1997, we studied a large family that came from a small town in Southern Italy in which PD was inherited from parent to child (dominant inheritance). We found the gene that caused their inherited Parkinson Disease and it coded for a protein called alpha-synuclein. If one studies the brains of people with PD after they die, one can see tiny little accumulations of protein called Lewy Bodies (named after the doctor who first found them). Research has shown that there is a large amount of alpha-synuclein protein in the Lewy Bodies of people who have noninherited PD as well as in the brains of people who have inherited PD. This immediately told us that alpha-synuclein played an important role in all forms of PD and we are still doing a lot of research to better understand this role.

Since 1997 four other genes have been found and they have been named parkin, DJ1, PINK1, and LRRK2. The first three genes were found in affected individuals who had siblings with the condition but whose parents did not have Parkinson disease (recessive inheritance). There is some research to suggest that these genes may also be involved in early-onset PD (diagnosed before the age of 30) or in dominantly inherited PD but it is too early yet to be certain. The most recently discovered gene (LRRK2) has been reported in families with dominant inheritance. Changes in this gene may account for 5–10% of dominantly inherited Parkinson disease.

What Determines Who Gets Parkinson Disease?

In most cases inheriting a nonworking copy of a single gene will not cause someone to develop Parkinson disease. We believe that many other complicating factors such as additional genes and environmental factors determine who will get the condition, when they get it, and how it affects them. In the families we have studied, some people who inherit the gene develop the condition and others live their entire lives without showing any symptoms. There is a lot of research on genes and the environment that is attempting to understand how all these factors interact.

Genetic Testing in Parkinson Disease

Genetic testing has recently become available for the parkin and PINK1 genes. Parkin is a large gene and testing is difficult. At the current stage of understanding, testing is likely to give a meaningful result only for people who develop the condition before the age of 30 years. PINK1 appears to be a rare cause of inherited Parkinson disease. A small percentage (about 2 percent) of those developing the condition at an early age appear to carry mutations in the PINK1 gene.

Chapter 8

Pain in PD

For most people with Parkinson's disease (PD), the most serious concern is with the motor system: stiffness, slowness of movement, impaired handwriting and coordination, poor mobility, and balance. Descriptions of PD do not generally include the mention of pain. And yet, when carefully questioned, more than half of all people with Parkinson's disease say that they have experienced painful symptoms and various forms of physical discomfort. Most people experience aching, stiffness, numbness, and tingling at some point in the course of the illness. For a few of them, pain and discomfort are so severe that they overshadow the other problems caused by the disease. This text will address these overlooked painful symptoms of PD, and describe an approach to diagnosing and treating the various pain syndromes that may occur.

Pain is described in textbooks as an unpleasant experience associated with physical injury or tissue damage. Pain can arise from anywhere in the body, of course. It goes without saying that people with Parkinson's are subject to all of the painful conditions—cardiac, gastroenterological, rheumatological, among others—that can affect people without PD. This discussion will focus on pain that is directly related to PD itself.

Pain syndromes and discomfort in Parkinson's usually arise from one of five causes: (1) a musculoskeletal problem related to poor posture, awkward mechanical function, or physical wear and tear; (2) nerve or root pain, often related to neck or back arthritis; (3) pain from dystonia, the sustained twisting or posturing of a muscle group or body part; (4) discomfort due to extreme restlessness and (5) a rare pain syndrome known as "primary" or "central" pain, arising from the brain.

It takes diagnostic skill and clinical experience to determine the cause of pain in someone with PD. The most important diagnostic tool is the patient's history. Where is the pain? What does it feel like? Does it radiate? When does it occur during the day? Does it occur in relation to any particular activity or medication? Perhaps the most important task for people with Parkinson's who experience pain is to describe as accurately as they can whether their medications induce, aggravate, or relieve their pain. To help your physician in diagnosing pain, refer to the questions listed on the back.

Musculoskeletal Pain

Aching muscles and joints are especially common in PD. Rigidity, lack of spontaneous movement, abnormalities of posture and awkward mechanical stresses all contribute to musculoskeletal pain in PD. One of the most common musculoskeletal complaints is shoulder stiffness, sometimes called a frozen shoulder (this may in fact be the first sign of PD). Hip pain, back pain, and neck pain are all common painful complaints in PD. With prolonged immobility of a limb, band-like tendons, termed contractures, may occasionally develop, usually in the hands or feet; one example is the clenched fist contracture that may occur with prolonged flexion of a hand.

An accurate diagnosis of musculoskeletal pain is based on a careful history and a physical examination that takes into account posture, limb, and trunk rigidity and gait. It can occasionally be challenging to distinguish between back pain due to PD and that caused by arthritis or scoliosis. Occasionally, further testing—including x-rays, bone scans, ultrasound, and rheumatologic or orthopedic consultation—will be needed. The proper treatment of musculoskeletal pain in PD depends upon the cause of the pain. If the pain is the result of excessive immobility or rigidity, a physician may prescribe dopaminergic therapy, physical therapy, and an exercise program. If the treatment is successful, patients should continue with an exercise program that strongly emphasizes range of motion, to prevent the development of further musculoskeletal problems.

Radicular and Neuritic Pain

Pain that occurs close to a nerve or nerve root is described as neuritic or radicular pain. The classic root-pain syndrome is sciatica, caused by compression or inflammation of the L5 lumbar root. Patients usually describe root pain as a sharp, lightning-like sensation that radiates towards the end of a limb. Of course, any nerve or root may be subject to injury or compression, and a careful neurological assessment is needed for the diagnosis. Electrodiagnostic studies and neuroimaging are occasionally required to confirm the location of the involved nerve or root, and to determine the cause of the problem. Radicular pain can usually be successfully treated with a mobility program and pain medication and rarely requires surgery.

Pain Associated with Dystonia

Dystonic spasms are among the most painful symptoms that a person with PD may experience. The pain arises from the severe, forceful, sustained twisting movements and postures that are called dystonia. This type of muscle spasm is quite different from the flowing, writhing movements described as dyskinesias, which are not painful. Dystonia in PD may affect the limbs, trunk, neck, face, tongue, jaw, swallowing muscles, and vocal cords. A common form of dystonia in PD involves the feet and toes, which may curl painfully. Dystonia may also cause an arm to pull behind the back, or force the head forward toward the chest.

The most important step in evaluating painful dystonia is to establish its relationship to dopaminergic medication. Does the dystonia occur when the medication is at peak effect? Or does it occur as a "wearing-off" phenomenon, when the benefits of medication are waning? The answers to these questions will usually clarify the nature and timing of the dystonia, and determine its treatment. Most painful dystonia represents an "off" parkinsonian phenomenon, and occurs early in the morning or during wearing-off spells. In uncertain cases, the neurologist should observe the patient in the office over a period of several hours in order to appreciate the relationship of the dystonia to the medication-dose cycle.

In terms of treatment, early-morning dystonia is typically relieved by physical activity, or by the first dose of dopaminergic medication, whether it be levodopa (Sinemet®) or a dopamine agonist. When dystonia occurs as the medications wear off, the problem can be corrected by shortening the "off" period. In some patients, the dystonia is so severe that subcutaneous injections of apomorphine, with its onset of action in minutes, may be necessary. Individuals with intractable dystonia may benefit from deep brain stimulation, a neurosurgical procedure that involves implanting and activating electrodes in the brain.

73

A few patients experience dystonic spasms as a complication of their medications. When they take their levodopa, these patients experience dystonic facial grimacing or uncomfortable limb posturing. The standard treatment approach for these individuals is to reduce the amount of dopamine medication, sometimes by substituting a less potent agent, or adding a medication for dystonia, such as amantadine.

Akathisia

No discussion of physical discomfort in PD is complete without a mention of akathisia, or restlessness, a frequent and potentially disabling complaint. Some patients with parkinsonian akathisia are unable to sit still, lie in bed, drive a car, eat at a table, or attend social gatherings. As a result of akathisia, patients may lose sleep or become socially isolated. In about half of the cases of parkinsonian akathisia, the symptom fluctuates with medications and may often be relieved by additional dopaminergic treatment.

Central Pain Syndromes

The most alarming pain syndrome in patients with PD is also one of the rarest: "central pain." This affliction—which is presumed to be a direct consequence of the disease itself, not the result of dystonia or a musculoskeletal problem—is described by patients as bizarre unexplained sensations of stabbing, burning, and scalding, often in unusual body distributions: the abdomen, chest, mouth, rectum, or genitalia. The treatment of central pain in PD is challenging, and usually begins with dopaminergic agents. Conventional painkillers, opiates, antidepressants, and powerful drugs for psychosis, such as clozapine, may also be helpful treatments for central pain.

Depression and Pain

It has long been known that chronic pain can induce depression, and depressed patients often experience pain. People who have PD are themselves at a higher-than-average risk for developing depression, which occurs in some 40 percent of patients at some point during the illness. It is therefore important that any assessment of pain in an individual with PD take into account the potential contributing role of depression, which may also require treatment.

Many patients with PD experience pain at some point during the illness. The complaint is often overlooked because PD is primarily a motor disorder. Yet, for a minority of patients, pain and discomfort can be so debilitating that they dominate the clinical picture. It is therefore important that individuals who experience pain discuss the problem with their neurologist. A careful history and examination— including, in some cases, additional diagnostic testing—can usually determine the cause of the pain. Depending on the category of painful complaint—musculoskeletal, root, or nerve pain, dystonic muscle spasm, akathisia, or central pain—it is usually possible for the physician to design an effective treatment plan.

Blair Ford, M.D., is Associate Professor of Clinical Neurology for the Center for Parkinson's Disease and Other Movement Disorders and Medical Director of the Center for Movement Disorders Surgery at Columbia University Medical Center. He serves as Scientific Editor for the *PDF News & Review* and is the author of the booklet *Deep Brain Stimulation for Parkinson's Disease.*

Chapter 9

PD: Treatments and Research

Chapter Contents

Section 9.1

All about PD Treatments and Research Developments

Excerpted from "Parkinson's Disease: Challenges, Progress, and Promise," by the National Institute for Neurological Disorders and Stroke (NINDS, www.ninds.nih.gov), part of the National Institutes of Health, November 2004. NIH Publication No. 05-5595.

Research Findings and New Directions

During the past 5 years, researchers have made substantial advances in our understanding of the biological factors involved in PD. They are beginning to decipher the roles of individual genes and environmental factors in PD and to learn how the interplay of these factors can lead to the disease. Each abnormal gene or environmental factor that is identified provides another clue to help solve the mystery of PD.

Genetics

Until the last decade, many researchers believed that PD was caused solely by environmental factors. However, the discovery of gene mutations in familial, or inherited, forms of PD has led to an explosion of research on PD genes and the function of the proteins that are encoded by these genes.

Although most people do not inherit PD, studying the genes responsible for the inherited cases can help researchers understand both inherited and sporadic (non-hereditary) cases of the disease. The same genes and proteins that are altered or missing in inherited cases may also be altered in sporadic cases by environmental toxins or other factors.

Identifying gene defects can also help researchers understand how PD occurs, develop animal models that accurately mimic the neuronal death in human PD, identify new drug targets, and improve diagnosis. The genetic approach has been very successful, with new discoveries occurring at an unprecedented pace. The following summary highlights current knowledge about the genes known to be involved in PD, and the functions of the proteins these genes produce.

Alpha-synuclein: The first PD-related gene to be identified was alpha-synuclein. Researchers at NIH and other institutions studied the genetic profiles of a large Italian family and three Greek families with familial PD and found that their disease was related to a mutation in this gene.

They found a second alpha-synuclein mutation in a German family with PD. These findings prompted studies of the role of alpha-synuclein in PD, which led to the discovery that Lewy bodies from people with the sporadic form of PD contained clumps of alpha-synuclein proteins. This discovery revealed a potential link between hereditary and sporadic forms of the disease and sparked investigations into the normal function of alpha-synuclein as well as the possible effects of alpha-synuclein mutations on normal cellular activity.

One theory about how alpha-synuclein is associated with PD holds that the mutated protein interferes with cell membranes. Within the cell body, individual molecules of alpha-synuclein join together to form tiny protein threads called fibrils; this process is called fibrillization. Investigators at the Brigham and Women's Hospital Udall Center and elsewhere have shown that mutations in the alpha-synuclein gene disrupt the fibrillization process and lead to the accumulation of protofibrils, an intermediate step in alpha-synuclein fibrillization. They found that alpha-synuclein protofibrils have protein structures which resemble bacterial and insect toxins that make membranes leaky. This could trigger cell death and may explain the toxicity of Lewy body proteins. This idea is supported by studies from the Massachusetts General Hospital and Massachusetts Institute of Technology Udall Center showing that alpha-synuclein is located near cell membranes in postmortem brain tissue from people with diffuse Lewy body disease.

Another study suggests that a buildup of normal alpha-synuclein may clog up the cell's protein disposal system and cause neurons to die. A group of researchers at NIH and other institutions investigated a rare familial form of early-onset PD and discovered that a multiplication of the normal alpha-synuclein gene, and a corresponding increase in alpha-synuclein protein, can cause the disease. The researchers analyzed blood samples from a family, the "Iowa kindred," in which many relatives developed PD or related neurological diseases. In the relatives with PD, the researchers found four copies of the alpha-synuclein gene—an abnormal triplication of three alpha-synuclein genes on one copy of chromosome 4 and one gene on the other chromosome 4—instead of the usual two copies of the alpha-synuclein gene. This multiplication resulted in an abnormally large amount of alpha-synuclein in the cells.

A third theory proposes that mutant alpha-synuclein interferes with the normal housekeeping functions of cells and lets proteins build up to toxic levels. Researchers at the Columbia University Udall Center, along with colleagues at Brigham and Women's Hospital and the Albert Einstein College of Medicine, have found that normal alpha-synuclein is broken down by lysosomes, which act as the cell's garbage disposal system. Mutant alpha-synuclein, however, blocks the pathway into the lysosomes. This inhibits the breakdown of alpha-synuclein as well as other proteins. This may trigger a toxic buildup of protein "garbage" inside the cell.

Researchers are continuing to study the alpha-synuclein gene to clarify how it affects PD. For example, Mayo Clinic Udall Center researchers are assessing the alpha-synuclein gene in a large group of people with PD, and in a control group of healthy people who match the PD patients in age, gender, and demographics, in order to look for variations in the gene that may affect susceptibility to the disease. Investigators at the Johns Hopkins University Udall Center have developed mice with alpha-synuclein gene mutations and found that the mice accumulate alpha-synuclein in the midbrain, cerebellum, brainstem, and spinal cord and develop an adult-onset neurodegenerative disease with symptoms resembling human PD, including motor dysfunction, bradykinesia, and dystonia.

The discovery of alpha-synuclein has paved the way for other genetic linkage studies in families with PD. Within the past 5 years, many regions of the genome have been linked to PD and four additional PD genes have been identified, including parkin, DJ-1, PINK1, and DRDN.

Parkin: Genetic studies on a rare, juvenile-onset form of PD led to the discovery of the parkin gene. Originally, this form of PD was not linked to Lewy bodies. However, Mayo Clinic Udall Center scientists have found parkin mutations that are accompanied by Lewy body pathology. Further studies have shown that parkin is a part of the so-called ubiquitin-proteasome system, which breaks down proteins in the cell. This suggests that parkin mutations may lead to accumulation of toxic proteins within neurons. Researchers also have shown that parkin interacts with synphilin-1 and alpha-synuclein and mediates an important step in protein handling. When alpha-synuclein, another protein called synphilin-1, and parkin are injected together into cells in culture, they form inclusions in the cell that are similar to Lewy bodies. This suggests that parkin may be important in both inherited and sporadic forms of the disease. Several studies have suggested that normal parkin protects neurons from diverse threats, including alpha-synuclein toxicity, proteasomal dysfunction, and excitotoxicity. Other evidence indicates that parkin degrades alpha-synuclein and that it accumulates on Lewy bodies in neurons within the substantia nigra, brainstem, and cortex of people with PD.

Findings from a different group of studies suggest that parkin may help to regulate the release of dopamine from substantia nigra neurons. In a mouse model for PD that is genetically engineered to lack the parkin gene, researchers found higher-than-normal levels of dopamine in the striatum. However, the neurons normally activated by dopamine required more stimulation to produce a response. The mice without parkin also had impairments in tests that require muscle coordination. These studies indicate that parkin may help to regulate the release of dopamine from nigral neurons.

Researchers at the Duke University Udall Center have shown that people with a parkin mutation in just one copy of the gene have a higher risk of getting PD as they get older than people without these mutations. Understanding why this happens could lead to strategies for preventing PD in people who are genetically predisposed to the disease.

DJ-1: The DJ-1 (PARK7) gene has been linked to another early-onset form of PD. This protein is involved in regulating gene activity and in protecting cells from a damaging process called oxidative stress. Mayo Clinic Udall Center researchers are screening patient samples for mutations in DJ-1, as well as other genes, to find out if these mutations are common among people with PD or restricted to just a few families. They also have evaluated DJ-1 in early-onset PD cases and identified a DJ-1 gene variation called R98Q.

Scientists at the Johns Hopkins University School of Medicine Udall Center have examined mutant DJ-1 genes in cultured human cells and found that the mutation reduces stability of the DJ-1 protein. These mutant proteins are degraded by proteasomes more quickly than usual and cannot form chains as the normal proteins do. Thus, the abnormal form of DJ-1 may not be able to perform its normal functions within the cell.

PINK1: Mutations in a gene called PTEN-induced kinase 1 (PINK1), also known as PARK6, have been identified in several families with PD. Kinases help to regulate protein function in both normal and disease

81

states. The PINK1 gene codes for a protein active in mitochondria, which convert food into energy inside the cell. Cell culture studies suggest that PINK1 may help to protect the cell and that mutations in this gene may increase susceptibility to cellular stress. The discovery of this gene provides a direct molecular link between mitochondrial dysfunction and the development of PD.

DRDN: Researchers at NIH and colleagues from several European institutions recently identified mutations in a gene called DRDN that appear to cause a late-onset form of PD. This gene, found in several English and Basque families, is located in a chromosomal region formerly called PARK8. DRDN codes for a protein called dardarin—a name derived from the Basque word for tremor. The function of this protein is still unknown.

Gene Discoveries

One of the most dramatic changes in PD research in the past decade has been the emergence of genetics as a major tool for understanding the disease. Until the mid-1990s, most researchers believed that PD was caused solely by environmental factors. However, researchers in New Jersey had identified an Italian family with what appeared to be an inherited form of PD. In 1995, they began to collaborate with researchers at the National Human Genome Research Institute (NHGRI), who analyzed DNA from these patients. Within a few years, the NHGRI researchers had traced the disease in this family to a mutation in the alpha-synuclein gene. Investigators soon identified alpha-synuclein mutations in several other families as well.

These findings touched off an explosion of work on the function of alpha-synuclein as well as intensive searches for other PD genes. Researchers soon discovered that alpha-synuclein is a major component of Lewy bodies, suggesting that it might play a role in sporadic forms of the disease as well as inherited ones. They also located four more PD genes—parkin, DJ-1, DRDN, and PINK1—and several other genes that appear to influence the disease, although their role is not yet clear. In 2003, investigators at the National Institutes of Health and elsewhere discovered that, in one large family, a triplication of the normal alpha-synuclein gene caused the disease. The extra genes cause overproduction of alpha-synuclein, which can accumulate inside brain cells.

Together, these studies have dramatically changed researchers' understanding of how PD develops. Hundreds of investigators are now looking for additional PD genes and studying how the proteins produced by these genes affect cells. Others are examining how genes and environmental factors may interact to produce the disease. These studies may lead to vastly improved treatments for the disease, or possibly even ways of preventing it.

Environmental Factors

Although the importance of genetics in PD is increasingly recognized, many researchers still believe that environmental exposures also increase a person's risk of developing the disease. Even when genes are a factor in the disease, as with many familial cases, exposure to toxins or other environmental factors may influence when symptoms of the disease appear and/or how the disease progresses.

One of the primary pieces of evidence that environmental factors play a role in the development of PD is that the relative risk of the disease is higher in industrialized countries than in less industrialized ones. In addition, studies have found that farmers and other agricultural workers have an increased risk of developing PD. Taken together, these studies suggest that toxic chemicals or exposure to other environmental factors present in industrial and agricultural areas might increase the risk of PD.

Another piece of evidence comes from observations of people who have been accidentally poisoned with the toxin MPTP (1-methyl-4-phenyl-1,2,5,6-tetrahydropyridine), which sometimes contaminates street drugs. MPTP is structurally similar to some pesticides. A breakdown product of MPTP, called MPP+, is toxic to substantia nigra neurons—the neurons that are affected in PD. MPTP produces a severe, permanent parkinsonian syndrome in affected people, and is now used to create animal models of PD. This discovery demonstrated that a toxic substance can damage the brain and produce parkinsonian symptoms.

A study of people in the World War II Veteran Twins Registry has suggested that genetic factors do not play a major role in causing sporadic PD that begins after age 50. However, genetic factors do appear to play a role when the disease begins at or before age 50. A number of other twin studies have found similar results. The chance that two siblings will both have PD is similar for fraternal and identical twins, suggesting that environmental exposures are more important than genetics in determining who will get the disease. Other studies have found that fraternal and identical twins of people with PD often have significant loss of dopamine neurons even when they don't experience any symptoms.

In another line of research, investigators are studying a disorder with a unique combination of parkinsonian symptoms, dementia, and motor neuron disease found in some people from the island of Guam to see if it might be due to an environmental factor or factors. A similar syndrome has been identified in people from the Kii peninsula in Japan. Researchers have long speculated that the disorder on Guam might be related to the consumption of animals that eat toxic cycad seeds found on that island. A 2002 study found neurotoxins in flour from cycad plants and showed that mice fed the cycad flour developed behavioral changes and neuron loss much like those seen in PD.

Viruses are another possible environmental trigger for PD. People who developed encephalopathy after a 1918 influenza epidemic were later stricken with severe, progressive Parkinson-like symptoms. A group of Taiwanese women developed similar symptoms after herpesvirus infections. In the latter case, the symptoms were linked to a temporary inflammation of the substantia nigra, and later disappeared. However, these cases showed that viruses can sometimes affect the region of the brain damaged in PD. Other studies have found evidence of activated immune cells and the accumulation of inflammation-associated proteins in PD. These changes might be triggered by viruses in some cases.

Scientists are continuing to study environmental toxins such as pesticides and herbicides that can cause PD symptoms in animals. Researchers supported by the NINDS and the National Institute on Aging have shown that exposing rodents to the pesticide rotenone can cause cellular and behavioral changes that mimic those seen in PD. Work supported by the National Institute of Environmental Health Sciences has shown that other agricultural compounds also can produce abnormalities in cells that are similar to those seen in PD. This research is supported through a program called the Collaborative Centers for Parkinson Disease Environmental Research (CCPDER) Consortium. This program sponsors a variety of projects to examine how occupational exposure to toxins and use of caffeine and other substances may affect risk, and whether inherited genetic mutations may predispose certain people to developing PD after exposure to certain chemicals.

Researchers at Rush-Presbyterian-St. Luke's Medical Center have examined whether prenatal exposure to toxins may increase the risk of PD. They found that exposure to a bacterial toxin called lipopolysaccharide during development in rats leads to the birth of animals with fewer than the normal number of dopamine neurons. This dopamine neuron loss persists into the animals' adulthood and increases with age, which mimics the course of human PD.

Along with genetic studies, these environmental studies lay the groundwork for a comprehensive understanding of how PD develops and how it might be prevented.

Neuroprotection

A major goal of PD research is the development of new therapies. Currently available treatments for PD can effectively control motor symptoms of the disease in the early stages, but they don't slow or halt the relentless progression of the disease. An explosion of discoveries during the past decade is now providing renewed hope of a therapy that will prevent the underlying nerve damage in this disease—a strategy known as neuroprotection.

The idea of neuroprotection for PD is not new. A number of clinical studies have tested different compounds to see if they might stop the disease progression. Some studies initially showed small positive effects, but most of these studies included a limited number of patients and did not examine the effects of these therapies over a long period of time. In addition, researchers have no good way of measuring whether these or other compounds truly prevent neuronal damage. Consequently, researchers cannot be sure that the positive effects seen in these studies are due to neuroprotection or if they represent short-term effects on symptoms.

Recently, a wealth of new information about how neurons may be damaged in PD has allowed investigators to identify many potential new ways of treating this disease, including nerve growth factors, anti-inflammatory drugs, and antioxidants. To overcome some of the problems that have plagued previous studies, in 2002 an NINDS-sponsored committee conducted a systematic review of data on 59 potential neuroprotective agents for PD. This committee ultimately selected four of the most promising drugs for study in a series of clinical trials known as Neuroprotection Exploratory Trials in Parkinson Disease (NET-PD). These drugs—coenzyme Q10, GPI-1485, creatine, and minocycline—are now being tested at more than 40 centers in the United States and Canada. Researchers hope that this new approach to selecting and testing compounds will lead to the first proven neuroprotective therapy or therapies for PD and revolutionize treatment of this disease.

Therapeutic Approaches

While levodopa and other drugs can provide initial relief from parkinsonian symptoms, none of these treatments halts the loss of dopamine neurons and nerve fibers. Thus, new treatments that slow the underlying disease are desperately needed. As knowledge about this disorder grows, potential new ways of preventing and treating the disease are being revealed. Promising treatments in development include new drug therapies (including neurotrophins, neuroprotectants, and immunotherapy), surgical therapies, cell transplantation, gene therapy, and transcranial magnetic stimulation.

Drug therapy: Current treatment for PD relies primarily on drugs to control the symptoms. While these drugs work well early in PD, they progressively fail as more nerve cells die. Drug-induced dyskinesias and fluctuations of motor symptoms also limit drug benefits in many cases.

Neurotrophic factors—molecules that support survival, growth, and development of brain cells—are one focus of new drug research. These chemicals are being studied as potential therapies for many neurological diseases. Researchers are investigating whether neurotrophic factors can halt dopamine cell degeneration and help to repair brain cells in PD. One such drug, glial cell line-derived neurotrophic factor (GDNF), has been shown to protect dopamine neurons and to promote their survival in models of PD. Researchers at the University of Kentucky Udall Center have helped to develop a technique for delivering these molecules directly into the brain. When GDNF was given for a period of 3 to 6 months, it prompted repair of dopamine neurons and improvement in their function. It also seemed to protect damaged dopamine cells from further degeneration. The researchers are now conducting an FDA-approved Phase I dose-escalation trial of chronic GDNF administration in 10 patients with advanced PD at the University of Kentucky Medical Center. The investigators also are studying the mechanisms by which neurotrophic factors affect the function of dopamine neurons and the long-term effects of these proteins on brain systems. Another clinical trial in the United Kingdom used tiny pumps implanted under the skin to deliver GDNF and has shown promising initial results.

GDNF is one of a family of compounds called neurotrophins or nerve growth factors. Many of these neurotrophins are potential therapies for PD. Examples include neurotrophin-4 (NT-4), brain-derived neurotrophic factor (BDNF), and fibroblast growth factor 2 (FGF-2). One study has shown that GDNF and NT-4 can protect dopamine neurons in culture from oxidative stress. Studies in mice have shown that BDNF can increase the number of dopamine receptors produced by brain cells. This may increase the brain's responsiveness to dopamine. Other studies have shown that BDNF protects dopamine neurons from damage in the 6-hydroxydopamine rat model for PD. FGF-2 is essential for the long-term survival of dopamine neurons, and impaired FGF-2 function may be a common underlying cause of the neuronal degeneration in PD. FGF-2 also stimulates the survival of dopamine neurons when they are transplanted into the brain.

Another developing area of PD drug research is neuroprotection—finding ways to prevent the ongoing degeneration of dopamine neurons that is a hallmark of PD. In 2002, a multicenter clinical trial suggested that a compound called coenzyme Q10 (also known as ubiquinone), which is believed to improve mitochondrial function, can slow the rate of deterioration in PD. Another early clinical trial tested a compound called GPI-1485, which acts as a neurotrophin, and found that it was well-tolerated and appeared to slow the loss of dopamine nerve terminals. A third drug, creatine, which affects mitochondrial function and acts as an antioxidant, prevents MPTP-induced neuronal damage in rats.

Investigators at the Harvard University Medical School and McLean Hospital Udall Center, along with other researchers, have identified genes that are neuroprotective in a variety of systems, from cell culture to primate models of PD. Increasing the expression of these genes, or mimicking their function with drugs, may be a new way to prevent brain damage in PD.

Therapies that change how the immune system reacts also may protect nerve cells in PD. For example, animal studies of the antibiotic minocycline, which has been used in humans for decades, have shown that it has anti-inflammatory effects in the brain and that it may prevent programmed cell death. In another study, researchers at the University of Nebraska Medical Center and the Columbia University Udall Center in New York have shown that an experimental vaccine using a drug called copolymer-1 can modify the behavior of supporting (glial) cells in the brain so that their responses are beneficial to the nervous system rather than harmful. The vaccine reduced the amount of neurodegeneration in a mouse model for PD. Another study by neurologists at the Columbia University Udall Center has shown that a drug called rofecoxib, which inhibits an inflammatory enzyme called COX-2, prevents about half of the dopamine neuron death in a mouse model for PD.

NINDS is now supporting a series of pilot clinical trials to test the effects of four of these potential neuroprotectants—coenzyme Q10, GPI-1485, creatine, and minocycline—in people with early, untreated PD. This series of clinical trials is called Neuroprotection Exploratory Trials in Parkinson Disease (NET-PD). NINDS is also supporting a network of Parkinson Disease Neuroprotection Clinical Centers to study these and other potential neuroprotectant drugs.

A variety of other compounds have been tested as potential therapies for PD. Some studies have found that proteins called alpha-2 adrenergic receptors play a role in the dyskinesias that commonly develop in PD patients treated with levodopa. Blocking these receptors has been successful in reducing dyskinesia in animal models of PD. An alpha-2 adrenergic receptor blocker called JP-1730 is now being studied in an NINDS-sponsored clinical trial to determine if it is safe and effective against dyskinesia and/or other PD symptoms. Another drug, levetiracetam, is also being tested in a controlled clinical trial to see if it can reduce dyskinesias in Parkinson patients without interfering with other PD drugs. Levetiracetam, which is approved by the FDA to treat epilepsy, is not an alpha-2 adrenergic receptor blocker. Instead, researchers believe it may work by interfering with the neurotransmitter GABA (gamma-amino butyric acid).

Another clinical trial is studying GM1 ganglioside, a chemical which contributes to cell growth, development, and repair, to determine if this drug can improve symptoms, delay disease progression, and/or partially restore damaged brain cells in PD patients. Preliminary studies have shown beneficial effects of this drug on the dopamine system in animal models. Several chemicals are being tested as potential treatments for the mood disorders that sometimes occur in people with PD. One clinical trial is investigating whether a drug called quetiapine can help to reduce psychosis and/or agitation in PD patients with dementia, and in dementia patients with parkinsonian symptoms. Another clinical study is examining whether s-adenosylmethionine (SAM-e), a food supplement that improves dopamine transmission, can help to alleviate depression in patients with PD.

A number of clinical studies have suggested that cholinesterase inhibitors, which are commonly used for Alzheimer disease, can also have a positive effect on cognition, psychiatric symptoms, and global function in patients with PD plus dementia. Additional clinical studies are now underway.

Surgical therapies: Surgical treatments for PD, especially pallidotomy and deep brain stimulation (DBS), are important options for improving the lives of people affected by this disease. Investigators are continuing to evaluate these procedures in patients.

NINDS is supporting a great deal of research about DBS, including studies that aim to improve the technology for DBS and a large-scale clinical trial done in collaboration with the Department of

Veterans Affairs that compares DBS to the best medical management with drugs. Investigators are studying normal brain circuits in order to find the best placement for the electrodes in the brain and the best stimulation patterns for DBS. In addition, they are working to develop a screening tool to identify PD patients who will get the most benefit from DBS.

Cell transplants: Cell replacement through transplantation is an emerging approach for repairing the damage PD causes in the brain. Many researchers are working to develop cell transplantation therapies. In addition to embryonic stem cells, which have the potential to become any kind of cell in the body, researchers are experimenting with adult neural stem cells, neural precursor cells, and fetal-derived dopamine-producing neurons. Even cells derived from non-neuronal tissue are being considered for PD research.

However, very little is known about these different types of cells, and researchers need to better understand the fundamental biology of stem cells and neural precursor cells before such technologies can be used to treat PD in a safe, effective, and predictable manner.

In several early clinical studies, grafting of fetal-derived dopamine tissue led to an increase in dopamine production in the brains of people with advanced PD. Unfortunately, these studies showed few long-term benefits and led to unanticipated side effects such as dyskinesias. These problems preclude widespread use of this particular approach.

Investigators at the Harvard University Medical School and McLean Hospital Udall Center have injected mouse embryonic stem cells directly into the rat brain and found that these cells can develop into dopamine neurons. They also have shown that they can generate dopamine neurons from rodent embryonic stem cells. They are now testing primate and human embryonic stem cells in animal models of PD with a goal of moving this therapy into human clinical trials.

Some researchers have found that muscle progenitor cells isolated from the muscle of adult rats can be induced to form cells with neuron-like properties. Although it is unclear whether these cells can actually function like neurons, this finding raises the possibility that muscle tissue may be a source of progenitor cells to treat diseases of the nervous system. In another study, researchers transplanted dopamine-producing brain cells from pigs into the brains of PD patients and found some evidence of clinical improvements. The immune systems of these patients had to be suppressed so that the grafted pig cells would not be rejected.

89

Yet another transplantation approach employs retinal pigment epithelial cells, which produce dopamine and can be cultivated in large numbers. These cells are attached to microscopic gelatin beads and implanted into the brains of PD patients as part of a clinical trial to determine if they can enhance brain levels of dopamine and thus reduce the symptoms of PD.

One of the key problems with stem cell transplantation is to control and manage how the cells become dopamine-producing neurons. Recently, investigators found that genetically engineering mouse embryonic stem cells to produce a protein called Nurr1 led to a four- to five-fold increase in the number of dopamine neurons produced in culture. Nurr1 also enhanced the neurons' ability to produce and release dopamine. The identification of this important factor in dopamine neuron development paves the way for new therapies that require management of stem cell differentiation.

Other studies have shown that embryonic stem cells also form dopamine cells if they are transplanted directly into the brain and that these cells can reduce motor dysfunction and normalize dopamine production in an animal model of PD. A low cell concentration of embryonic stem cells increases the influence of the host brain, increasing the number of dopamine cells produced and reducing the likelihood that the stem cells will develop into tumors.

Researchers at NINDS are studying signals that control the proliferation and differentiation of stem cells. Along with other researchers, they have shown that stem cells can generate nerve cells that are capable of establishing connections (synapses) with other neurons. They also have shown that mouse embryonic stem cells can be manipulated to generate central nervous system stem cells.

The NIH has established an NIH Stem Cell Unit to help characterize stem cells for future clinical use and to learn how to control differentiation in federally approved stem cell lines.

Gene therapy: Gene therapy offers great potential for PD and many other brain disorders. With this type of therapy, viruses are engineered to deliver genes that increase the supply of dopamine, prevent cell death, or promote regeneration of neurons. Although this approach is promising, researchers need to develop efficient and safe means to deliver genes to brain cells in order for gene therapy to be used in humans. Many researchers are working to develop better viral vectors—viruses that can carry genes into the targeted cells—and to find ways of improving the transfer of these vectors to the brain. As researchers accumulate more information about the safety and efficacy of different delivery systems, research on gene therapy for PD can move forward.

The NINDS is supporting a consortium called the Parkinson Disease Gene Therapy Study Group, which is investigating dopaminergic enzyme gene therapy and neurotrophic gene therapy in animal models of PD. This consortium includes many Parkinson experts from research centers across the country. The investigators are comparing different genes and testing different gene delivery approaches. As part of this project, researchers at Northwestern University in Illinois have developed a viral gene vector with a special modification that allows the introduced gene to be temporarily "turned off" when the patient is given a small dose of a specific antibiotic. The development of this vector should permit researchers to better control the delivery of genes once the vector is in the host. The researchers are now conducting safety and toxicity studies of this new vector with the hope that it will prove safe enough for testing in humans.

NINDS-funded investigators have found that using a genetically modified virus to deliver specific growth factors to primates with a parkinsonian condition leads to dramatic improvements in symptoms. Another group of researchers has shown that engineering a virus to deliver enzymes important for the production of levodopa can have beneficial effects in a rat model of PD.

Investigators also are experimenting with the gene for 1-amino acid decarboxylase (AADC), an enzyme that converts levodopa into dopamine. Research in animal models has shown that neurons in the striatum can be given the AADC gene using a viral vector, causing them to convert levodopa to dopamine. This essentially mimics the function of the dopamine neurons that are lost in PD and may reduce the need for drugs that increase the level of dopamine in the brain.

Researchers also are experimenting with gene therapy to deliver the GDNF gene to the brain. In a monkey model, GDNF prevented dopamine neurons from dying, and the monkeys regained some of their lost motor skills.

Transcranial magnetic stimulation: Transcranial magnetic stimulation (TMS) is a technique that uses an insulated wire coil placed on the scalp to create a magnetic pulse that stimulates the brain. Investigators at NINDS are conducting clinical studies of TMS and a related technique called transcranial electrical polarization to learn if they might have beneficial effects for people with PD. Studies have suggested that these techniques might be able to alter brain circuits in beneficial ways. Some studies of TMS have shown small effects on bradykinesia. TMS also may be able to produce beneficial effects on gait and freezing.

Section 9.2

Skin Patch Used to Treat PD

"Skin Patch Delivers Dementia Drug," from the U.S. Food
and Drug Administration (FDA, www.fda.gov), August 6, 2007.

A patch that delivers medication through the skin has been approved to treat the symptoms of dementia in both Alzheimer and Parkinson diseases.

The Exelon Patch (rivastigmine transdermal system), approved in July 2007, provides another form of delivering the drug rivastigmine, which FDA previously approved in the form of a capsule and an oral solution. All three formulations are for use in treating mild-to-moderate dementia of people with Alzheimer or Parkinson disease. Dementia is a slowly worsening decline in mental abilities, such as thinking, remembering, and reasoning, that interfere with a person's daily functioning.

The patch continuously delivers medication through the skin, maintaining steady levels of the drug in the bloodstream. The patch can be applied to the back, chest, or upper arm, and should be replaced every 24 hours. It comes in two strengths: one strength delivers 4.6 mg of rivastigmine every 24 hours and the other, 9.5 mg of rivastigmine every 24 hours. An initial dose of 4.6 mg delivered every 24 hours is to be used for at least 4 weeks before increasing to the maintenance dose of 9.5 mg, delivered every 24 hours.

The Exelon Patch is manufactured by LTS Lohmann Therapie-Systeme AG, Andernach, Germany. It is distributed by Novartis Pharmaceuticals Corporation, East Hanover, New Jersey.

Effectiveness

FDA's approval of the Exelon Patch is based on results from a large study of the patch used in people with Alzheimer disease and several smaller studies of the Exelon capsule used in people with Alzheimer disease and people with Parkinson disease who had dementia. In the large study of nearly 1,200 people with mild-to-moderate Alzheimer disease, the Exelon Patch showed effectiveness similar to that of Exelon capsules. The side effects of nausea and vomiting were lower in people treated with the patch than with the capsules.

Side Effects

Exelon belongs to a class of drugs called cholinesterase inhibitors, whose most common side effects include:

- nausea;
- vomiting;
- diarrhea;
- loss of appetite; and
- weight loss.

Precautions

Before using the Exelon Patch, tell your doctor if you currently have, or have a history of:

- stomach ulcers;
- taking NSAIDs (nonsteroidal anti-inflammatory drugs);
- a heart condition; or
- asthma or pulmonary (lung) disease.

Your doctor may need to monitor you more closely while you are on this medicine.

About Alzheimer Disease

This gradually occurring brain disorder starts with mild memory loss, changes in personality and behavior, and a decline in thinking abilities (cognition). It progresses to loss of speech and movement, then total incapacitation, and eventually death. According to the National Institute on Aging, up to 4.5 million Americans suffer from Alzheimer disease.

About Parkinson Disease

The main symptoms of this disorder of the nervous system affect movement and posture. However, the Exelon Patch is approved to treat only dementia, which can affect some people with Parkinson disease.

The main symptoms of Parkinson disease are:

- trembling in the hands, arms, legs, jaw, and face (tremor);
- stiffness of the limbs and trunk (rigidity);
- slowness of movement (bradykinesia); and
- impaired balance and coordination (postural instability).

The features of dementia in Parkinson disease may resemble those of Alzheimer disease. According to the Parkinson Action Network, more than 1 million Americans live with Parkinson disease and 60,000 new cases are diagnosed each year. Two of five people with Parkinson disease are estimated to have dementia.

Section 9.3

Vaccine Reduces PD Neurodegeneration in Mice

"Vaccine Reduces Parkinson's Disease Neurodegeneration in Mice," from the National Institute of Neurological Disorders and Stroke (NINDS, www.ninds.nih.gov), part of the National Institutes of Health, updated April 2008.

For the first time, researchers have shown that an experimental vaccine can reduce the amount of neurodegeneration in a mouse model for Parkinson disease. The finding suggests that a similar therapy might eventually be able to slow the devastating course of Parkinson disease in humans.

The experimental treatment in this study is among the first to show potential for slowing brain degeneration in this disease, the researchers say. Currently available therapies can treat symptoms of the disease, but they do not prevent the loss of brain cells.

"This is a novel therapeutic approach to stop the damaging inflammation associated with neurodegeneration. It is exciting because an approach like this may be beneficial in a variety of neurodegenerative diseases in addition to Parkinson disease," says Diane Murphy, Ph.D., a National Institute of Neurological Disorders and Stroke (NINDS) program director for Parkinson disease research. The research was funded in part by the NINDS and appeared in the June 22, 2004 issue of the Proceedings of the National Academy of Sciences (PNAS).

Studies in the last decade have shown that inflammation is common to a variety of neurodegenerative diseases, including Parkinson disease, Alzheimer disease, HIV-1 [human immunodeficiency virus] associated dementia, and amyotrophic lateral sclerosis (ALS or Lou Gehrig disease). The inflammation in these diseases involves activation of microglia—specialized support cells in the brain that produce immune system signaling chemicals called cytokines. Although inflammation can be damaging, Michel Schwartz, Ph.D., and colleagues at the Weizmann Institute in Rehovot, Israel, have pioneered research which shows that activating immune cells in specific ways also may lead to neuroprotective responses in animal models of spinal cord and brain injury.

In the new study, Howard E. Gendelman, M.D., of the University of Nebraska Medical Center in Omaha, along with graduate student Eric Benner and colleagues, experimented with a drug called copolymer-1 (Copaxone). Previous studies have shown that Copaxone, which is commonly used to treat multiple sclerosis, increases the number of immune T cells that secrete anti-inflammatory cytokines and growth factors. The researchers took immune cells from mice that had received Copaxone immunization and injected them into mice which had received injections of a drug called MPTP [1-methyl-4-phenyl-1,2,3,6 tetrahydropyridine]. MPTP leads to Parkinson-like neuronal degeneration in the brain.

Mice that received the Copaxone-treated immune cells had significantly less degeneration of dopamine-producing neurons in their brain than mice that did not receive the treated cells. These mice also lost fewer dopamine-transmitting nerve fibers than control mice and had only a small decrease in the amount of dopamine produced in the brain. Dopamine is a nerve signaling chemical (neurotransmitter) that controls movement; a loss of dopamine-producing neurons is the central problem in Parkinson disease.

The researchers found that T cells in the treated mice migrated to the damaged area of the brain, reduced the harmful reactions of the microglia, and triggered a neuroprotective response. In addition, the vaccine dramatically increased the amount of a growth factor called GDNF (glial-derived neurotrophic factor) that helps prevent neurodegeneration.

"This study provides a proof of concept," says study coauthor Serge Przedborski, M.D., Ph.D., of Columbia University in New York. The vaccination modifies the behavior of the glial cells so that their responses are beneficial to the nervous system rather than harmful, he explains.

The researchers injected Copaxone-treated cells in this study because MPTP destroys the mouse immune system, Dr. Gendelman says. The MPTP mice needed replacement immune cells in order to respond to the drug. However, Copaxone could be given to humans directly, he says.

The researchers are now planning follow-up studies to confirm their results and to identify the specific cytokines, nerve growth factors, and other proteins that play a role in the protective response. Other work is needed to determine how to translate the study results into a therapy for humans and to make sure the treatment is safe for patients with Parkinson's, who may not react to the drug in the same way that MS [multiple sclerosis] patients do, Dr. Przedborski says.

While Copaxone is currently approved by the U.S. Food and Drug Administration for use in treating multiple sclerosis, the dose needed to treat Parkinson will probably be quite different from the dose used in treating MS, says Benner. The timing of treatment may also prove critical. Therefore it is premature for patients with Parkinson disease to begin taking the drug. Currently available doses of the drug could be ineffective or even harmful for these patients, he adds.

Reference: Benner EJ, Mosley RL, Destache CJ, Lewis TB, Jackson-Lewis V, Gorantia S, Nemacheck C, Green SR, Przedborski S, Gendelman HE. "Therapeutic immunization protects dopaminergic neurons in a mouse model of Parkinson's disease." *Proceedings of the National Academy of Sciences,* June 22, 2004, Vol. 101, no. 25, pp. 9435–9440.

Section 9.4

Neural Transplants to Treat PD May Not Function Long-Term

Neurons grafted into the brain of a patient with Parkinson disease fourteen years ago have developed Lewy body pathology, the defining pathology for the disease, according to research by Jeffrey H. Kordower, Ph.D., and associates and published in the April 6 [2008] issue of *Nature Medicine.*

The findings suggest that Parkinson disease [PD] is an ongoing process that can affect cells grafted into the brain in the same way the disease affects host dopamine neurons in the substantia nigra of the brain, according to Kordower, who is the lead author of the study and a neuroscientist at Rush University Medical Center.

"These findings give us a bit of pause for the value of cell replacement strategy for Parkinson disease," said Kordower. "We still need to vigorously investigate this approach among the full armament of surgically delivered Parkinson disease therapies. While it is not clear to us whether the same fate would befall stem cell grafts, the next generation of cell replacement procedures, this study does suggest that grafted cells can be affected by the disease process."

The collaborative research study described in the article involves Rush, Mt. Sinai School of Medicine, New York, and the University of South Florida, Tampa, In it, individuals with Parkinson disease received fetal cell transplants to reverse the loss in the brain of striatal dopamine.

The individual described in this article was a woman with a 22-year history of Parkinson disease who underwent transplantation in 1993. After transplantation she experienced improvements in disease symptoms as measured by the Unified Parkinson Disease Rating Scale (UPDRS) and required substantially lower doses of antiparkinsonian medications. Her UPDRS scores remained improved into 1997, but by 2004, she experienced progressive worsening of Parkinson disease symptoms. She died in 2007 and her brain and that of two other patients in the study were comprehensively processed and analyzed. She had the longest survival after transplantation that had been reported to date among this study's participants.

Double-blind, sham-controlled studies that followed did not establish clinical benefit although significant improvement was observed in a subpopulation of patients. Postmortem studies of individuals in these studies showed a robust survival of grafted neurons, suggesting that the cells were not affected by Parkinson disease as Kordower explains: "Because Parkinson disease pathology progresses over decades, we think that the individuals did not live long enough for the Parkinson disease pathology to develop in the grafted cells."

Scientists have long debated whether Parkinson disease results from an acute insult or event, or whether it is an ongoing pathological process that continues to affect healthy neurons, according to Kordower. This research indicates that mechanisms and molecules responsible for initiating the degenerative process are still present at a late stage and are capable of affecting grafted neurons. In addition, the processes that destroy dopamine neurons are not restricted to the midbrain.

"The findings also suggest that there may be either a pathogenic factor in the brain that affects dopamine producing neurons or a pathological process that can spread from one cellular system to another," said Kordower. "These findings have striking implications for understanding what causes PD and the potential for cell replacement strategies to reverse the motor symptoms."

Chapter 10

Deep Brain Stimulation for PD

Introduction

Surgery for Parkinson's disease (PD) was developed decades before the advent of any of the effective medications that we use today. For most of the past century, innovative surgeons worked to refine surgical treatments for PD. During the 1940s and 1950s, these procedures consisted of surgically created lesions in deep parts of the brain to control symptoms of tremor and rigidity. In one frequently performed procedure, the pallidotomy, a surgeon created a tiny lesion in an area of the brain known as the globus pallidus. When levodopa was introduced as a treatment for PD in the late 1960s, interest in surgical approaches waned dramatically. For the next 30 years, medications dominated the treatment of PD.

Unfortunately, clinical experience has since shown that medical therapy for PD has significant shortcomings. After several years of taking medications, including levodopa (the current "gold standard" of antiparkinsonian agents), many patients with PD experience a shortening of benefit following each oral dose, a problem called "wearing-off." Many of them also develop drug-induced, involuntary writhing and twisting movements, known as dyskinesias. It was these limitations of medical therapy that reawakened a strong interest in developing effective, surgically based techniques for the treatment of PD.

From "Deep Brain Stimulation for Parkinson's Disease," by Blair Ford, M.D. © 2002 Parkinson's Disease Foundation (www.pdf.org). Reprinted with permission. Reviewed by David A. Cooke, M.D., October 5, 2008.

The new techniques of deep brain stimulation are the products of several advances: improved understanding of brain electrical circuitry, developments in brain imaging techniques, improvements in neurosurgery, and innovations in medical technology. DBS is the state-of-the-art surgical treatment for Parkinson's disease, and has replaced all earlier types of surgery, including pallidotomy. The goal of this text is to describe DBS and to address some of the issues that patients and their families should consider.

Historical Perspective

It may not be intuitive that shutting down brain cells using an electrode, or destroying brain cells using earlier surgical interventions, will help symptoms of PD. It is even more surprising that scientists discovered the basis for these approaches before they understood how the brain controls body movement. As with many important discoveries, surgery for PD began by trial and error, not according to a predetermined theory.

The basis for surgery in the treatment of PD began in the early 1900s, when researchers first began to perform neurosurgery guided by brain maps, known as stereotactic surgery, in animals. Neurosurgeons Horsley and Clark developed techniques that allowed them to place lesions—surgically created holes—deep in the brain with great accuracy by injecting tiny amounts of corrosive chemicals. Over the next 40 years, neurosurgeons applied lesion-making techniques to the human brain but no surgeon was able to relieve parkinsonism without injury to the motor system, resulting in weakness.

In the 1940s, Dr. Russell Meyers was the first to perform surgery in the basal ganglia, a deep brain region that is responsible for controlling movement. He found that he could reduce the tremor and rigidity of PD in almost half his patients without causing weakness or other motor deficits. This crucial observation led to the development of all of modern neurosurgery for PD, including DBS.

In subsequent decades, surgeons perfected the techniques of placing lesions in the brain. Many different brain sites were targeted: the globus pallidus, the thalamus, the subthalamic nucleus, and individual fiber tracts connecting different parts of the basal ganglia. Lesions were created using thermal electrodes that heated brain tissue at their tips, enabling the precise destruction of a small volume of brain tissue.

The accuracy of surgical targeting was improved by electrophysiological recording techniques, first developed in the 1960s. Using tiny electrodes inserted deep into the brain, Dr. Hirotaro Narabayashi was able to find cells in the thalamus that fired in synchrony with the tremor of Parkinson's disease. This site was later confirmed to be the key brain target for tremor control. The procedures for making lesions in the thalamus and in the globus pallidus, respectively, were given the names of thalamotomy and pallidotomy.

These early approaches were followed by the development of our current state-of-the-art procedure: deep brain stimulation (DBS), pioneered in France in the early 1990s by Dr. Alim-Louis Benabid. While preparing to create a lesion in the thalamus of a patient, Dr. Benabid noticed that he could stop the tremor simply by giving an electrical stimulation to the same area. He speculated that a wire providing continuous electrical stimulation would be an effective treatment for Parkinson's tremor.

This idea led to the development of the deep brain stimulator, a device that has proven superior to all earlier surgical approaches that were based on creating lesions. Within less than 10 years from its development, deep brain stimulation replaced the thalamotomy and pallidotomy operations, both of which were less effective and carried an increased operative risk.

Deep brain stimulation on one side of the brain was first approved by the U.S. Food and Drug Administration (FDA) in 1997 for the treatment of tremor. It was approved for implantation on both sides of the brain in 2002 as a treatment for other parkinsonian symptoms—specifically, rigidity, slowness of movement, and dystonia. In the years since then, thousands of patients worldwide have undergone this treatment. Deep brain stimulation continues to evolve and further improvements are likely as time goes on.

How Does Deep Brain Stimulation Work?

When an electrical signal is given to the deep brain structures, normal electrical activities of brain cells are shut down. Why does this help PD? The answer relates to the nature and design of the human motor system. Normal muscle tone, speed of movement, and coordination all depend upon a complex flow of signals in electrical pathways of the brain. The parts of the motor system are arranged in connected loops that maintain continuous cycles of electrical activity. An electrical signal that begins in one part of the loop goes back to its starting point, establishing a feedback mechanism that prevents excessive activity from developing.

In patients with PD, the electrical feedback loops of the deep brain structures cycle abnormally. Normal movement is replaced by unwanted tremor, rigidity, and slowness. By using a deep brain electrode that provides an electrical current, it is possible to jam abnormal signaling between brain structures. This does not remove PD from the brain but it shifts the electrical activity of the system toward the normal state and thereby reduces the main motor symptoms of PD.

Unlike the earlier pallidotomy, which created a permanent lesion in the brain, DBS produces electrical effects that are largely reversible and can be varied by programming. DBS can be applied to several sites including the thalamus, the globus pallidus and the subthalamic nucleus. DBS on one side of the brain generally reduces symptoms of PD only on the opposite side of the body. For patients with symptoms on both sides of their body, DBS must be done on both sides of the brain.

Approaches to Deep Brain Stimulation

Deep brain stimulation can be delivered to any desired brain structure. In PD, three targets have consistently shown the most important antiparkinsonian effects: the ventral intermediate (VIM) thalamus, the subthalamic nucleus (STN), and the globus pallidus (GPi). These brain structures were the targets of earlier procedures: the thalamus was the site of the thalamotomy and the globus pallidus, the site of the pallidotomy. But procedures that involved creating permanent lesions, despite their effectiveness, were replaced in the late 1990s by deep brain stimulation, which had the advantages of safety, reversibility, and adjustability. A summary of neurosurgical procedures for PD is described in Table 10.1.

In the following section, specific operations are described in detail.

Thalamic Stimulation

Thalamic stimulation is for tremor. The thalamus is a large, round, oblong mass of cells that acts as a relay station for many important functions including motor control. A region on the undersurface of the thalamus called the ventral intermediate (VIM) nucleus is the critical center for all types of tremors. Electrical stimulation of the VIM thalamus can completely and reliably stop a tremor on the opposite side of the body. Thalamic stimulation on both sides of the brain will reduce tremors on both sides of the body, as well as midline tremors of the jaw, neck, and trunk.

Thalamic stimulation will suppress tremor of any cause: Parkinson's tremor, essential tremor (ET), multiple sclerosis, and dystonic tremors.

In patients who have both essential tremor and Parkinson's disease tremor (ET-PD), thalamic stimulation may provide control of tremor that is superior to deep brain stimulation in other targets. Sometimes patients with bilateral thalamic stimulation experience slurred speech or poor balance as an adverse effect, but these symptoms can be reversed through adjustments in stimulator settings.

Subthalamic Nucleus Stimulation

The subthalamic nucleus (STN) is a small lens-shaped structure of about 6 mm in length located right beneath the much larger thalamus. The STN can be identified accurately using mapping techniques and a DBS electrode can be placed right through it—much like a toothpick skewers an olive. Stimulation of the STN influences its connections to the globus pallidus and can have broad antiparkinsonian effects. It can improve not only tremor, but also slowness, rigidity, dyskinesias, speech, handwriting, and dystonia. The antitremor effect of STN stimulation is comparable to that of thalamic stimulation.

STN stimulation has been performed in thousands of patients at many medical centers around the world and is now considered the most effective surgical intervention for PD. The largest single-center clinical experience is held by the surgical group in Grenoble, France, where the technique of DBS was pioneered. In carefully selected patients, STN stimulation can reduce parkinsonian symptoms in the unmedicated state by 30 to 60 percent, as measured by standard rating scales. With this degree of improvement, patients who suffer from disabling wearing-off periods may experience a significant reduction in the severity and duration of these episodes. In some patients, the wearing-off periods can be completely eliminated, enabling them to function independently throughout the day.

Many patients find that they require less antiparkinsonian medication after STN stimulation. Some can stop their medication altogether. As a result of the decreased need for medication, and also because of a direct stimulation effect, there may be a dramatic reduction—or even elimination—of dyskinesias. As noted earlier, the beneficial effects of STN stimulation generally parallel those of levodopa, but do not surpass the best result of medication treatment. Its main advantage, therefore, is improvement in wearing-off spells and dyskinesias.

Most patients with advanced PD require STN stimulation on both sides of the brain to control symptoms on both sides of the body. STN stimulation on one side generally helps parkinsonian symptoms only on the opposite body side. For patients who have tremor or other symptoms on only one side, one-sided STN stimulation may be considered. Gait and speech problems generally require STN stimulation on both sides of the brain. STN stimulation can also improve parkinsonian symptoms in patients who have undergone previous pallidotomy or thalamotomy surgeries.

More research on outcomes will be needed before we know which patients will benefit the most from STN stimulation. Some patients who undergo DBS have developed problems with memory and thinking, but those with a good cognitive baseline before surgery are less likely to experience these symptoms.

Parkinson's disease is a progressive disorder. No medical or surgical therapy to date has been able to prevent the development of late symptoms that do not improve with medication, such as memory problems or lack of balance.

Globus Pallidus Stimulation

The globus pallidus, named for its pale appearance, is a dense wedge of nerve tissue that occupies the center of the basal ganglia region. The deepest portion of the globus pallidus, named the posteroventral medial globus pallidus interna (GPi), is the site of the pallidotomy operation, and represents the main outflow connection from the globus pallidus to the thalamus. The globus pallidus is a larger and more complex structure than the STN, with a complicated internal circuitry. Like STN stimulation, globus pallidus stimulation has broad beneficial antiparkinsonian effects. Because the globus pallidus is so large, the entire deep brain electrode resides within it as contrasted with the STN, a much smaller structure in which the electrode protrudes out both sides.

Globus pallidus stimulation has effectiveness similar to that of STN stimulation but the operation is performed less frequently due to the surgeon's preference or training. In randomized comparisons between the two techniques, the result of bilateral globus pallidus stimulation is the same as that for STN stimulation, a 30 to 60 percent improvement in parkinsonian symptoms in the unmedicated state. Globus pallidus stimulation can also have an important benefit on parkinsonian dyskinesias and dystonia.

An important advantage of surgery at the STN site is that patients who go through surgery are usually able to reduce their medications by a greater amount than those who go through stimulation of the globus pallidus. Based on this observation, it has been argued that

Table 10.1. Summary of Neurosurgical Treatments for PD

Type of Surgery	Deep Brain Structure	Effects and Outcome
Lesion-Based Surgery	Thalamotomy	• Lesion is created in VIM thalamus. • Effective treatment for tremor on the opposite body side. • No effect on slowness or rigidity. • Effectiveness may decrease over time. • Bilateral thalamotomy not advisable because of potential adverse effects on speech.
	Pallidotomy	• Lesion is created in globus pallidus. • The state-of-the-art surgical treatment for PD up until 1990. • Reduction in tremor, slowness, rigidity and dyskinesia on the opposite body side. • Beneficial antiparkinsonian effects decrease over time. • Bilateral pallidotomy is associated with cognitive and behavioral impairments.
Deep Brain Stimulation	Thalamus	• Deep brain electrode in VIM thalamus. • Effective treatment for tremor on the opposite body side. • Benefit appears to be longer lasting than thalamotomy. • Bilateral thalamic stimulation can be accomplished without significant adverse effects.
	Subthalamic Nucleus (STN)	• Deep brain electrode in subthalamic nucleus (STN). • Effective treatment for tremor, slowness, rigidity, dystonia, and dyskinesia on the opposite body side. • Bilateral procedures well tolerated. • Usually allows patients to decrease medications by a greater amount than those who undergo GPi stimulation.
	Globus Pallidus (GPi)	• Deep brain electrode in globus pallidus. • Effective treatment for tremor, slowness, rigidity, dystonia, and dyskinesia on the opposite body side. • Bilateral procedures well tolerated.

the reduction in dyskinesias following globus pallidus stimulation is a direct effect of the procedure whereas with STN stimulation, the dyskinesias are improved mainly as a result of the decreased medication requirement.

The Key Issues

Who Should Consider Surgery, and Who Should Not?

Surgery is not for everyone.

The best candidate for deep brain stimulation is someone who has had Parkinson's disease for 10 to 20 years, and experiencing wearing off motor fluctuations, episodes of extreme slowness and stiffness caused by a failure of medications, and dyskinesias, twisting movements that are caused by excessive medication. A smaller group of patients who undergo surgery do not have severe fluctuations but do suffer with tremors that cannot be stopped using medication.

Perhaps the most important determinant of a successful outcome is the patient selection. Patients who are younger and whose primary symptom is tremor have better results than do older patients who have balance impairment.

Table 10.2. Patient Selection Determines Outcome

Good Candidate for DBS	Poor Candidate for DBS
Typical PD with tremor	Atypical parkinsonism
Good response to levodopa	Poor response to levodopa
Dyskinesias	Memory problems, apathy, or confusion
Wearing-off spells	Severe depression or anxiety
Good general health	Severe medical problems
Excellent family support	No social support

The best candidates for deep brain stimulation have:

- typical "classical" PD, defined by the presence of tremor at rest, rigidity, and slowness

- symptoms that still respond to antiparkinsonian medications even if the response is brief

- disabling parkinsonian symptoms in the "off" state

- uncontrollable medication-induced movements called dyskinesias

- severe tremors

- a good understanding of the potential benefits and risks of the operative procedures and evaluation procedures and the ability to give informed consent

- good general health

- a good emotional support network of family and friends

Patients with these problems are not good candidates for surgery, and will likely not benefit from the procedure:

- atypical or rare forms of parkinsonism, such as progressive supranuclear palsy (PSP), multiple system atrophy (MSA), corticobasoganglionic degeneration (CBGD), or a known acquired cause of parkinsonism such as stroke or brain trauma

- failure to experience any benefit from antiparkinsonian medications

- severe memory loss, confusion, hallucinations, or apathy (these problems may actually get worse as a result of brain surgery)

- experience of freezing, balance problems, and frequent falling

- a severe chronic psychiatric disorder such as psychosis, depression, bipolar disorder, alcoholism, or a personality disorder

- inability to understand the potential benefits and risks of the operative procedures or to give informed consent

- significant medical problems that would unacceptably increase the surgical risk, such as cancer or serious heart disease

Note that age is not an essential criterion for surgery. An otherwise healthy older patient with PD can safely undergo and benefit from this type of surgery. While advanced age does not preclude surgery, the best results are obtained in younger patients.

How to Predict If You Will Benefit from DBS

It is important to recognize that some symptoms of PD respond better to surgery than others. The effect of surgery on slowness and stiffness can generally be predicted from the response to medication.

Some patients have an excellent response to levodopa and other medications, with almost complete suppression of symptoms, but suffer from spells of wearing-off during which they become stiff, immobile, and frozen. These individuals will do well with surgery because at least some of the time, their parkinsonism is levodopa-responsive.

Other patients have an incomplete response to levodopa. Even when experiencing their maximal medication effect, they have some gait or balance or speech impairment. These patients, who do not do as well on regular antiparkinsonian medications, will not do as well with surgery. They will probably only experience relief of those symptoms that are eased by their medication. Patients who cannot walk independently at their best on levodopa will still not be able to walk after surgery.

Table 10.3. Predicting Benefit from Deep Brain Stimulation

DBS helps with:	DBS does not help with:
Tremor	Freezing
Rigidity	Backwards falling
Hand function	Tachyphemia: rapid, soft, stuttering speech
Dyskinesias	Flexed neck or posture
Wearing-off spells	Dementia or apathy; Anxiety or depression

When should surgery be considered? Some have argued that surgery should be performed on patients with mild PD in order to delay the progression of disease or forestall complications of medication usage. This notion is not justified because there is no evidence that earlier surgery would accomplish these goals. Current surgical techniques, along with medications, provide benefit only by suppressing the symptoms of PD. There is no evidence that DBS is neuroprotective. The risks and inconveniences of surgery underscore its role as a treatment of last resort, after medication options have been thoroughly tried.

At some centers, patients who are considered candidates for deep brain stimulation undergo a simple test that can help predict the result of surgery. The test consists of observing a patient after a moderately large dose of dopamine medication. The usual procedure involves a dose of levodopa, and the test is called a "levodopa challenge." At other centers, the test involves an injection of the dopamine drug apomorphine. In either case, the improvement that follows a dose of levodopa or apomorphine tends to correlate well with the effects of deep brain stimulation.

Each patient is unique, and the goals of surgery are different for each individual. With some, the most pressing requirement is tremor control. With others, it is the need to reduce dyskinesias. It is very important that every patient contemplating surgery have a clear idea about what can and what cannot be accomplished by using this powerful intervention.

Long-Term Results

What happens in the years after DBS surgery? According to scientists at the medical centers with the longest follow-up data, patients with advanced PD continue to experience marked benefits for many years after the operation. Tremor, especially, remains well-controlled but rigidity and dyskinesias are also improved and do not return to the levels that they were before the surgery. A patient's ability to perform activities of daily living may gradually decline after the first year following surgery but remains 50 percent improved even after 5 years or more, according to long-term studies. Many patients can reduce their medications after surgery and this reduction can persist.

In the early months after surgery, patients typically return to the medical center for frequent stimulator adjustments. After the initial adjustment period, the stimulator settings tend to remain stable, and only limited additional programming is required to keep symptoms under control. Depending on the settings, the system battery, which is implanted in the chest like a pacemaker, will deplete and require replacement in three to five years.

Unfortunately, PD is a progressive condition. DBS does not prevent later complications of the disease, such as poor posture, speech impairment, gait freezing, balance problems, backwards falling, or dementia. If these problems develop in a patient treated with DBS, the overall gains in quality of life after surgery may be lost even if tremor and dyskinesias remain well-controlled.

Effects of Deep Brain Stimulation on Thinking and Mood

Most individuals tolerate brain surgery and deep brain stimulation without noticeable effects in their memory or thinking ability; in some studies, mood and behavior have improved.

Unfortunately, there is a small group of patients who experience cognitive decline after surgery. These individuals are typically more elderly and have pre-existing dementia that may include word-finding difficulty, inability to carry out a sequence of tasks, problems with judging space, and apathy. The presence of dementia at baseline is not an absolute disqualification to DBS if the patient has tremor and other symptoms that would otherwise benefit. However if the results of pre-operative neuropsychological tests are poor, the appropriateness of DBS may be questioned.

A very small group of patients have become seriously depressed after surgery and several suicides have been reported. Such individuals invariably had pre-existing depression, a frequent problem in PD that requires careful attention and expert treatment. In most centers, the presence of depression is a disqualifying factor for surgery.

Surgery—The Process

The prospect of having an operation of any kind is anxiety-provoking. To think of having brain surgery for Parkinson's disease is enough to tax the emotional resources of even the strongest patient and the most supportive of families.

Preparing for Surgery

Before surgery, the patient and family should educate themselves about the procedure. Deep brain stimulation is an elective procedure and, ultimately, the decision to proceed must be that of the patient. He or she should read the available literature and become acquainted with the practical aspects of deep brain stimulation. It can be helpful and reassuring to meet someone who has already gone through the experience. And of course, the patient and family must meet the surgeon.

After detailed discussions with the treating neurologist and the surgeon, the patient must undergo preoperative screening tests. The tests include a brain imaging study, a general medical examination, blood tests, an electrocardiogram, a chest X-ray, neuropsychological testing, and any other data collection required by the institution's protocol. If everything turns out right, the next step is scheduling the surgery.

The Brain Operation in Stages

DBS involves the placement of an electronic device in stages. Each piece of the apparatus must be fitted into the patient and the procedures can be done in any order. A stimulator consists of three parts: (1) DBS electrode, or lead, (2) connecting wire, and (3) battery.

1. The DBS electrode is an insulated wire with four contacts at its end. The electrode is inserted deep into the brain so that its tip directly stimulates the target site. Its other end, near the surface of the brain, is anchored to the inside of the skull.

2. The connecting wire runs under the skin from the DBS lead at the scalp site, behind the ear, and down the neck into the chest where it connects to the battery pack, or implantable pulse generator (IPG).

3. The battery, or implantable pulse generator (IPG), resides like a pacemaker beneath the skin of the chest wall under the collar bone. The IPG is a metal disc about two inches in diameter and one-half inch thick. It contains a small battery and a computer chip. The IPG sends electrical impulses through the connecting wire to the DBS electrode implanted in the brain.

By far the most complicated and time-consuming part of the operation is placement of the DBS lead, which requires careful brain mapping. Patients with symptoms on both sides require bilateral operations. Sometimes the two DBS leads are implanted in the same operation; at other times, they are staged over two operations that are weeks or months apart. Similarly, some surgeons place the entire apparatus—DBS lead, connector, and IPG—in a single, marathon procedure while others first perform only the DBS lead insertion and delay the rest of the work to a second, outpatient procedure the following week. Some patients prefer the idea of staged procedures so they can recover between steps, while others "just want to get it over."

The Day of Surgery

The day of brain surgery may seem endless. Procedures vary from hospital to hospital but the operations generally take 3 to 6 hours and are usually performed while patients are awake, without medication and experiencing PD symptoms at their worst. Thankfully, most patients lose track of the passing hours as they lie immobile on the operating table while the surgeons perform their delicate work.

The first step of the operation is placement of the stereotactic head frame, a large, open casing made of metal bars that is screwed into the patient's skull at several points. This procedure is done under local anesthesia and is not painful, though some patients complain of headache afterward. Sometimes, the head frame is placed on the patient's head the day before the operation, but it is usually done on the morning of surgery. Some surgeons insert the skull screws days in advance to facilitate attachment of the head frame on the day of the surgery.

The goal of the operation is to place, with millimeter accuracy, an electrode deep within the brain. The successful outcome and the risks of the procedure depend critically upon accurate targeting. After the head frame is attached, the patient undergoes a brain imaging scan while wearing the apparatus. The calibrations on the head frame are merged with the brain image to form a computerized map of the brain. This map becomes the blueprint for planning and measuring the trajectories of the electrodes into the deep brain regions of the basal ganglia. The entire head frame structure is then bolted to the operating table to maintain the head in a fixed position throughout the operation.

The surgeon next creates an operative field by drilling a burr hole (a small opening in the skull made with a surgical drill) into the top of the skull—the passageway for the insertion of the stimulating electrode into the brain. The burr hole is made under local anesthesia, and since the brain is completely anesthetic (has no sensation), the rest of the operation is painless. Because of the need to communicate with the operative team, patients undergo surgery while awake. During the procedure, the neurosurgeon asks the patient a number of questions.

Table 10.4. Step-By-Step Plan of Operation for DBS

1. Head frame is attached to skull

2. Magnetic resonance imaging is done for brain mapping

3. Burr hole is drilled in scalp under local anesthesia

4. Electrophysiological brain mapping using microelectrode is done

5. Deep brain stimulator electrode is inserted in brain

6. Implantable pulse generator (IPG) is placed in chest wall

7. Connecting wire is attached to IPG in the chest, and tunneled under skin of neck to deep brain electrode at the scalp site

As an additional means to ensure the accuracy of the surgical probe, some hospital centers perform electrical brain mapping during surgery. This technique uses tiny electrodes that can record electrical activity from individual brain cells within deep brain regions. The microelectrodes are much smaller and more delicate than the electrodes that provide the deep brain stimulation. They are used to identify cells within the thalamus, globus pallidus, subthalamic nucleus, and adjacent brain structures, and help steer the main probe toward the desired surgical target.

For patients who have symptoms on both sides of their body, electrode insertions need to be performed on both sides of the brain. After the first DBS electrode has been placed, the procedure is repeated on the opposite side. Another burr hole is made, the brain mapping is done all over again and the second-side insertion of the deep brain electrode is accomplished—all within the same operation.

After the Operation

The hospitalization required for a deep brain stimulator implantation is usually 2 or 3 days. Patients usually tolerate the procedure very well. Sometimes symptoms are dramatically improved after the DBS electrode is in position, even though the battery has not been attached and the system has not yet been activated. This effect is usually attributed to brain swelling at the tip of the electrode. After the operation, many patients find themselves exhausted, and perhaps slightly confused. Some complain of mild headache. These symptoms usually resolve within 24 hours. Most patients recover quickly and can be safely discharged from the hospital just 1 or 2 days after the surgery. Most patients should remain on their preoperative medication at discharge, although some centers begin a medication reduction protocol at this point. Typically, patients return home with scalp staples or stitches in place, to be removed 1 week later in the surgeon's office once the scalp heals.

Placing the Battery

The DBS electrode requires a power source. Once the deep brain electrode has been inserted, the remaining surgical task is implanting the extension wire and the battery, or implantable pulse generator (IPG). This may be done at the same time as the brain implant or may be deferred to a later date—usually, 1 week after the brain operation. The operation is relatively simple; the surgeon makes an incision under the collarbone, creates a small pocket in the muscle, and inserts the IPG. The IPG is attached to the connecting wire, which is tunneled up the neck, behind the ear and to the scalp site where the external end of the DBS electrode was implanted previously. The connecting lead is attached to the DBS lead. At this point, the entire apparatus is in place under the skin. The chest wall pocket is closed using stitches or staples. The battery produces a visible bump on the chest, especially in patients who are lean.

Patients with electrodes on both sides of the brain have a choice: each electrode can be connected to its own battery, one on each side of the chest or both electrodes can be connected to a single, larger generator implanted on one side. Both options are acceptable, but there are practical and cosmetic differences. Having two batteries means two protrusions, one on each side of the chest. Having one battery means a protrusion on only one side—but the battery is larger and more noticeable. In the rare case of a battery failure or infection, individuals with a single battery will lose power in both stimulators.

The battery implants are performed under general anesthesia. The procedure can be performed during hospitalization or as an outpatient procedure. When patients wake up after the procedure, they may experience chest or neck discomfort and require mild painkillers. Once the batteries and wires are connected, the deep brain stimulation system can be activated. Sometimes, the initial programming is done immediately after the batteries are implanted, but often, this step is deferred. After the batteries are implanted, patients are discharged from the hospital, returning to the office the following week to have the stitches or staples removed. After the incision heals, most patients report that they do not feel the battery or the wires.

After the operation, patients usually resume their preoperative medications, although, in some centers, doctors begin to reduce the PD medications at this point. All postoperative medication adjustments must be carefully supervised by the treating neurologist.

Programming the Stimulator

For patients who undergo deep brain stimulation, the surgical operation is just the beginning.

Years ago, the notion of a patient coming to the office to have deep brain electrodes programmed by a physician or nurse would have seemed like science fiction. Now this scenario happens on a daily basis at busy centers where many such procedures are performed.

After the operation, patients are discharged to home. They must now begin a period of stimulator adjustments, performed over the course of several outpatient visits. The stimulator adjustments and settings are different for every patient. Some undergo surgery believing they will be immediately much better after the stimulator devices are activated. In practice, this improvement may take several weeks, even months, while the stimulator settings are being improved and the medications adjusted to an appropriate level.

Physicians and nurses who program the stimulator work with several variables at once: the way the electrode contacts are turned on, the frequency, the pulse width, and the voltage. In the first months following implantation, patients may require frequent adjustments. After this period, the electrical settings usually stabilize.

Patients may check their deep brain stimulators using a handheld device that resembles a television remote control. Provided by the stimulator manufacturer, the handheld device is called Access Review. By holding the lightweight plastic remote over their implanted battery for a second and pressing a button, patients can determine whether their stimulators are in the "on" or "off" position. If the stimulator has inadvertently been turned off, pressing another button on the remote will turn it back on. The Access Review device does not permit patients to adjust their stimulator parameters themselves or perform any troubleshooting, although future versions will allow this. Any problems with the stimulator require a visit to the medical center to have the device checked.

The life expectancy of the stimulator battery varies with output settings but is estimated at 3 to 5 years. As the energy in the battery becomes depleted, the efficacy of the stimulation starts to decline and PD symptoms increase. Patients can check the battery status using the handheld device or the neurologist can do this in the office. When the battery is depleted, the implantable pulse generator (IPG) will require replacement under local anesthesia in an ambulatory surgical procedure that takes about one hour. The old IPG is removed from the chest wall site by reopening the incision. The device is disconnected from the connecting lead, the new IPG is inserted and hooked up and the incision is again closed with stitches or staples. The procedure is done under general anesthesia. In the near future, it is expected that externally rechargeable batteries will eliminate the need for battery replacement.

Risks of Deep Brain Stimulation

Risks of Surgery

Potential complications of surgery for Parkinson's disease range from mild headache or drowsiness to more serious or irreversible effects, such as infection, stroke, or hemorrhage. Some patients, especially those who are already suffering from mild cognitive problems, may experience postoperative sleepiness, disorientation, slowness of mental processing, hallucinations, poor motivation, or depression. These events typically resolve within 24 or 48 hours but may last longer. After bilateral STN stimulation, some patients have experienced difficulty opening their eyes. To remedy this, some may need injections of botulinum toxin, a muscle relaxant.

115

At the medical centers that have the most experience with DBS, the risk of stroke or bleeding is less than 5 percent. The earlier lesion-based techniques, pallidotomy and thalamotomy, had a slightly higher incidence of permanent complications than deep brain stimulation because direct destruction of brain tissue was part of the operation.

Because deep brain stimulation requires implanted hardware, there is a risk of infection, sometimes requiring antibiotics or even replacement of an infected device. Despite every precaution, a skin infection can sometimes occur at the battery site in the chest wall, in the neck or at the scalp. Like all types of surgery, operator experience is the most important determinant of risk. The lowest complication rates are at major centers that perform this type of highly specialized surgery on a weekly basis.

Adverse Effects of Stimulation

The process of programming the device is tedious and sometimes uncomfortable for the patient. Patients are often asked to withhold their medication for several hours while the stimulator personnel determine the optimal device settings. It may take hours of testing different electrode combinations before the best setting is determined. Sometimes, during a programming session, patients may experience temporary tingling or shocking sensations, and uncomfortable muscle spasms or contractions.

Additional stimulator-induced problems may include balance impairment, dizziness, speech difficulties, or a general vague sensation of "not feeling right." There are rare reports of stimulation-induced feelings of depression or despair. Deep brain stimulation can also

Table 10.5. Reversible Adverse Effects of Stimulation

- Jolting or shocking sensations
- Numbness or tingling, often in the face or hand
- Dizziness or balance impairment
- Twisting movements that resemble dyskinesias
- Muscle spasms, usually in the face or hand
- Slurred speech
- Double vision
- Depression

induce dyskinesias that resemble the dyskinesias caused by levo-dopa.

All stimulator-induced effects are temporary and reverse promptly with a change in the stimulator output. After a programming session, it is a good idea for patients to wait at the center for an hour or so before returning home just to make sure that the new stimulator settings are well-tolerated and free of adverse effects.

Patients with implanted deep brain stimulators are generally free to participate in any physical activity they choose. However, it is important to use common sense and not to engage in activities that could subject the device or wires to a direct physical blow or acceleration. Examples of specific activities that could potentially harm the stimulator include contact sports or chiropractic neck manipulation. Sometimes, with repeated trauma, the connecting lead or the battery erodes through the skin, requiring replacement.

Deep brain stimulators may switch off by accident if patients walk through a magnetic field, such as a security device or theft detector. This is simply an inconvenience and carries no permanent risk to the patient or stimulator device. When the stimulator switches off, however, PD symptoms can immediately return. If this happens, the patient may reactivate the stimulator using the handheld device. The manufacturer provides a list of appliances that may cause interference with deep brain stimulation.

There is an important warning for patients with implanted brain electrodes not to undergo ultrasound diathermy, a treatment that involves applying a heating coil to the skin. It is also recommended that patients with deep brain stimulators check with their neurologist before undergoing magnetic resonance imaging (MRI) scans, a technique that uses a powerful magnetic field. In theory, the DBS electrode is unaffected by magnetic fields, but some of the larger MRI scanners are very powerful.

In case of questions about the stimulator, patients should always contact their treating neurologist, who may recommend a return visit to the medical center for a device check.

Future Perspectives on Surgery for PD

Deep brain stimulation is the most advanced surgical approach currently available for Parkinson's disease. For some patients, the procedure is miraculously effective. People who once experienced disabling tremors, severe dyskinesias, or paralyzing wearing-off episodes may find themselves free of their former disabilities. For many others, however, deep brain stimulation does not solve their problems.

Deep brain stimulation is in its infancy and will almost certainly improve over time. Anticipated improvements include batteries that are smaller, last longer, and are rechargeable. The original battery packs were capable of providing an electrical current only to a single electrode but now patients may choose a single side battery that is capable of powering both stimulators. Someday, the entire apparatus, including the generator, will be implanted in the skull, eliminating wires and batteries in the neck and chest. Other anticipated changes include an alarm feature that lets the patients know when the device is malfunctioning; advanced troubleshooting features; and the ability to program the deep brain stimulator over the telephone or internet so that patients do not have to return to the office for these adjustments.

It seems likely that the numbers of effective brain targets will rise. As deep brain stimulation becomes more sophisticated, the stimulating electrode will have motion sensors that allow it to detect when a patient wants to make a specific movement. The stimulation electrode in current use has four electrical contacts arranged in a line. Electrodes of the future will have more contacts, and improved ability to direct electrical current into brain tissue. Someday, the stimulators will have branch leads implanted in other parts of the basal ganglia to produce network effects that more closely resemble the physiology of the person's motor system.

Other futuristic possibilities beyond DBS may include the surgical implantation of cells with regenerative capacity; gene therapies; and other treatments that can prevent or reverse the cell loss in PD.

Ten Commonly Asked Questions

Who is the ideal candidate for surgery?

The ideal candidate for surgery is a patient with PD who responds well to levodopa and other antiparkinsonian medications but who experiences dyskinesias or wearing-off spells. Such patients usually have had PD for 10 years or more and have reached a stage where even a complicated medication schedule, sometimes requiring pills every 2 hours or less, is not sufficient to control the wearing-off episodes.

People who never experience clear benefit from levodopa are unlikely to improve with deep brain stimulation, and therefore should not consider this approach. People who have an atypical form of parkinsonism, such as progressive supranuclear palsy (PSP), will also not benefit from surgery. To be a candidate for the operation, people must be in good general physical and psychiatric health, have no cognitive impairment, and have a good support system of family or friends to help them through the ordeals of surgery and subsequent postoperative management.

Does surgery help all symptoms of Parkinson's disease?

Surgery for PD helps many, but not all, symptoms of PD. As a general rule, the symptoms that respond best to medication respond best to surgery. Tremor and rigidity can greatly improve with surgery, but slowness improves as well. Dystonic posturing of the limbs, often present in the early morning or during "off" spells, also responds well to surgery. Drug-induced dyskinesias may completely resolve after surgery. On the other hand, patients who experience stooped posture, poor balance, cognitive impairment, or rapid stuttering speech, sometimes called tachyphemia, may not experience benefit in these symptoms after a surgical procedure.

Which is the best choice of deep brain stimulation for me?

The choice of which surgical technique is best for a given patient—and indeed, the decision to have surgery at all—depends on many factors. No two patients are alike. For most people with PD, the chance of significant benefit must clearly outweigh the operative risks. The choice of surgical approach is best determined through careful discussions involving the patient, the family, the neurologist, and the neurosurgeon.

The choice of surgery may depend on the patient's specific symptoms. Is the main issue a disabling tremor? Or is drug-induced dyskinesia the biggest problem? Other pertinent questions include: Has the patient had previous brain surgery? Does he or she live in an area that offers ready access to the medical center for DBS programming or troubleshooting? The techniques with the most benefit appear to be deep brain stimulation in the subthalamic nucleus or globus pallidus but there are patients for whom a different approach may be preferable.

Where is the best place to have surgery?

Although enthusiasm for surgery is widespread, the techniques are very specialized and the surgical skills and support systems that are necessary are not available everywhere. For this reason, patients and their families would be wise to seek out a center that has long-standing experience with DBS as well as resources specifically dedicated to the surgical treatment of PD. As with any complicated technical procedure, there is a learning curve, and surgeons with the most experience have the lowest complication rates.

The ideal center should have a clinical team devoted to the surgical treatment of PD, with a neurosurgeon specially trained in stereotactic surgery and an electrophysiologist to perform intra-operative brain mapping. There should be experienced neurologists and nursing personnel skilled in preoperative screening and postoperative care, including programming the deep brain stimulator. It is essential that center personnel be available for immediate advice and evaluation should the need arise.

Considering the rapid pace of technological advance in this field, it may be worth considering whether the surgical center has a serious commitment to PD research, or whether the surgery is being offered simply to provide a clinical service. One telling question may be: does the surgical team regularly publish and report its results and complications to the medical community?

Does my insurance cover the cost of the surgery?

To date, most private insurers, as well as Medicare and Medicaid, have approved the surgery for PD and have covered all expenses completely. This is fortunate as the cost of the procedures is extremely high, running to as much as $100,000 for the surgery, anesthesia, stimulator devices, and hospital care. The FDA gave a general approval for deep brain stimulation in 2002, so this advanced treatment is now considered standard therapy, and not experimental.

Will surgery enable me to stop my antiparkinsonian medications?

For many patients, DBS surgery will reduce the dependency on medication. Individuals who undergo bilateral subthalamic nucleus stimulation, for example, may reduce their medication by 50 percent or more in the months following surgery. For patients who experience adverse effects of their medications, such as hallucinations or dyskinesias, limiting medication intake is an important secondary benefit of the operation. Patients whose main problem is severe tremor may find their tremor so well controlled by surgery that medication becomes unnecessary.

What is the effect of surgery on the long-term course of PD?

The effect of surgery on the prognosis of PD is unknown. Most investigators believe that a surgical intervention will have little or no effect on slowing the progression of the disease even though relief of symptoms may be dramatic and long-lasting. Studies have shown benefits lasting at least 5 years. Tremor and dyskinesia are two symptoms of PD that may be permanently stopped by surgery. But other disabling symptoms of PD—gait impairment, falling, poor posture, soft speech—may worsen with time, despite surgery. As for the possibility of dementia, the long-term effect of surgery is unknown.

Will a decision to undergo surgery now disqualify me from better treatments that might be available in the future?

It is impossible to predict what new or improved therapy might be coming in the near future or who will be eligible for it. Deep brain stimulation, unlike earlier techniques, does not destroy significant amounts of brain tissue and is therefore, in theory, a reversible treatment. As such, having DBS done now should not exclude an individual from a future, more promising therapy.

Is surgery for Parkinson's disease a cure?

No—at least, not yet. A cure for PD would be a treatment that can stop the disease from progressing and even reverse it. Neither deep brain stimulation, nor the older lesion-based techniques, nor medications, can provide this at present. At best, surgery may be able to control some or all of the disabling problems of PD, such as drug-induced dyskinesias, tremor, wearing-off fluctuations, slowness of movement, rigidity and tremor—but the disease remains progressive.

What are the chances of finding a cure for PD?

Many scientists believe that the cure for PD will come from a deeper understanding of what causes the disease. What is the reason that dopamine neurons in the basal ganglia begin to degenerate and die? If the cause of the neurodegeneration can be identified, perhaps a specific treatment could be applied to slow, stop, or reverse its process.

Strategies of treatment in the future may include the delivery of substances or genetic material directly to degenerating brain cells. Future treatment may involve replacing dying cells using an alternative source of brain tissue, such as stem-cell lines or embryonic tissue. However, these techniques are in the earliest stages of development.

For sufferers of Parkinson's disease and their families, the progress is always too slow. But there are reasons to be optimistic. DBS revolutionized the treatment of PD and has improved the quality of life for thousands of patients. It is anticipated that many scientific advances will be translated into benefits for people with Parkinson's, and so the hope for a cure is linked with true promise and great optimism.

Chapter 11

Complementary and Alternative Medicine and PD

In the last decade or so, great strides have been made in the treatment of Parkinson disease (PD). New dopamine agonists and COMT [Catechol O-methyltransferase] inhibitors have improved motor function, and several new medications will soon become available. The treatment of other symptoms that may be present in PD, such as depression and sleep disorders, also has improved.

A select group of patients may benefit from surgical therapy for PD. At a minimum, the addition of an exercise program is vital to maintaining good health.

Though significant, these developments are insufficient in treating every aspect of the disease. Unfortunately, there still exist many symptoms and medication side effects for which current "traditional" treatments are unsatisfactory or incomplete.

Because persons with PD generally tend to be well-educated and quite proactive about the care they receive, many have chosen to explore treatment options outside the realm of "Western" medicine. Alternative therapies have been slow to gain favor with some practitioners of more traditional medicine because there is little research to demonstrate their effectiveness. This is beginning to change, due in part to the establishment of The National Center for Complementary and Alternative Medicine, a government organization that will fund and carry out such studies. Many universities have established similar departments.

For some patients and caregivers, alternative or complementary approaches to treatment are completely novel. Others have been raised in cultures where the use of herbal medicines or acupuncture are commonplace. In fact, many of these modalities have been in use for thousands of years. In the treatment of PD, a number of complementary therapies, such as yoga and tai chi, are well-established companions to traditional medications. Acupuncture and therapeutic massage also have become popular in some PD centers, as have herbal therapies and dietary supplements (though self-prescription of supplements can be dangerous in some cases).

The intention of this text is to provide a summary overview of various complementary therapies, and how some can be useful in the treatment of PD.

Diet

The choices we make about food—what we consume, its quality and quantity—are crucial to our health and well-being. Of course, conflicting information abounds concerning what constitutes a healthy diet: Are fats and carbohydrates "good" or "bad" dietary components? This may depend on which fad diet is currently in vogue. There is some agreement that it is generally wise to consume a varied diet high in fruits and vegetables and to avoid excessive saturated fats, especially trans fats. There is also some evidence that the so-called Mediterranean diet, a diet high in monounsaturated fats, such as olive oil, may be beneficial in reducing blood pressure and cardiovascular disease. The diet also emphasizes fish, especially those high in omega-3 fatty acids, such as salmon, and foods containing antioxidants.

Persons with PD are often particularly concerned about the possibility that protein intake can decrease the effectiveness of carbidopa/levodopa, one of the common medications used to treat PD. While it is true that levodopa absorption into the brain can be slowed by a high protein meal, most patients do not notice that their motor function varies along with their diet. Since PD can affect digestive function, many patients do notice symptoms such as constipation and early satiety (the sensation of feeling very full after consuming a small amount of food). Since these changes can be of long-term duration, it may be advisable to treat them with dietary modifications such as frequent, small meals and increased fiber intake to avoid or delay the need for additional medications.

Antioxidants

Antioxidants are substances that can detoxify free radicals, which are reactive particles involved in certain types of cell death. Since there is evidence that free radical damage is involved to some extent in PD, vitamin E, a moderately potent antioxidant, was studied in people with early PD in a large study in the 1980s. The study did not demonstrate benefit in slowing the disease or "neuroprotection." However, it is possible that dietary vitamin E may be used more easily by the body than the supplements used in the study. This might be another reason to consider the Mediterranean diet. Another antioxidant substance that has achieved importance in PD treatment is coenzyme Q10. In a relatively small but well-designed study in early PD, CoQ10 appeared to have some effect on disease progression at doses of 1200 mg/day. This is a much larger dose than most people were taking prior to the release of the study data, a deliberate choice designed to avoid the risk of missing a significant effect by giving too low a dose. In fact, the study showed no benefit from the lower doses, possibly because only a small amount of the ingested dose (10–15 percent) is actually absorbed by the body. The researchers involved in the study did not recommend that all persons with PD begin taking this compound and, in fact, there is no information on the effects of CoQ10 in more advanced disease. It is also very expensive and, as a nonprescription agent, is not covered by insurance, although it is covered by health saving accounts. However, it does appear to be safe and well-tolerated.

Ayurvedic Medicine

One of the oldest systems of medicine is Ayurveda, which has been practiced in India for thousands of years. The practice is concerned more with establishing and maintaining one's health in terms of body, mind, and spirit than in treating a particular disease entity. However, the principles of Ayurveda have been found to be useful by some practitioners for treating various conditions. The initial step is to determine the metabolic type of an individual. Then the practitioner looks at environmental factors, such as season and time of day. Diseases are diagnosed by assessing various pulse points and their relationship to internal organs.

Treatment of disease consists of detoxification (shodan) through various cleansing therapies, then restoring balance through palliation (shaman) with such modalities as yoga and meditation. Finally, a process of tonification, called rasayana, is initiated. Interestingly, one of the medications used in Ayurveda was derived from a legume, *Mucuna pruriens*, which has been found to contain levodopa. The condition for which it was used, as described many centuries ago, most likely was Parkinson disease.

Yoga

Yoga is an ancient practice associated with Ayurvedic medicine. A complete practice of yoga integrates mind, body, and spirit in a process involving one's complete lifestyle. The most popular form of yoga is asana or Hatha yoga, which involves execution of a series of postures with attention to breathing (pranayama), meditation, and proper execution of the poses. Like tai chi, the practice of yoga has been shown to improve various aspects of health such as blood pressure, digestion and asthma. Most yoga centers offer a range of classes and list them as to level of experience required. Yoga classes are also offered at many senior centers, park districts, and fitness enters. Most instructors inquire about any physical limitations at the beginning of the class. As with any form of exercise, it is important to start slowly and build up gradually to a more advanced level to avoid injury. Since exercise is so important in the treatment of PD, patients are seeking to improve their strength, balance, and flexibility. Yoga and tai chi are both excellent for this. In addition to more traditional fitness programs such as walking and weight lifting, classes in yoga and tai chi have become standard offerings in senior centers, gyms, and park districts.

Traditional Chinese Medicine (TCM)

Like Ayurveda, Chinese or Oriental Medicine has been in practice for thousands of years and also is concerned with maintaining health instead of just reacting to disease. Much emphasis is placed on maintaining a balance between opposites within the body as well as with the natural world. These opposites are termed the yin and the yang. According to Roger Jahnke, O.M.D., Chairperson of the National Qigong Association (quoted in Alternative Medicine; The Definitive Guide, 2nd Edition, edited by Burton Goldberg), "yin refers to the organ, while yang refers to its activity." Disease results from a disturbance in this balance. The concept of qi (pronounced "chee") is also important; this refers to life force and energy within the body. The energy flows in channels or "meridians" along the surface of the body and through the internal organs for which they are named.

A condition described in the text *Principles of Medicine,* written in 1565, sounds very much like PD; "Wind tremors are (caused by) by Wind entering the Liver and the Qi of the channels rebelling upward, (causing) tics of the face and tremors of the limbs." In this context, Liver refers to the organ itself as well as the associated meridian and sphere of influence. The Liver is believed to rule coordination and smooth movement. Parkinson disease is thought to represent a defective Liver (yin) and the invasion of Wind (yang), which is thought to result in tremor. Imbalances between yin and yang are treated with modalities such as acupuncture and herbal medicine. There are many variants of TCM practices, some involving the practice of martial arts such as tai chi.

Tai Chi

Tai chi, both a form of martial arts and a system of meditation, is part of an ancient Chinese system of healing called qigong. In tai chi classes, participants follow a teacher in performing a choreographed series of movements. There are various styles and levels of difficulty, including some classes performed while practitioners are seated. Tai chi has been shown in several studies to improve balance in older patients as well as persons with PD. There may be other benefits as well, including reduction of stress and improvements in digestion and arthritis pain.

Acupuncture

One of the methods used to help restore the balance of yin and yang is acupuncture, a technique developed over 2,500 years ago in China. The treatment involves inserting hair-like needles into certain points on the body, known as acupoints. This is done to restore the flow of qi to the organ system associated with that acupoint. It is important to choose a practitioner who is licensed in acupuncture and is recommended either by another trusted physician or by the National Certification Commission for Acupuncture and Oriental Medicine (NCCAOM). As with most areas of complementary medicine, there is a paucity of data in the use of acupuncture in PD. Some persons with PD describe temporary relief from symptoms such as tremor and rigidity.

Herbal Medicine

Herbal medicine refers to compounds made from plants or plant components such as flowers, leaves, or roots. In addition to being an important component of TCM, herbal medicine exists in many forms in many cultures. In many Spanish-speaking countries, for example, it is common to visit the local herbal practitioner for an infusion designed to treat a particular ailment. Symptoms of PD might be treated with a preparation to treat "nerves." Consulting a traditional physician such as a neurologist might happen later, or not at all. It has also become relatively common for people to self-prescribe herbal remedies based upon their own research on the internet or the advice of the sales staff at a health food store. This can be expensive and is potentially dangerous. These products are not regulated by the FDA [U.S. Food and Drug Administration], and many of them are imported from countries where there may be no quality control or guarantee of purity. It is also important to realize that many of these agents have distinct pharmacologic properties with the potential to be harmful on their own or to interact with medications the patient is already taking. Therefore, it is strongly recommended that the use of herbal treatments be supervised by a competent specialist and that all prescribing physicians be informed of these additions.

In TCM, herbs are chosen by a trained practitioner as part of a comprehensive treatment plan and prescribed in combination based on their properties related to specific organ systems.

Body Work/Massage Therapy

Body work comprises a group of "touch therapies" such as reflexology, Rolfing, and therapeutic massage. Massage therapy in particular has become very popular because of its beneficial effects on the muscle stiffness and aching that may accompany PD. Massage may also help with associated conditions such as arthritis and sleep and digestive disorders. In addition, a well-executed massage can be an extremely relaxing and enjoyable experience.

Of the many different styles of massage therapy, two in particular may be useful in PD. Shiatsu, or acupressure, uses touch rather than needles to treat the same pressure points as acupuncture. Swedish massage consists of gently kneading the muscles of the back, neck, scalp, and limbs. It is not uncommon for people to feel a bit awkward about letting a stranger touch their bodies, especially if they are asked to disrobe for the treatment.

It is worth noting that the client will be covered by a sheet or blanket; only the part of the body being massaged will be uncovered at any one time. If this is still an intimidating concept, it might be helpful to start out by having a chair massage first. This is done while the client is seated in a specially designed chair while fully clothed. This may allow one to experience the benefits of the massage in a less stressful setting while getting to know the therapist. Some therapists are able to do a full body massage on a person who is wearing clothes, but it is wise to ask in advance, if this is an issue. This is another treatment that should only be performed by a licensed massage therapist or by a physical therapist with training in this area. In some cases, massage therapy will be reimbursed by insurance or Medicare, especially when performed as part of a physical therapy program.

In summary, many of these therapies are becoming accepted by patients and practitioners in the contemporary treatment of Parkinson disease and can work well in complement with medications and other so-called traditional treatments. Diet and exercise are proving to be extremely important in maintaining good health, and this may be augmented by practices such as yoga, tai chi, or the addition of appropriate supplements or herbs. It is important to find practitioners who are well-trained and appropriately certified, and who have been recommended by a trusted source, such as one's primary care physician, neurologist, or the regulatory board for that discipline. Herbal agents and supplements should be used cautiously, preferably under the supervision of a trained professional in the use of these drugs.

A list of physicians, specially trained in alternative medicine, can be found at www.integrativemedicine.arizona.edu.

By Melanie M. Brandabur, M.D., Medical Director, Parkinson's Disease and Movement Disorders Center, Alexian Neuroscience Institute, Chicago-Hoffman Estates, Illinois, a National Parkinson Foundation Center of Excellence. The author wishes to thank Patrick Massey, M.D., Ph.D., and David Bates for their assistance in writing this text.

Chapter 12

Choosing the Right Doctor If You Have PD

I was 44 years old when I first noticed a slight tremor in my left pinky. My internist attributed it to my being "a middle-aged woman about to become an empty nester." Why then, I wondered, in the immortal words of Jerry Lee Lewis, didn't I see "a whole lot more shakin' goin' on" among my friends?

A few months later, with my tremor worsening, I went to a general neurologist for a second opinion. His diagnosis—based on my age—was essential tremor. He obviously had not read his office copy of *People* magazine featuring Michael J. Fox's "coming out" story on the cover (after all, Michael was only 30 when he was diagnosed!).

My extensive online research had already convinced me I had Parkinson's, and I set out to find the right doctor to guide me on what I knew would be a long, difficult journey. I needed someone with a good bedside manner who was on top of the latest research and treatment strategies. Not knowing where else to turn, I called PDF for a referral. What I got was "a match made in heaven."

Research says that the better the relationships patients have with their doctors, the more likely they are to follow their treatment plans and improve their health and/or quality of life. In this column, I address several ways to find the right doctor for you.

MDS or General Neurologist?

While there is yet no cure for Parkinson's, there is a growing line-up of medications that provide significant, long-term symptomatic relief. The challenge for doctors and patients is to decide together when to introduce which PD medications and, as the disease progresses, how to adjust the combination and doses of treatments to optimally control PD symptoms and to minimize side effects.

This is where movement disorder specialists (MDS)—neurologists who have additional training in this subspecialty, which includes Parkinson's— have an advantage over general neurologists. Because they treat a greater number of patients with Parkinson's, MDS tend to be more experienced in diagnosis and treatment than do most general neurologists or internists. Often connected to major medical institutions, they also may be involved in research and/or teaching, which keeps them up-to-date with clinical trial opportunities for which their patients may be eligible.

Although you may have to travel farther to find a MDS, most people with Parkinson's say it is worth it—especially because you usually need to make the trip only two or three times a year. Your general neurologist can continue to take care of your overall healthcare needs, and consult by phone, fax, or mail with your MDS as necessary.

Finding Your Doctor

I have found through experience that there are several ways to find a doctor with a good reputation to treat your Parkinson's. First, ask friends, family, and co-workers for referrals. Second, attend educational sessions and support groups for people with Parkinson's and their families, and ask for recommendations.

Another approach is to go to the experts, by telephone or online. Several of the national Parkinson's organizations maintain lists of specialists. Start by calling PDF 800-457-6676; the American Parkinson Disease Association 800-223-2732; or the National Parkinson Foundation 800-327-4545.

Be sure to check which physicians are in your health insurance network and whether they accept Medicare. And, lastly, contact your state department of insurance to see if the doctors whom you are considering have any complaints filed against them.

The Initial Meeting

Review the referrals that you have obtained and the information you have collected about each doctor. Schedule an exam with your top choice and prepare written questions to bring to your appointment. The information below provides a list of questions to ask yourself after the appointment to help you decide if you have found a doctor who is the right fit.

Whatever may be the diagnosis of the first doctor, you may want to seek a second opinion. A good doctor will never be offended by this, and may even provide you with a referral. And if you like this first doctor, you can return to him or her to continue treatment after obtaining a second opinion. (Confirm that the second-opinion visit is covered by your insurance.)

On BrainTalk, an online support group for people with Parkinson's, a man named Todd made an astute observation: "You either have a good relationship with your doctor or you don't. You have to trust your physician and feel like they respect you as a person and a patient."

Five Questions to Ask

Does your doctor:

- Put you at ease when discussing your concerns?
- Take your opinions and questions seriously?
- Answer questions to your satisfaction?
- Encourage your input into decision making and treatment?
- Invite e-mail contact between visits?

Sheryl Jedlinski is a self-employed writer and desktop publisher. She is the Communication Coordinator for the Parkinson Pipeline Project. Sheryl is married, has two adult sons, and lives in Palatine, IL.

Chapter 13

Treating PD:
The Role of the Patient

Treating Parkinson's disease (PD) is not exclusively the doctor's job; there are many things a person with Parkinson's can do to contribute. Regular exercise, joining a support group, maintaining a healthy diet, and taking part in a clinical trial are just some of the things you might consider.

A Healthy Patient/Doctor Relationship

Making an accurate diagnosis of Parkinson's—specifically in its early stages—is difficult, but a skilled practitioner can come to a reasoned conclusion that it is Parkinson's. Every person diagnosed with Parkinson's should consider getting a second opinion from a neurologist who specializes in movement disorders and is up-to-date on research and approaches to therapy.

Locating a qualified physician is a first step; next is considering whether the physician is the right one. A person with Parkinson's will work with a physician for many years. Consider these questions:

- Are you comfortable speaking with your physician?
- Do you feel respected by your doctor?
- Are questions answered to your satisfaction or do you come away from a visit feeling that you have not been taken seriously?

- Can you get in touch with the doctor between visits?

To find a neurologist or movement disorder specialist in your area:

- Ask your primary care physician for a referral.
- Seek referrals from others living with Parkinson's.
- Contact your insurance provider for a list of neurologists or movement disorder specialists in your network.
- Contact PDF for a referral.

Exercise

For people with Parkinson's, regular exercise or physical therapy is crucial for maintaining and improving mobility, flexibility, balance, range of motion, and for warding off many of the disease's secondary symptoms such as depression and constipation. PDF offers Motivating Moves for People with Parkinson's, a unique program of 24 seated and stimulating exercises that were created especially for people with Parkinson's. Copies are available for ordering through the website, or you can call or e-mail PDF for more information. As with every aspect of your care, always consult your doctor before starting an exercise program.

Diet

Many people with Parkinson's lose weight because of poor appetite and inadequate food intake. It is recommended to maintain a full diet that contains all the daily nutritional requirements, including extra fresh fruits and vegetables for fiber to help prevent constipation and plenty of fluids to keep hydrated.

Some people who take levodopa find that protein may interfere with the medication's effect. Limiting protein intake or staggering the medication dosing to avoid conflicts with meals can help this problem. However, adjustments in protein intake are only worthwhile for those very few people whose response to levodopa is indeed sensitive to dietary protein.

People with Parkinson's who lose weight for no clear reason should discuss this with a physician.

Please go to www.pdf.org/Publications/factsheets/PDF_Nutrition_Fact_Sheet_Web.pdf to view a copy of PDF's fact sheet, Nutrition and Parkinson's Disease, written by a registered dietitian.

Support Groups

For many people, support groups play an important role in the emotional well-being of patients and families. They can provide a caring environment for asking questions about Parkinson's, for sharing stories and advice, and for creating friendships with people who have experienced similar problems. PDF keeps a listing of nationwide Parkinson's support groups. To find one your area, please call or e-mail PDF at 800-457-6676. In addition to in-person support groups, many people also find online groups and listservs helpful. For a listing of listservs that serve the Parkinson's community, please request our publication, Web Resources for People with Parkinson's Disease [www.pdf.org/Publications/Web_Resources.pdf].

Physical, Speech, and/or Occupational Therapy

These therapies can help Parkinson's patients control their symptoms and make daily life easier. Physical therapy may increase muscle strength and flexibility and decrease the incidence of falls. Speech therapy can increase voice volume and assist with word pronunciation. The Lee Silverman technique is a special speech therapy that can be very beneficial to people with Parkinson's—for further information see www.lsvt.org.

Occupational therapy gives people alternative methods of doing tasks that they can no longer perform with ease. These options may provide a stronger sense of control when living with Parkinson's disease. A neurologist should be able to provide recommendations for these therapies and, if needed, a referral. These therapies may or may not be covered by insurance.

Clinical Trials

Clinical trials (also called medical research, clinical research, or a clinical study) help researchers answer specific questions about the safety and efficacy of new treatments by studying its effects in people. They are an essential and necessary component of the scientific research process. Simply put, there is no other way for research to show that a proposed treatment works. In addition to contributing to research, joining a clinical trial can provide a person with early access to potentially helpful Parkinson's treatments and drugs that are not yet on the market.

PDtrials was created in 2004 to increase the PD community's awareness of clinical trials and provide up-to-date information on trials enrolling participants. For more information on clinical trials and how you can get involved, visit www.PDtrials.org. This project is led by the Parkinson's Disease Foundation, in cooperation with the following organizations: American Parkinson Disease Association, Inc., The Michael J. Fox Foundation for Parkinson's Research, National Parkinson Foundation, Parkinson's Action Network, The Parkinson Alliance, and WE MOVE.

Chapter 14

Five Frequently Asked Questions about Hospitalization for PD

Most people with Parkinson disease [PD] will need to be hospitalized at some time. Hospitalization can be stressful for a number of important reasons. The neurologist who takes care of you and manages your Parkinson disease medications may not have privileges at the hospital where you are admitted, and the physicians and nursing staff responsible for your care in the hospital may not know a lot about Parkinson disease. If you need to undergo surgery or other invasive medical procedures, you may not be able to take any medications until the surgery or procedure is complete.

It is important for the patient and the caregiver to plan and anticipate what is likely to happen. This text will answer five of the most frequently asked questions about hospitalization for people with Parkinson disease.

When I am in the hospital, why don't I always get my medications on time?

It is important to realize that hospitals and hospital pharmacies have their own dosing schedules. For example, if a medication is written for "QID" (four times a day [in Latin: *quater in die*]), the standard

"Five Frequently Asked Questions about Hospitalization: For Patients with Parkinson Disease," by Kelvin Chou, M.D., Michael Okun, M.D., Hubert Fernandez, M.D., Diane Breslow, MSW, LCSW, Joseph Friedman, M.D. From Parkinson Report, Summer 2007. © 2007 National Parkinson Foundation (www.parkinson.org). Reprinted with permission.

hospital schedule may be 8 AM—1 PM—6 PM—11 PM or some similar variation. A medication written for "TID" (three times a day [in Latin: *ter in die*]) may be given at 7 AM—3 PM—11 PM or some other standard schedule. Furthermore, many hospitals may have a policy that permits nurses to give medications at times different (generally, one hour before or after) from the scheduled time. This window is provided as a practical compromise because nursing staffs are busy, and each nurse usually cares for multiple patients. Such a policy provides the nurse time to complete his/her scheduled duties, and provides flexibility in case of emergency on the ward. As a result, patients with Parkinson disease will in most cases receive their medications at seemingly random times.

How can such a situation be remedied? First, make sure that the drug schedule, with specific times, is written into the doctor's orders. For example, if carbidopa/levodopa (Sinemet) is given four times a day, but at 6 AM—10 AM—2 PM—6 PM, make sure that the physician taking care of you knows that it should be given at those specific times. Also make sure that you bring with you the complete list of your medications and the dose of each medication is correct. When you first arrive in your room, talk with your nurse about the importance of receiving your medications on time. Explain that without the medications you can be immobile or uncomfortable and that the medications allow you to move around independently. You may know more about Parkinson disease than the doctor and the staff, and it is your job to help them understand your situation. While you will still need to be somewhat flexible (there are many other important things that may occupy a nurse's time), sharing your knowledge with the staff can alleviate many problems. All hospital staffs want their patients to be well cared for during their stay.

Why can't I take my own medications in the hospital? Why do they substitute some medications for me?

While you are hospitalized, the nursing staff must have control of your medications. This is a safety issue and is standard hospital policy. It is not a reflection of what the staff thinks of you, so don't take it personally. In some cases, patients may be taking medications that are not stocked in the hospital pharmacy. In such situations, the physician taking care of you in the hospital may have to prescribe substitute medications. If you want to take your own medications, you need to bring them from home in their original bottles and give them to the nursing staff. They will then dispense your medications while you are admitted, and there will be no need for substitution. If you are enrolled in an experimental drug protocol, it is even more important that you follow this practice. In some hospitals and outpatient surgical facilities, the doctor can write an order to allow patients to take their own medicines; however, the doses and times must be written in the chart, and the pill ingestion must be supervised and documented.

My mother has Parkinson disease and was recently hospitalized. However, she seems to be moving much worse in the hospital than at home. Why is that?

Several explanations are possible. When patients with Parkinson disease have an infection of some kind, whether it is the common cold, pneumonia, or a urinary tract infection, they often feel like their symptoms worsen. Increased tremor or more difficulty walking may be noted. When the infection is treated and resolves, their symptoms generally return to baseline. Another symptom that may worsen when patients with Parkinson disease have an infection is swallowing. When swallowing is impaired and patients are weak, the food may go down into the lungs, causing an "aspiration pneumonia," which, in turn, may further impair swallowing ability. In these situations, a speech pathology consultation can be useful to formally assess swallowing and make dietary recommendations. In addition, a respiratory therapist consultation for "chest PT" [physical therapy] may be helpful. Chest PT consists of several minutes of chest clapping to help mobilize the sputum and make it easier to cough.

Another possibility is the addition of a new medication. Common offenders include antipsychotic drugs or antinausea drugs. Haloperidol (Haldol) is a common antipsychotic drug that is used in hospital settings. This drug blocks dopamine receptors and worsens PD. Other commonly used antipsychotics include risperidone (Risperdal), olanzapine (Zyprexa), and aripiprazole (Abilify). The only antipsychotics that can be used safely in PD patients are clozapine (Clozaril) and quetiapine (Seroquel). Common antinausea medications that can worsen symptoms of Parkinson disease include prochlorperazine (Compazine), promethazine (Phenergan), and metoclopramide (Reglan). These medications have similar structures to the antipsychotics and should not be used. Trimethobenzamide (Tigan) and ondansetron (Zofran) are suitable alternatives that can be used without fear of worsening symptoms.

Regardless of the cause, all patients with Parkinson disease should be as active as possible while in the hospital. Moving around not only tones muscle, it allows faster recovery and prevents decomposition of the skin, which can happen when staying in one position for too long. Depending upon your condition, however, you may not have a choice as your doctor may order you to bed rest. In that case, physical therapy should be ordered as soon as possible. Some patients may also need rehabilitation at a rehabilitation hospital or a nursing facility before being discharged to home.

My husband has Parkinson disease and became confused in the hospital last time he was there. How can I prevent this?

Many things happen in the hospital that can contribute to confusion. Any infection in a patient with Parkinson disease can be enough to tip a patient "over the edge" mentally. Similarly, infections can adversely affect motor function as we discussed above.

The introduction of new medications, especially pain medications, frequently results in disorientation and memory problems. Lack of sleep while in the hospital can also contribute to a confusional state. Continuous alarms from IV [intravenous] machines and hallway lights can all result in frequent awakening. Nurses also may regularly enter the room overnight to take vital signs, give medications, or check on a patient. In some patients, especially in the elderly with intermittent confusion at home, the mere fact that they are placed in a different and unfamiliar environment may tip them into a delirious state. Finally, confusion is commonly seen following a surgical procedure. The combined effects of anesthesia and medications to treat surgical incision pain are contributing factors in this situation.

Confusion will often disappear once the underlying cause is treated, whether it is addressing the infection or withdrawing the offending medications. Diagnostic testing is rarely necessary. Frequent reassurance, support, and comfort may be all that is needed to assist the patient through this period. However, sometimes confusion can lead to behavioral problems, such as aggression, refusal to take pills, and even hallucinations or delusions. In these cases, physical restraints are sometimes necessary to prevent self-injury. Some hospitals have bed or wheelchair alarms to alert nurses when patients attempt to wander, while other hospitals may use a sitter to promote safety. If there are psychotic symptoms, such as visual hallucinations, antipsychotics may be used. Remember, in nearly all cases, clozapine (Clozaril) and quetiapine (Seroquel) are the only antipsychotics that should be used in patients with Parkinson disease.

In very severe cases of confusion with hallucinations and behavioral changes, it may be necessary to temporarily discontinue dopamine agonists, MAO inhibitors, amantadine, benzodiazepines, and pain medications if possible. Treatment with carbidopa/levodopa and either clozapine or quetiapine will usually result in improvement. Later, once patients are stable, they may be slowly titrated back onto previous doses if tolerated.

I had deep brain stimulators (DBS) placed 2 years ago. I now need to have knee replacement surgery. Will the doctors know how to take care of me?

While thousands of patients worldwide have had deep brain stimulation treatment for Parkinson disease and other movement disorders, many medical professionals and hospitals may still not be familiar with this treatment. Many patients with DBS undergo knee replacement surgery and other procedures without difficulty. However, there are a few things you and your doctors should be aware of. First, if you have had DBS surgery, you can only get an MRI [magnetic resonance imaging test] of the brain, and it must be done with something called a head-receive coil. You cannot get an MRI of any other part of the body. This situation exists because the DBS device can become heated and damage the brain tissue during MRI. There are also certain precautions that the radiologists must be aware of while performing a brain MRI. These are available from the FDA [U.S. Food and Drug Administration]. Furthermore, the voltage on your stimulator should be turned down to 0 prior to having an MRI performed. Only an experienced programmer should supervise the procedure. If there is not an experienced member of the DBS team available in the hospital where you are being treated, and/or if the institution is not familiar with performing MRIs in DBS patients, it is probably best not to have the MRI or to wait and have it at an experienced center.

The stimulators can sometimes interfere with the ability to obtain an electrocardiogram (EKG). This test may be important if you happen to have cardiac problems before, during, or after surgery. Therefore, you should bring your portable Medtronic Access Device or Access Review Device (or a magnet that comes with the device) to turn off your stimulator in the hospital. Make sure you know how to turn your stimulators on and off before going to the hospital, and before having any type of surgery. (Again, do not assume that the medical staff will be able to turn them off for you.) Similarly, if you need a brain wave test called an electroencephalogram (EEG), or will simply be monitored during an inpatient or outpatient procedure, you will need to know how to turn your device off.

If you are undergoing surgery and you have DBS, most anesthetics are safe. However, some precautions need to be taken when using electrocautery. Electrocautery stops bleeding during surgery and could potentially reset your stimulator to its factory settings. As a precaution, only bipolar electrocautery is recommended (with grounding placed below the level of the device). If your neurologist is on staff at the hospital where you are getting surgery, he/she should confirm that your stimulator is on and that the correct settings are reset following surgery. If your neurologist is not at the hospital where you are being operated, you should schedule a follow-up appointment soon after you are discharged from the hospital to recheck your settings.

The above tips and scenarios will hopefully aid in minimizing problems for patients with Parkinson disease who are hospitalized. Be aware that, for unclear reasons, some symptoms worsen following general or local anesthesia, and some patients have even reported feeling as if they never return to their baseline. In general, local anesthesia is thought to be safer than general anesthesia, and if you have problems with thinking and memory, they should be evaluated prior to surgery as they may also worsen.

Finally, it is important for you to have discussions with close family members about what you would like to have done in case of a life-threatening emergency. They and the medical staff should be aware of your medical wishes. You should choose an advocate who can ask questions and act as your spokesperson. If you have a living will or a durable health care power of attorney, these documents should be brought to the hospital and placed in the medical chart.

In the following text are two checklists for you to take with you to the hospital: one for you and one for your doctor/nurse. You can play an important role in easing the stress of your hospital stay, which can, in turn, help other patients with Parkinson disease who will follow you.

Information Checklist for Hospital Stays

General Points to be Aware of When Entering the Hospital

- Provide a list of your medications with exact times, frequencies, and dosages. Be prepared to share your knowledge about Parkinson disease, including on-off fluctuations and the importance of taking medications at specific time intervals.

- Bring medication in original bottles.

- Know which drugs can worsen the symptoms of Parkinson disease.

- Research study participants should provide information explaining the experimental drugs and phone the study coordinator to let them know you are in the hospital.

- Speak up when medications are wearing off.

- Do not take medication on your own. Unless you have prearranged permission, the staff should administer all medication.

- Let the staff know if you have a deep brain stimulation (DBS) implant. Bring the access review or magnet device to turn the stimulator on and off for procedures.

- Contact your neurologist letting him/her know you are in the hospital and give the phone number of your neurologist to your doctor in the hospital.

Be mobile, especially during prolonged stays.

- Walk around as much as possible.

- Inquire about physical therapy or occupational therapy. Even passive range of motion exercises can help prevent contractures if you are not mobile.

If you have difficulty swallowing:

- Sit up while eating.

- Ask for a speech-swallowing therapist.

- Alert staff that your medications may need to be crushed and administered through a tube. Make sure medications are administered 1 hour prior to meals or feedings, especially if medications are crushed.

- There is a dissolvable form of carbidopa/levodopa called Parcopa® that can be given by placing on the tongue.

Know what factors may make your symptoms worse:

- Failing to get medications at specific times and coordinated with meals.

- Dopamine-blocking drugs such as haloperidol (Haldol), risperidone (Risperdal) and olanzapine (Zyprexa) can worsen symptoms. If absolutely necessary because of hallucinations, behavior, or sleep, only quetiapine (Seroquel) or clozapine (Clozaril) should be used.

- Anxiety, stress, and sleep deprivation.

- Urinary tract, lung, or other infections (and antibiotics).

Provide advance directives:

- Provide power of attorney for health care and living will. Choose an advocate who can ask questions and act as your spokesperson. Make sure this person is aware of your medical wishes so (s)he can assist in speaking for you if needed.

Information for Your Nurse and Doctor when You Enter the Hospital

The following are some suggestions to make the hospitalization of this person with Parkinson disease smoother:

- Parkinson disease medications often need to be given at specific times of the day. Therefore, when writing medications in the orders, instead of writing TID or QID, please write specific times (e.g., q8AM, q11AM, etc.).

- Patients with Parkinson disease should resume medications immediately following procedures unless vomiting or severely incapacitated.

- If there is confusion, consider urinary or lung infections. Also consider pain medications or benzodiazepines as a potential cause.

- In cases of prolonged confusion, and an antipsychotic is necessary, quetiapine (Seroquel) and clozapine (Clozaril) are the best options. These two drugs minimally affect symptoms. Avoid using haloperidol (Haldol), risperidone (Risperdal), olanzapine (Zyprexa), aripiprazole (Abilify), and ziprasidone (Geodon).

- If the patient has nausea, please avoid the use of prochlorperazine (Compazine), promethazine (Phenergan), or metoclopramide (Reglan), as they can worsen symptoms. Trimethobenzamide (Tigan) and ondansetron (Zofran) are alternatives that can be used safely.

- Do not mix selegiline or rasagiline (MAO [monoamine oxidase inhibitor]-B inhibitors) with meperidine (Demerol), as it can precipitate a serious reaction characterized by blood pressure fluctuations, respiratory depression, convulsions, malignant hyperthermia, and excitation.

- Do not stop carbidopa/levodopa (Sinemet) abruptly, as this can lead to neuroleptic malignant-like syndrome.

- If medications have to be crushed and administered through a tube, give them at least one hour prior to meals and be aware that CR [controlled-release] formulations may not work as well. Protein in meals may interfere with the absorption of carbidopa/levodopa (Sinemet). There is a dissolvable form of carbidopa/levodopa called Parcopa® that may be useful in some patients.

- If you are having trouble getting an EKG, EEG, or using heart rate monitors, consider that the patient may have a deep brain stimulator. You may need to ask the patient or family member to turn the device off to avoid electrical interference.

Chapter 15

Nutrition and PD

Chapter Contents

Section 15.1

Eating Right If You Have PD

"Nutrition and Parkinson's Disease: What Matters Most?,"
By Karol Traviss. © 2006 Parkinson's Disease Foundation
(www.pdf.org). Reprinted with permission.

Navigating the maze of nutrition information and advice available to the public is challenging, even for a healthy consumer. Add Parkinson's disease to the mix and the challenges spiral higher. The nutritional issues faced by people with PD are complex and diverse, and many of the issues do not have clear answers.

When it comes to nutrition, what matters most? Here we help you to answer that question.

Eat a Balanced Diet

It is difficult for a person to feel well and maintain energy when he or she is not eating properly. Eating properly involves eating regularly (no meal skipping), eating a variety of foods from all of the food groups (grains, vegetables, fruit, milk/dairy, meat/beans) and eating prudently to maintain a healthy weight. Although this sounds like simple advice, implementing it can be a challenge, particularly if you have a hectic lifestyle or if the symptoms of Parkinson's are affecting your ability to shop, prepare food, and eat.

If you are not eating as well as you should, you may wish to consult a registered dietitian who can help assess your food intake and discuss with you strategies for improving your diet. It is also helpful to seek the assistance of others for shopping and meal preparation, and to keep easy-to-eat, nutritious foods on hand. If you have any problems with depression, this can interfere with appetite; be sure to discuss the problem with your doctor.

Maintain Bone Health

People with Parkinson's are prone to osteoporosis, a disease caused by low bone-mineral density. Risk factors for osteoporosis include older age, low body weight, smoking, excessive alcohol intake, limited exposure to sunlight, inadequate intake of vitamin D and calcium, and lack of weight-bearing exercise.

Osteoporosis can be especially worrisome to a person with Parkinson's who faces an increased risk of falling. The inevitable result is an increased risk of fractures, which are dangerous and painful and tend to be detrimental to one's quality of life. Ask your doctor about having your bone-mineral density checked. If it turns out to be low, medical treatments may be available.

To maintain bone health, make sure your diet includes plenty of calcium and vitamin D. People who are over the age of 50 should consume 1500 mg of calcium and 800 IU [international units] of vitamin D daily. Milk and milk products are the richest dietary source of calcium. Three servings per day are recommended (one serving is one cup of milk or yogurt, or one and one-half ounces of hard cheese). Although there are other calcium-containing foods (e.g., tofu, calcium-fortified soy-based beverages, orange juice, and dark leafy greens), calcium from non-dairy sources may not be well-absorbed.

You can also obtain vitamin D by getting outdoors regularly and consuming foods rich in vitamin D (e.g., vitamin D–fortified milk, yogurt, or breakfast cereals and fatty fish). If you live in a region with limited sunshine and/or do not consume many vitamin D–rich foods, use of a nutritional supplement is recommended. Supplements come in several forms. Some are easier to tolerate than others. Your pharmacist will be able to advise you on the different kinds available.

Maintain Bowel Regularity

Constipation is common in Parkinson's disease. While this can be an embarrassing issue to raise with your healthcare provider, prevention and treatment of constipation is critical, as severe constipation can lead to bowel obstruction, a potentially life-threatening condition. Although the constipation observed in Parkinson's is due in large part to the disease itself, lifestyle measures can be useful for managing it. These include eating foods high in fiber (whole grain bread, bran cereals or muffins, fruits and vegetables, beans and legumes, and prunes) and drinking plenty of fluid. Then there is exercise, which helps maintain bone density as well as eases constipation.

If you are not able to achieve bowel regularity through lifestyle alone, laxatives and other bowel interventions may be required. Make sure to see your doctor if constipation persists.

Balance Medications and Food

The medications used for Parkinson's can themselves cause nutrition-related side effects, such as nausea and poor appetite. Typically these side effects are most severe when a medication is first prescribed but some individuals have continuing problems with them. Taking a small snack (such as ginger ale and a few crackers) along with medications may help to control these side effects. If nausea or poor appetite persist, contact your doctor, as these symptoms can lead to undesired weight loss.

Amino acids (from dietary protein) can interfere with the uptake of levodopa into the brain. If you find (not everyone experiences this) that eating high-protein food (such as meat, fish, poultry, and dairy products) decreases the effectiveness of levodopa, keep the meat portion of your meal to about the size of a deck of cards and take your Sinemet® half an hour prior to a protein-containing meal.

Do not use a restricted-protein diet; the problem, if you find you have one, is usually with the timing of the protein intake, not its total quantity over the course of the day.

Do "Wonder" Foods or Supplements Delay Progression of Parkinson's?

Supplements (both nutritional and herbal) and dietary therapies are high on the list of complementary therapies used by people with Parkinson's. In spite of compelling theories about the effectiveness of various supplements or dietary factors in delaying progression of the disease, we lack definitive, evidence-based answers. Some therapies have been studied only in test tubes or with laboratory animals. Few human trials have been done (e.g., those examining antioxidant vitamin supplements), and most have produced disappointing results. Coenzyme Q10 is one nutritional supplement that is of considerable interest to the scientific community and is under study to determine if it has any potential benefit in Parkinson's disease.

Some foods that are in the "won't hurt and might help" (at least in theory) category include coffee (several population studies have suggested that coffee may be protective against Parkinson's, particularly in men); green tea; a variety of fruits and vegetables; foods rich in vitamin E such as wheat germ; nuts and seeds; and vegetable oil. If the antioxidants present do not help with Parkinson's symptoms, they may help with some other aspect of health so there is certainly no reason not to use them.

When thinking about the potential value of using this or that supplement, consider the factors of cost, safety, and effectiveness and be sure not to be "taken in" by hyped headlines. For example, a recent headline read, Vitamin B6 May Cut Risk of Parkinson's Disease. Behind the headline: this study finding, while interesting, was only observed among smokers and the study addressed only the onset, and not the progression, of Parkinson's. However tempting it may be to seek out "wonder" foods and supplements, at this time there is not enough evidence to suggest that they play a major role.

Adjust Nutritional Priorities for Your Situation and Stage of Disease

Parkinson's symptoms vary from person to person and by stage of disease. Each person must set nutritional priorities based on the issues they face. In early Parkinson's, we should all emphasize eating well and maintaining a healthy weight. As the disease progresses, we should adjust our diets to manage specific new symptoms as they emerge (such as swallowing difficulties, medication side-effects, bowel issues, and eating challenges). The goal of thoughtful nutrition is not just to ease PD symptoms; it is also to allow you to continue to use food as a source of pleasure in your life.

Karol Traviss, M.Sc., R.D., is a registered dietitian on faculty at the University of British Columbia in Vancouver, Canada. She has worked collaboratively with the British Columbia Parkinson's community for many years and spoke on complementary nutritional therapies at the 2006 World Parkinson Congress.

Section 15.2

Swallowing Problems Sometimes Associated with PD

From "Dysphagia," from the National Institute on Deafness and Other Communication Disorders (NIDCD, www.nidcd.nih.gov), part of the National Institutes of Health, October 1998. Reviewed and revised by David A. Cooke, M.D., August 26, 2008.

What is dysphagia?

People with dysphagia have difficulty swallowing and may also experience pain while swallowing. Some people may be completely unable to swallow or may have trouble swallowing liquids, foods, or saliva. Eating then becomes a challenge. Often, dysphagia makes it difficult to take in enough calories and fluids to nourish the body.

How do we swallow?

Swallowing is a complex process. Some 50 pairs of muscles and many nerves work to move food from the mouth to the stomach. This happens in three stages. First, the tongue moves the food around in the mouth for chewing. Chewing makes the food the right size to swallow and helps mix the food with saliva. Saliva softens and moistens the food to make swallowing easier. During this first stage, the tongue collects the prepared food or liquid, making it ready for swallowing.

The second stage begins when the tongue pushes the food or liquid to the back of the mouth, which triggers a swallowing reflex that passes the food through the pharynx (the canal that connects the mouth with the esophagus). During this stage, the larynx (voice box) closes tightly and breathing stops to prevent food or liquid from entering the lungs.

The third stage begins when food or liquid enters the esophagus, the canal that carries food and liquid to the stomach. This passage through the esophagus usually occurs in about 3 seconds, depending on the texture or consistency of the food.

How does dysphagia occur?

Dysphagia occurs when there is a problem with any part of the swallowing process. Weak tongue or cheek muscles may make it hard to move food around in the mouth for chewing. Food pieces that are too large for swallowing may enter the throat and block the passage of air.

Other problems include not being able to start the swallowing reflex (a stimulus that allows food and liquids to move safely through the pharynx) because of a stroke or other nervous system disorder. People with these kinds of problems are unable to begin the muscle movements that allow food to move from the mouth to the stomach. Another difficulty can occur when weak throat muscles cannot move all of the food toward the stomach. Bits of food can fall or be pulled into the windpipe (trachea), which may result in lung infection. In some cases, there may be poor coordination of muscle movements, which prevents proper forward movement of food during swallowing. This may be seen in a condition known as esophageal dysmotility, as well as a number of other neurologic disorders.

Dysphagia can also occur when the esophagus is blocked. In a condition known as achalasia, muscles at the bottom of the esophagus fail to relax and prevent food from entering the stomach. Tight narrowing (strictures) of the esophagus can also prevent passage of food and may occur due to acid reflux and other conditions. Rarely, the esophagus can be compressed from the outside by a mass or a blood vessel.

What are some problems caused by dysphagia?

Dysphagia can be serious. Someone who cannot swallow well may not be able to eat enough of the right foods to stay healthy or maintain an ideal weight.

Sometimes, when foods or liquids enter the windpipe of a person who has dysphagia, coughing or throat clearing cannot remove it. Food or liquid that stays in the windpipe may enter the lungs and create a chance for harmful bacteria to grow. A serious infection (aspiration pneumonia) can result.

Swallowing disorders may also include the development of a pocket (Zenker diverticulum) outside the esophagus caused by weakness in the esophageal wall. This abnormal pocket traps some food being swallowed. While lying down or sleeping, a person with this problem may draw undigested food into the pharynx. The esophagus may be too narrow, causing food to stick. This food may prevent other food or even liquids from entering the stomach.

What causes dysphagia?

Dysphagia has many causes. Any condition that weakens or damages the muscles and nerves used for swallowing may cause dysphagia. For example, people with diseases of the nervous system, such as cerebral palsy or Parkinson disease, often have problems swallowing. Additionally, stroke or head injury may affect the coordination of the swallowing muscles or limit sensation in the mouth and throat. An infection or irritation can cause narrowing of the esophagus. People born with abnormalities of the swallowing mechanism may not be able to swallow normally. Infants who are born with a hole in the roof of the mouth (cleft palate) are unable to suck properly, which complicates nursing and drinking from a regular baby bottle.

In addition, cancer of the head, neck, or esophagus may cause swallowing problems. Sometimes the treatment for these types of cancers can cause dysphagia. Injuries of the head, neck, and chest may also create swallowing problems.

Acid reflux is a very common cause of dysphagia. Acidic fluid from the stomach washes up and burns the lining of the esophagus. This can result in pain, swelling, and scarring of the esophagus.

How is dysphagia treated?

There are different treatments for various types of dysphagia. First, doctors and speech-language pathologists who test for and treat swallowing disorders use a variety of tests that allow them to look at the parts of the swallowing mechanism. One test, called a fiberoptic laryngoscopy, allows the doctor to look down the throat with a lighted tube. Other tests, including video fluoroscopy, which takes videotapes of a patient swallowing, and ultrasound, which produces images of internal body organs, can painlessly take pictures of various stages of swallowing.

Once the cause of the dysphagia is found, surgery or medication may help. Treating acid reflux with medication or surgery often improves matters considerably. Obstructions in the esophagus are often stretched out with procedures using a fiberoptic scope that extends into the esophagus.

If treating the cause of the dysphagia does not help, the doctor may have the patient see a speech-language pathologist who is trained in testing and treating swallowing disorders. The speech-language pathologist will test the person's ability to eat and drink and may teach the person new ways to swallow.

Treatment may involve muscle exercises to strengthen weak facial muscles or to improve coordination. For others, treatment may involve learning to eat in a special way. For example, some people may have to eat with their head turned to one side or looking straight ahead. Preparing food in a certain way or avoiding certain foods may help other people. For instance, those who cannot swallow liquids may need to add special thickeners to their drinks. Other people may have to avoid hot or cold foods or drinks.

For some, however, consuming foods and liquids by mouth may no longer be possible. These individuals must use other methods to nourish their bodies. Usually this involves a feeding system, such as a feeding tube, that bypasses the part of the swallowing mechanism that is not working normally.

What research is being done on dysphagia?

Scientists are conducting research that will improve the ability of physicians and speech-language pathologists to evaluate and treat swallowing disorders. All aspects of the swallowing process are being studied in people of all ages, including those who do and do not have dysphagia. For example, scientists have found that there is great variation in tongue movement during swallowing. Knowing which tongue movements cause problems will help physicians and speech-language pathologists evaluate swallowing.

Research has also led to new, safe ways to study tongue and throat movements during the swallowing process. These methods will help physicians and speech pathologists safely reevaluate a patient's progress during treatment. Studies of treatment methods are helping scientists discover why some forms of treatment work with some people and not with others. For example, research has shown that, in most cases, a patient who has had a stroke should not drink with his or her head tipped back. Other research has shown that some patients with cancer who have had part or all of their tongue removed should drink with their head tipped back. This knowledge will help some patients avoid serious lung infections and help others avoid tube feedings.

Where can I get help?

If you have a swallowing problem, you may need to consult with an otolaryngologist (physician with special training in disorders of the ear, nose, and throat) or a speech-language pathologist trained in dysphagia.

You may need to consult with a neurologist if a stroke or other neurologic disorder causes the swallowing problem. Other trained professionals who may provide treatment are occupational therapists and physical therapists.

Chapter 16

Can Exercise Reverse Symptoms of PD?

Why Exercise?

Some people turn away from exercise because they think that it will be too difficult, or that they can't fit it into their busy schedules. Others simply do not understand how exercise can help them. Exercise is important for everyone. It is the foundation for fitness, and it also helps us fight the effects of aging.

If you have Parkinson disease (PD), exercise is even more important. Recent research shows that regular exercise can help people with PD stay more flexible, improve posture, and make overall movement easier.

While medication has long been the most promising treatment available, a regular exercise program should always be part of managing PD. Exercise is one of the few treatments available that is free, has no bad side effects, and can actually be enjoyable. Though exercise is not a cure, it can help you to stay ahead of the changes that take place in your body and can help you feel more in control of your condition.

Physical and Occupational Therapy

This information is designed to provide general information and suggestions regarding exercise to all people living with PD. Specific

From Parkinson Disease: Fitness Counts, 3rd Ed., by Heather Cianci, PT, MS, GCS. © 2005 National Parkinson Foundation (www.parkinson.org). Reprinted with permission.

questions or problems should be dealt with by a licensed physical therapist (PT) or occupational therapist (OT).

Physical or occupational therapists can:

- Design or modify an exercise program to meet your particular needs.

- Evaluate and treat mobility and walking problems.

- Evaluate and treat joint or muscle pain which interferes with the activities of daily living.

- Help with poor balance or frequent falling.

- Teach care partners proper body mechanics and techniques for assisting someone with PD.

- Refer to movement and exercise programs in the community.

- Treat difficulties performing activities of daily living (ADL) such as eating, dressing, bathing, and handwriting.

- Recommend and teach the use of appropriate adaptive equipment.

Your doctor or other health care professional should be able to refer you to a therapist in your area. When possible, it is best to see a therapist that has special training and/or experience with PD. Visits to a physical or occupational therapist are usually covered by medical insurance with referral by a physician.

To build a foundation for fitness you will need three main components: stretching, strengthening, and aerobic conditioning. Each component on its own is important, but together they can help you remain as active as possible and better equipped to deal with the changes that PD can bring.

Stretching

Regular stretching is the first step in your exercise program, and it can be one of the most enjoyable. Stretching helps you combat the muscle rigidity which comes with PD. It also helps your muscles and joints stay flexible. People who are more flexible tend to have an easier time with everyday movement.

Why Should I Stretch?

You should stretch because it:

- Increases range of motion of joints.

- Helps with good posture.

- Protects against muscle strains or sprains.

- Improves circulation.

- Releases muscle tension.

Dos and Don'ts of Stretching

- Do stretch until you feel a gentle pull.

- Don't stretch to the point of pain.

- Don't bounce while you stretch. Bouncing can cause small tears in muscle fibers. This can actually lead to less flexibility.

- Don't hold your breath while you stretch. Breathe evenly in and out during each stretch.

- Don't compare yourself to others. Everybody varies in how far they can stretch.

When Should I Stretch?

A good thing about stretching is that you can do it at any time. Get your day off to a good start by stretching before getting out of bed. Try to stretch throughout the day. For example, you can stretch while you watch television or ride in a car. Choose a time for exercise when you are well-rested and your PD medications are working.

How Often Should I Stretch?

Every day.

How Many Times Should I Do Each Stretch?

Each stretch should be done three times. If you can't do the entire series of stretches at one time, select a few stretches to do at different times throughout the day.

How Long Should I Hold Each Stretch?

For at least 3–5 breath counts. One breath count = 1 full breath in and out.

A Note about Deep Breathing

Learning how to breathe deeply will not only help you get more oxygen, but will help you relax. Often times, people with PD take shallow breaths. Taking a shallow breath means we are not fully using our lungs or diaphragm. Shallow breaths only use the upper part of the lungs and overwork the upper chest muscles. This can lead to tension and fatigue. It can also affect the quality of your speech. Full, deep breaths allow the diaphragm to lower and the lungs to expand more deeply, ensuring more oxygen is taken in with each breath.

This simple exercise can help you practice breathing deeply:

1. In a lying or sitting position, gently place your palms over your lower abdomen.

2. Take in a full breath through your nose, allowing the diaphragm to expand. You will feel your abdomen lift out if you are doing this correctly.

3. Slowly breathe out through the mouth. Your out breath should last longer than your in breath.

4. Perform this exercise for 5 minutes a day, or at any time you need help to feel relaxed.

Breathing exercise:

1. Stand tall with feet hip width apart.

2. Cross arms over one another.

3. Take in a deep breath and begin lifting arms up and open.

4. Breathe out and lower hands to starting pose.

5. Perform for 5 deep breaths.

Strengthening

Strengthening is another important part of a PD exercise program. Strengthening certain muscles can help you stand up straighter and can make tasks like getting up from a chair easier. Strengthening exercises also helps to make bones stronger, so if you fall, you are less likely to get a fracture.

Strength training is more than just lifting weights. If you have access to handheld weights or a gym with weight machines, by all means, use them. However, you can build strength by using your own body weight as resistance. Like stretching, you can do strengthening exercises in the privacy of your home. The trick is to find out what kind of strengthening exercises work best for you.

What Tools Do I Need to Do Strengthening Exercises at Home?

There are many tools available that you can use to build strong muscles and bones. Choose the one that best suits your situation and surroundings. Here are some examples:

- Small hand weights (commonly available in sporting goods departments).
- Wrist and ankle weights with Velcro® closures.
- Elastic resistance bands, such as TheraBands®.
- Common household items:
  - Soup cans.
  - Plastic shampoo or milk bottles filled with water or sand.
  - Laundry detergent bottles.
- Some exercises use your body weight as resistance. A few examples are squats and prone on elbows.

Dos and Don'ts for Strengthening

- Do work one muscle group at a time.
- Do stop any exercise that causes pain.
- Do perform the movements slowly.
- Do concentrate on standing up straight while doing the exercises.
- Do breathe in while performing the movement, breathe out while relaxing the movement.
- Don't grip hand weights too tightly.
- Don't do rapid or "jerky" movements.
- Don't hold your breath. Breathe evenly throughout each exercise.

How Much Weight Should I Use?

Use a technique known as the 10 Rep Max. This means that you use the maximum amount of weight you can lift for 10 repetitions.

For example, if you can lift 3 pounds 10 times with no difficulty, the weight is too light for you. You could try 5 pounds. If you can only do 10 repetitions with 5 pound weights before getting too tired to continue, 5 pounds is a good weight for you to use.

How Often Should I Perform Strengthening Exercises?

You shouldn't perform strengthening exercises on the same muscles two days in a row. So, you could strengthen your arms one day, and your legs the next, but you shouldn't strengthen your arms on both days.

How Many Repetitions Should I Perform?

- Begin by performing 1 set of 10 repetitions of the exercise. Slowly increase to 3 sets of 10 repetitions.

- Increase the amount of weight once you can perform 2–3 sets with no difficulty.

- If you are unable to perform the entire series of strengthening exercises at one time, select a few to perform at different times throughout the day.

Aerobic Conditioning Exercise

Aerobic, or conditioning, exercise includes any nonstop activity that uses the entire body, working the heart and lungs as well as muscles. Examples of aerobic activities include:

- Walking
- Swimming
- Water aerobics
- Biking
- Dancing

Even some regular daily activities have an aerobic, or conditioning, benefit, including:

- Household chores such as mopping or vacuuming.
- Walking the dog.
- Gardening and yard work.

A program of regular aerobic exercise performed 3 or more times per week can:

- Strengthen the heart and lungs.
- Improve stamina and endurance.
- Reduce stress.
- Improve mood and combat depression.
- Help control high blood pressure, high cholesterol, and diabetes.

Aerobic, or conditioning may also be done from a seated position. Armchair aerobics exercise videos can be found at many sporting goods stores or video areas of department stores.

How Often Should I Perform Aerobic Exercise?

Your goal should be at least 20 minutes of aerobic exercise 3 times per week. Start slowly and gradually increase the time until you reach 20 minutes or more.

- Begin by performing a 3–5 minute warmup. This does not necessarily have to be the same as the activity you are going to perform. Example: Walk around the block or march in place for 3–5 minutes before swimming or biking.

- Finish your routine with a 3–5 minute cool down. This can be done by continuing your activity for an additional 3–5 minutes at a lesser intensity, or switching to a different activity. Example: If you were biking, either take a gentle walk or sit and perform leg kicks.

You should get approval from your doctor before beginning an aerobic, or conditioning, program. This is especially important if you are over 50 years of age, or have a history of cardiovascular disease.

How Hard Should I Work When Performing Aerobic Exercise?

There are two methods to rate how hard you are working.

The first is the Target Heart Rate method. This method helps you keep track of your heart rate while exercising. For the best benefit, you should keep your heart rate between 60% and 80% of your maximum heart rate. For beginners, it is good to start out at 60%.

To calculate your Target Heart Rate, subtract your age from 220. This is the maximum number of times your heart can beat in a minute. This number is then multiplied by the percentage of your maximum heart rate that you want to exercise. If you are just starting your aerobic program, your target heart rate should be between 60 to 75% of your maximum heart rate. Generally, after 6 months at this rate, you may increase to 85%.

For example, if you are 65 years old: 220 - 65 = 155: This is your maximum heart rate. If you want to exercise at 60% of your maximum heart rate: 155 x .60= 93: This is your target heart rate. If you want to exercise at 80% of your maximum heart rate: 155 x .80=124: This is your target heart rate if you want to exercise at 80% of your maximum heart rate.

You can periodically check your heart rate by counting your pulse for 6 seconds and multiplying by 10. If the total is lower than your target heart rate, you can increase how hard you are working. If the total is higher, you should work less hard.

Caution: Do not use the target heart rate method if you:

- Take any medications that change your heart rate.

- Have a pacemaker.

- Have atrial fibrillation.

Chapter 17

Voice Treatment for People with PD-Associated Speech Difficulties

Lorraine Olson Ramig, Ph.D., has been telling her patients to speak up for the past 15 years. But her hearing is fine.

Ramig and her colleagues are using a behavioral treatment for people with Parkinson disease (PD) who have an accompanying voice disorder. A professor in the department of speech, language, and hearing sciences at the University of Colorado at Boulder and a senior scientist at the National Center for Voice and Speech in Denver, Ramig asserts that by speaking more loudly, individuals with PD will gain control of their speech and improve their ability to communicate with others. More than 75 percent of individuals with PD have voice and speech disorders, yet historically, only three to four percent receive any type of speech therapy and an even smaller percentage of these individuals are successful at improving their speech over the long run.

Ramig hopes to change that statistic. An NIDCD grantee, she and her colleagues are the developers of the Lee Silverman Voice Treatment (LSVT) program, an approach designed specifically to address the challenges faced by people with PD who also have voice disorders. She knows too well what these individuals face. "Many of my PD patients with voice disorders speak with a soft, breathy, hoarse voice and have reduced loudness and imprecise articulation, all of which affect speech intelligibility and oral communication."

From "Say It Loud: NIDCD Grantee's Innovative Voice Treatment Gives People with Parkinson's Disease a Voice," from the National Institute of Deafness and Other Communication Disorders (NIDCD, www.nidcd.nih.gov), part of the National Institutes of Health, April 1, 2008.

PD affects about 1.5 million Americans and belongs to a group of motor system disorders marked by tremors in the extremities and face, rigidity of the limbs and trunk, slow movement, and impaired balance and coordination. As these symptoms become more pronounced, patients may have difficulty walking, talking, and performing other simple tasks. Problems with voice and speech are believed to be related to the motor and sensory deficits of the disease, but the neural mechanisms behind these problems are not well understood.

Traditional methods of speech therapy, namely those focusing on articulation and rate of speech, largely have been unsuccessful in PD patients, especially in the long run.

Enter Lee Silverman—a woman with speech and voice deficits accompanying PD. In 1987, Silverman's family mused to Dr. Ramig, "If only we could hear and understand her." Inspired by Lee, the Silverman family established the Lee Silverman Center for Parkinson Disease in Scottsdale, AZ. It was at this center that Ramig and her colleague, Carolyn Mead Bonitati M.A., began to develop the innovative treatment that now is known globally as LSVT.

"The development of LSVT was motivated by the recognition that the reduced ability to communicate is one of the most difficult aspects of PD," says Ramig. "For those with PD, voice disorders can contribute to their isolation from others and can adversely affect their social, economic, and psychological well-being."

How LSVT Works

In a manner of speaking, LSVT is to the voice what sit-ups are to the abdominals: a focused workout. LSVT concentrates on a simple set of tasks designed to improve voice and respiratory functions. Speech-language pathologists instruct and constantly stimulate patients to produce a louder healthy voice by using increased effort. Patients also are continually reminded to monitor the loudness of their voice and the effort it takes to produce it. The treatment is intensive, requiring four 1-hour sessions per week for 4 consecutive weeks.

The loud and effortful tasks are aimed at stimulating increased movement in the respiratory and laryngeal systems to improve air movement and vocal fold closure as well as vocal tract function involved in speech. The physiological changes that take place as a result of the treatment have been found to improve voice quality and loudness, articulation, and speech intelligibility. When coupled with appropriate feedback and auditory self-monitoring, LSVT can help those with PD retrain motor output during speech production and learn the relationship between increased loudness and improved speech.

According to Ramig, it is challenging for individuals with PD who normally speak softly to comprehend fully the impact of their reduced loudness and to learn to regulate this in normal conversation. Patients often feel as if the whole world needs a hearing aid and that they are shouting. However, during the course of daily treatment, they learn that if they don't feel as if they are talking too loudly they are not talking loudly enough. Patients learn that what feels "too loud" to them is a level that helps listeners hear and understand them.

Ramig adds that by targeting loudness, people with PD are tapping into well-established centrally stored areas of motor control in the brain involved in speech production. Increasing loudness to improve speech is a common and natural function of normal speech, she says, and does not require concentrating on rate of speech, pauses, or precision in articulation, all of which may be more difficult for persons with PD. The patient has one simple target with a functional impact—to "be loud"—with the benefits extending across the entire speech production system.

Research on LSVT Shows Benefits

In various clinical studies, LSVT has been shown to be an effective speech treatment for persons with PD. LSVT works well with patients who have cognitive impairments as a result of their PD. "On the surface, the treatment is redundant, simple, and intensive and thus may help compensate for the processing, speed, memory, and executive function problems seen in patients with PD and allow them to learn," says Ramig.

Other areas of improvement that have been found through LSVT are:

- more stable motor speech output;

- improved ability to convey emotion through facial expression and voice;

- stimulation of right-brain activity as well as of the centers of the brain known as the limbic system, a driving mechanism behind the ability to speak; and

- improved swallowing ability in a number of patients.

So far, efficacy studies on just under 100 patients have shown LSVT to be effective over the short and long term. While LSVT is being used effectively today in 30 countries, large-scale, multisite clinical trials looking at the effects of different variables such as age, stage of disease, time since diagnosis, and cognitive abilities need to be conducted to provide a more complete picture of LSVT. More comparison studies with persons receiving alternative treatments also need to be done.

Research so far has not been able to isolate the exact reason for LSVT's success: Is it due to the focus on phonation, the intensity of the treatment, or the sensory awareness training? Researchers are exploring ways to improve methods to assist with at-home use and practice of LSVT, thus potentially extending its positive long-term outcomes. Through support from NIDCD, Ramig and her colleagues are turning to technology, including the use of webcam, software programs, and a virtual therapist to help patients receive additional access to treatment that may help improve their communication abilities.

Ramig emphasizes that in speech therapy for PD patients, control rests with the patient. "Effective speech therapy carries the added benefit of improved self-confidence and better quality of life, and some measure of control over a significant symptom of PD." As more information is obtained on LSVT, researchers can find new ways to help people with PD improve their communication abilities.

Chapter 18

Driving and PD

As baby boomers age and life expectancy rises, increasing attention is turning on how to determine when and if older people—and people with health problems—should stop driving. The issue hits home for people with Parkinson's since both the symptoms of the disease and the medications designed to ease them can affect driving ability. If you are struggling with the decision of whether or not to stop driving, or if you are a caregiver for someone who is wrestling with this problem, this text may help you explore your options.

How Does Parkinson's Disease Affect Driving?

People with Parkinson's disease [PD] may eventually experience a decline in both motor skills and cognition. These problems can make driving unsafe. For example, a decrease in visuospatial skills—the kind that are necessary to determine distance and distinguish shapes—is not uncommon in PD. A driver with decreased visuospatial skills may be unable to gauge the distance to a stop sign or a traffic light or keep a car in the correct lane. Some people with Parkinson's also may have cognitive difficulties and at times become confused. Unfortunately, patients with dementia may not realize that their driving has become a problem and must rely on a physician, family members, and friends to bring it to their attention. Another common symptomatic problem for people with Parkinson's is muscle tightness, which can make reacting quickly difficult. Delayed reaction time is dangerous because drivers need to be able to react swiftly, both mentally and physically, to avoid accidents and adapt to changing traffic patterns.

Additional complications come from the medications that are used to treat PD. Common medications—including carbidopa/levodopa (Sinemet®), amantadine, dopamine agonists, and anticholinergics—may produce side effects such as sleepiness, dizziness, blurred vision, and confusion. Anticholinergics are especially dangerous as they can cause confusion and sedation along with memory impairment. However, not every patient experiences these side effects and they may be decreased with simple adjustments in dosage. You should note any changes and report these to your physician.

Assessment Options for People with Parkinson's

It is important to remember that while not every person with Parkinson's experiences problems with driving, disease symptoms and treatments can make driving dangerous for you and others. Driving is a sign of independence and freedom and you may be reluctant to stop, but being responsible is also important. To help you determine your driving risk, the American Medical Association (AMA) offers *The Physician's Guide to Assessing and Counseling Older Drivers*. It includes extensive information about diseases that may affect driving ability, such as Parkinson's. This guide, accessible at www.ama-assn.org/ama/pub/category/10791.html, is an outstanding resource. Although it was developed primarily for doctors, it will help laypersons make their own assessment of their driving ability and determine a course of action.

The guide features a questionnaire, Am I a Safe Driver? [see Appendix B], to help you evaluate your driving. If you score poorly on this and are still reluctant to stop driving, refer to the Tips for Safe Driving sheet [see Appendix B] and consider speaking with a doctor about the issue. The guide includes suggested tests on cognition, mobility, reaction time, and visual ability for physicians to perform on patients to determine if a person is driving safely.

During an examination to determine medical fitness for driving, your doctor may discuss several options. One is to visit a Driver Rehabilitation Specialist (DRS). The Association for Driver Rehabilitation Specialists (ADED) certifies a DRS to assess driving skills with on-road tests, provide rehabilitation based on the results of the on-road tests, and recommend modifications on your vehicle to help you drive more safely. This service can be costly, averaging $200 to $400 for an assessment and about $100 an hour for rehabilitation. Expenses increase substantially if you decide to include adaptive equipment for a vehicle, and Medicare may not cover any of this. Before signing up for services, talk with the DRS and your insurance company to determine what will be covered. To find a DRS near you, call ADED at (877) 529-1830 or check the directory at www.driver-ed.org. You can also inquire at hospitals, driving schools, rehabilitation facilities, and state motor vehicle departments in your area.

A less costly, although less thorough, option is to enroll in a driver safety class, such as the AARP 55 ALIVE Driver Safety Program [http://www.aarp.org/families/driver_safety], and the AAA Safe Driving for Mature Operators

Program (contact your local AAA for details). While these classes are not specifically tailored for people with Parkinson's, they can provide helpful tips for safe driving. An instructor will lead the class through various ways of enhancing driving skills and safety but often will not make individual assessments. One potentially useful resource is the National Older Driver Research and Training Center, a joint project of the University of Florida and the American Occupational Therapy Association. The center works to train Driver Rehabilitation Specialists and develop better off-road tests for driver safety.

Finally, you can always visit the Department of Motor Vehicles and ask to take a driving test. Of course, if you were to fail the test, your license would be revoked.

What Can Family Members and Friends Do to Help?

Understandably, most people are reluctant to give up the opportunity to drive. Because of this, it is often up to family members and caregivers to spot a problem first. If you are a family member or caregiver for a person with Parkinson's and you think it may be time for them to stop driving, remember that this is a very sensitive issue and you must help the person see that his or her driving has become dangerous. The AMA doctor's guide features several helpful materials to make it easier to approach a person about his or her driving. Before bringing up the subject, look at the How to Help the Older Driver tip sheet [Appendix B], which is extremely relevant for Parkinson's patients. This can help you determine if your concerns are valid and if so, how you might address them.

Another way to help your loved one with this decision is by stressing that giving up driving does not mean giving up mobility. Your support is crucial in helping a person with Parkinson's admit that his or her skills have decreased without feeling stripped of power. To help people with Parkinson's with their decision to stop driving, provide them with transportation alternatives. The Getting by Without Driving tip sheet [Appendix B] in the AMA guide identifies other possible modes of transportation, including taxis, buses, subways, and getting a ride from family members. Some cities also provide travel assistance for people unable to use public transportation. If you know someone with Parkinson's who has had to give up driving, provide him or her with bus routes, taxicab phone numbers, and offer to give rides. For more transportation alternatives, call the ElderCare Locator at (800) 677-1116 and ask for your local Office on Aging, or visit the website at www.eldercare.gov. This may help a person with Parkinson's adjust and realize that stopping driving does not mean losing independence.

What's the Bottom Line?

Having Parkinson's does not necessarily result in giving up driving. However, whether you are a person with Parkinson's or a loved one, it is important to be responsible and remember the potential dangers that Parkinson's presents to driving. Ignoring the effects of the disease and its medications on driving will only create a more dangerous environment for you and other drivers. The best way to be a responsible driver is by paying attention to your driving skills and reporting any changes to your physician. If you have concerns, don't avoid voicing them out of fear of losing your license. Doctors and family members are often happy to help you exhaust rehabilitation options before asking you to give up driving. If it does come to the point where family, doctors, and driving coaches ask you to give up your keys, realize that it is in your best interest to stop driving and explore other transportation options.

Chapter 19

Employment with PD

One of the first questions a newly diagnosed person will likely ask is, "How long will I be able to work?" This question is especially important to young onset patients, who may be many years from retirement age, and who are often raising families and facing numerous financial responsibilities.

As with most aspects of this "designer disease," there are no standard answers; they vary from person to person. Factors in the decision-making mix include the nature and physical demands of a job, the acceptance and support offered by employers and coworkers, the individual' s response to medication, financial issues, and the rate of disease progression. Some people continue to work for many years after a Parkinson's diagnosis, while others may find that the physical and mental stresses of their job become too challenging, too quickly.

It is important to recognize that a diagnosis of PD does not mean that your career is automatically over. I was diagnosed in 1995 at the age of 45, and have continued working as a college librarian for 10 years since then. Here I will share my experiences working with Parkinson's, in the hope that the information may be helpful to others who are facing similar decisions about jobs and careers.

"Employment with PD: Working it Out," By Linda Herman. © 2007 Parkinson's Disease Foundation (www.pdf.org). Reprinted with permission.

To Tell or Not to Tell?

Should a person newly diagnosed with Parkinson's tell his or her employer about the disease? For many, the symptoms can be effectively controlled by medications for several years, and colleagues at work may not even know that you have Parkinson's disease. Your symptoms may not interfere with your ability to do your job, and—because in most cases your medical records are confidential—it is entirely your decision as to whether or not your Parkinson's diagnosis is made public.

How comfortable are you with keeping your condition a secret at work? The answer will be influenced by such factors as your existing relationship with your employer and coworkers, and your instincts about how they will respond to the news. Ideally, employers would do whatever they can to help employees continue working. Besides being the right thing to do, and being required under the Americans with Disabilities Act (ADA), it also makes good business sense for an employer to try to keep experienced and valued workers. Unfortunately, not all employers are of this mindset.

My own decision was to tell most of my coworkers about my illness soon after receiving my diagnosis. People's responses varied; a few individuals seemed to avoid me from that day on, but most have been supportive and have even become well-educated about Parkinson's. I have also been able to enlist their support in writing to Congress to support increases in federal funding for Parkinson's research. I found that involving friends and coworkers in PD advocacy efforts helped them to understand my illness and also provided them with a way to support me. In fact, my library director has been a shining example of what should—and can—be done to help people with disabilities in the workplace.

Workplace Accommodations

By law, people with Parkinson's disease are protected under the ADA against discrimination in employment practices. This law requires employers to make reasonable accommodations for employees, as long as they do not impose an "undue hardship" on the employer's business. A reasonable accommodation is defined as "any modification or adjustment to a job or the work environment that will enable a qualified applicant or employee with a disability to participate in the application process or to perform essential job functions."

As my symptoms progressed and medication became less effective, my job responsibilities have been adjusted to be more manageable.

For example, as teaching became more difficult for me, my class load was reduced. In place of these responsibilities, I have taken on other duties that can be performed in my office by computer, helping me cope on my own schedule with my now longer and less predictable "off" periods. I type all of my written communications, rather than expecting others to decipher my typical Parkie handwriting. I take shorter lunch breaks, so that I am able to leave work early if fatigue becomes a problem by the end of the day.

Some other examples of workplace accommodations that can be helpful for people with Parkinson's include the provision of adaptive computer equipment, such as an ergonomic work station, voice recognition software, or a trackball. Mobility devices, such as a scooter or cane, or speech amplifiers, might be requested. Depending on the nature of the job and company, requests for a more flexible work schedule, or reversion to a part-time arrangement, or telecommuting might be options. Accommodations to help deal with cognitive problems could include arranging for a workspace away from noise or other distractions, and the use of such memory aids such as schedule planners and written instructions.

One outside source of information about the workplace is the Job Accommodations Network (JAN). JAN is a free consulting service that is provided by the U.S. Department of Labor. Its services are "designed to increase the employability of people with disabilities by 1) providing individualized worksite accommodations solutions, 2) providing technical assistance regarding the ADA and other disability related legislation, and 3) educating callers about self-employment options."

Visit the JAN homepage at www.jan.wvu.edu and be sure to check out the "Accommodation and Compliance Series: Employees with Parkinson's Disease" at www.jan.wvu.edu/media/PD.html. The staff at JAN is also available for free consultations by phone at 800-526-7234.

Making the Choice

Part of working with Parkinson's is also knowing when it is time to stop working. In my situation, I have slowly realized that even with accommodations, I am no longer able to do my job as I would like to, with fatigue a constant problem. So after 22 years as an academic librarian, 10 of them with PD, I have concluded that fall 2005 will be my last semester working. Difficult as the decision certainly was, it helps me to know that my volunteer advocacy work on behalf of the

Parkinson's community will continue to make good use of my research skills.

Linda Herman is a Librarian at Medaille College. She is active in Parkinson's advocacy and is the Upstate New York State Coordinator for the Parkinson's Action Network. She also works with the New Yorkers for the Advancement of Medical Research (NYAMR). Linda resides in Amherst, NY.

Chapter 20

Helping Your Children Cope with Your PD

When I was diagnosed with Parkinson's [disease, PD] in 2000, I first thought of my three children and of how my diagnosis would impact them. How would I tell them? Would I be able to help my daughter fix her hair and makeup? Would I be able to walk at their weddings?

At first, I chose not to share my diagnosis with my children but I soon realized that I had to tell the older two—Kyle (9) and Erik (6). Their first question was, "Are you going to die?" I reassured them that this disease was not fatal, but told them that sometimes I might need help with small tasks. At the time, neither child asked many questions and seemed relieved to know that I was technically "okay."

As time went on, I could see small but distinct ways that my announcement changed their behavior. When my son Kyle and I would go shopping, he would hold only my left hand. When I asked him why, his reply was that he was trying to stop the shaking. Then Erik decided suddenly that he would become a scientist, and create a bracelet and anklet that would stop people with Parkinson's from shaking.

As I considered how to help my boys understand my disease, I got some wonderful suggestions from my movement disorders specialist. Upon his request, my husband and I brought the boys on a "special" doctor's appointment. The doctor showed us pictures of the brain, explained the disease in simple terms and told us—and the boys—what it is like to live with PD.

"Helping Your Children Cope with Your PD," By Michelle Lane. © 2007 Parkinson's Disease Foundation (www.pdf.org). Reprinted with permission.

While this visit was invaluable to me and my children, I continued to see signs of their struggle with my diagnosis. They were unsure how to answer children at school when they were asked why their mom shakes so much, and I continually had to reassure them that I was not going to die. At one point we decided to seek outside counseling from a psychologist for one of the boys who was having a particularly difficult time adjusting. We found him to be helpful in teaching us how to cope.

For my daughter, Rachel, who was only two years old when I was first diagnosed, living with Parkinson's has raised different issues. Rachel and I both had a hard time dealing with my inability to pull up her long, thick brown hair in a ponytail and have her look like the other girls her age. At first I asked the stylist to cut her hair short, but now, with adjustments and help from other family members, Rachel is learning to make her own ponytails. It's just one of the many examples of simple things that Parkinson's can take away from you, but which you can take back with a little teamwork.

This problem turned out to be minor compared to what was to come. Just this year, at age 7, Rachel hit me with a bombshell that I will never forget. I was sitting on my porch enjoying a cool day when she sat on my lap, placed her arms around my neck and asked, "Why do you have to have Parkinson's?" I tried to explain, but she kept saying, "I want you to be like you were before. It just isn't fair because Kyle and Erik got to see you like you were before and I never have." It made me realize that my daughter had many questions going through her mind. We held each other, and she asked what the word "cure" meant. We talked about this, and then she asked the inevitable question—was Parkinson's contagious? I told her that it was not, and that I would be around for a long time to answer any other questions that she may have. I also set up a phone call with my doctor so that he could have the same conversation with Rachel that he had with my boys.

Of course my children continue to have questions. Just last month Rachel asked me how old I was when I started shaking. I replied that I was 30, whereupon she asked if she too would start shaking when she turns 30. As I assured her that she would not, it reminded me that the questions about my Parkinson's disease probably will not end. But at least I know I am here for my children, and plan to be for a long time.

My overall advice in dealing with this disease is to keep the faith and recognize the strength of your family. Expect that they will have questions, and be open to suggestions for dealing with these questions from your doctor, friends, and other family. Remember that we are all in this together, and that only together will we win this war on Parkinson's disease.

Michelle Lane is an advocate and founder of the Parkinson's Association of Louisiana.

Part Three

Other Hypokinetic Movement Disorders: Slowed or Absent Movements

Chapter 21

Amyotrophic Lateral Sclerosis (ALS)

What is amyotrophic lateral sclerosis?

Amyotrophic lateral sclerosis (ALS), sometimes called Lou Gehrig disease, is a rapidly progressive, invariably fatal neurological disease that attacks the nerve cells (neurons) responsible for controlling voluntary muscles. The disease belongs to a group of disorders known as motor neuron diseases, which are characterized by the gradual degeneration and death of motor neurons.

Motor neurons are nerve cells located in the brain, brainstem, and spinal cord that serve as controlling units and vital communication links between the nervous system and the voluntary muscles of the body. Messages from motor neurons in the brain (called upper motor neurons) are transmitted to motor neurons in the spinal cord (called lower motor neurons) and from them to particular muscles. In ALS, both the upper motor neurons and the lower motor neurons degenerate or die, ceasing to send messages to muscles. Unable to function, the muscles gradually weaken, waste away (atrophy), and twitch (fasciculations). Eventually, the ability of the brain to start and control voluntary movement is lost.

ALS causes weakness with a wide range of disabilities. Eventually, all muscles under voluntary control are affected, and patients lose their strength and the ability to move their arms, legs, and body. When

From "Amyotrophic Lateral Sclerosis Fact Sheet," National Institute of Neurological Disorders and Stroke (NINDS, www.ninds.nih.gov), part of the National Institutes of Health, February 2008.

muscles in the diaphragm and chest wall fail, patients lose the ability to breathe without ventilatory support. Most people with ALS die from respiratory failure, usually within 3 to 5 years from the onset of symptoms. However, about 10 percent of ALS patients survive for 10 or more years.

Although the disease usually does not impair a person's mind or intelligence, several recent studies suggest that some ALS patients may have alterations in cognitive functions such as depression and problems with decision-making and memory.

ALS does not affect a person's ability to see, smell, taste, hear, or recognize touch. Patients usually maintain control of eye muscles and bladder and bowel functions, although in the late stages of the disease most patients will need help getting to and from the bathroom.

Who gets ALS?

As many as 20,000 Americans have ALS, and an estimated 5,000 people in the United States are diagnosed with the disease each year. ALS is one of the most common neuromuscular diseases worldwide, and people of all races and ethnic backgrounds are affected. ALS most commonly strikes people between 40 and 60 years of age, but younger and older people also can develop the disease. Men are affected more often than women.

In 90 to 95 percent of all ALS cases, the disease occurs apparently at random with no clearly associated risk factors. Patients do not have a family history of the disease, and their family members are not considered to be at increased risk for developing ALS.

About 5 to 10 percent of all ALS cases are inherited. The familial form of ALS usually results from a pattern of inheritance that requires only one parent to carry the gene responsible for the disease. About 20 percent of all familial cases result from a specific genetic defect that leads to mutation of the enzyme known as superoxide dismutase 1 (SOD1). Research on this mutation is providing clues about the possible causes of motor neuron death in ALS. Not all familial ALS cases are due to the SOD1 mutation, therefore other unidentified genetic causes clearly exist.

What are the symptoms?

The onset of ALS may be so subtle that the symptoms are frequently overlooked. The earliest symptoms may include twitching, cramping, or stiffness of muscles; muscle weakness affecting an arm or a leg; slurred and nasal speech; or difficulty chewing or swallowing. These general complaints then develop into more obvious weakness or atrophy that may cause a physician to suspect ALS.

The parts of the body affected by early symptoms of ALS depend on which muscles in the body are damaged first. In some cases, symptoms initially affect one of the legs, and patients experience awkwardness when walking or running or they notice that they are tripping or stumbling more often. Some patients first see the effects of the disease on a hand or arm as they experience difficulty with simple tasks requiring manual dexterity such as buttoning a shirt, writing, or turning a key in a lock. Other patients notice speech problems.

Regardless of the part of the body first affected by the disease, muscle weakness and atrophy spread to other parts of the body as the disease progresses. Patients have increasing problems with moving, swallowing (dysphagia), and speaking or forming words (dysarthria). Symptoms of upper motor neuron involvement include tight and stiff muscles (spasticity) and exaggerated reflexes (hyperreflexia) including an overactive gag reflex. An abnormal reflex commonly called Babinski sign (the large toe extends upward as the sole of the foot is stimulated in a certain way) also indicates upper motor neuron damage. Symptoms of lower motor neuron degeneration include muscle weakness and atrophy, muscle cramps, and fleeting twitches of muscles that can be seen under the skin (fasciculations).

To be diagnosed with ALS, patients must have signs and symptoms of both upper and lower motor neuron damage that cannot be attributed to other causes.

Although the sequence of emerging symptoms and the rate of disease progression vary from person to person, eventually patients will not be able to stand or walk, get in or out of bed on their own, or use their hands and arms. Difficulty swallowing and chewing impair the patient's ability to eat normally and increase the risk of choking. Maintaining weight will then become a problem. Because the disease usually does not affect cognitive abilities, patients are aware of their progressive loss of function and may become anxious and depressed. A small percentage of patients may experience problems with memory or decision-making, and there is growing evidence that some may even develop a form of dementia. Health care professionals need to explain the course of the disease and describe available treatment options so that patients can make informed decisions in advance. In later stages of the disease, patients have difficulty breathing as the muscles of the respiratory system weaken. Patients eventually lose the ability to breathe on their own and must depend on ventilatory support for survival. Patients also face an increased risk of pneumonia during later stages of ALS.

How is ALS diagnosed?

No one test can provide a definitive diagnosis of ALS, although the presence of upper and lower motor neuron signs in a single limb is strongly suggestive. Instead, the diagnosis of ALS is primarily based on the symptoms and signs the physician observes in the patient and a series of tests to rule out other diseases. Physicians obtain the patient's full medical history and usually conduct a neurologic examination at regular intervals to assess whether symptoms such as muscle weakness, atrophy of muscles, hyperreflexia, and spasticity are getting progressively worse.

Because symptoms of ALS can be similar to those of a wide variety of other, more treatable diseases or disorders, appropriate tests must be conducted to exclude the possibility of other conditions. One of these tests is electromyography (EMG), a special recording technique that detects electrical activity in muscles. Certain EMG findings can support the diagnosis of ALS. Another common test measures nerve conduction velocity (NCV). Specific abnormalities in the NCV results may suggest, for example, that the patient has a form of peripheral neuropathy (damage to peripheral nerves) or myopathy (muscle disease) rather than ALS. The physician may order magnetic resonance imaging (MRI), a noninvasive procedure that uses a magnetic field and radio waves to take detailed images of the brain and spinal cord. Although these MRI scans are often normal in patients with ALS, they can reveal evidence of other problems that may be causing the symptoms, such as a spinal cord tumor, a herniated disk in the neck, syringomyelia, or cervical spondylosis.

Based on the patient's symptoms and findings from the examination and from these tests, the physician may order tests on blood and urine samples to eliminate the possibility of other diseases as well as routine laboratory tests. In some cases, for example, if a physician suspects that the patient may have a myopathy rather than ALS, a muscle biopsy may be performed.

Infectious diseases such as human immunodeficiency virus (HIV), human T-cell leukemia virus (HTLV), and Lyme disease can in some cases cause ALS-like symptoms. Neurological disorders such as multiple sclerosis, postpolio syndrome, multifocal motor neuropathy, and spinal muscular atrophy also can mimic certain facets of the disease and should be considered by physicians attempting to make a diagnosis.

Because of the prognosis carried by this diagnosis and the variety of diseases or disorders that can resemble ALS in the early stages of the disease, patients may wish to obtain a second neurological opinion.

What causes ALS?

The cause of ALS is not known, and scientists do not yet know why ALS strikes some people and not others. An important step toward answering that question came in 1993 when scientists supported by the National Institute of Neurological Disorders and Stroke (NINDS) discovered that mutations in the gene that produces the SOD1 enzyme were associated with some cases of familial ALS. This enzyme is a powerful antioxidant that protects the body from damage caused by free radicals. Free radicals are highly reactive molecules produced by cells during normal metabolism. If not neutralized, free radicals can accumulate and cause random damage to the DNA and proteins within cells. Although it is not yet clear how the SOD1 gene mutation leads to motor neuron degeneration, researchers have theorized that an accumulation of free radicals may result from the faulty functioning of this gene. In support of this, animal studies have shown that motor neuron degeneration and deficits in motor function accompany the presence of the SOD1 mutation.

Studies also have focused on the role of glutamate in motor neuron degeneration. Glutamate is one of the chemical messengers or neurotransmitters in the brain. Scientists have found that, compared to healthy people, ALS patients have higher levels of glutamate in the serum and spinal fluid. Laboratory studies have demonstrated that neurons begin to die off when they are exposed over long periods to excessive amounts of glutamate. Now, scientists are trying to understand what mechanisms lead to a buildup of unneeded glutamate in the spinal fluid and how this imbalance could contribute to the development of ALS.

Autoimmune responses—which occur when the body's immune system attacks normal cells—have been suggested as one possible cause for motor neuron degeneration in ALS. Some scientists theorize that antibodies may directly or indirectly impair the function of motor neurons, interfering with the transmission of signals between the brain and muscles.

In searching for the cause of ALS, researchers have also studied environmental factors such as exposure to toxic or infectious agents. Other research has examined the possible role of dietary deficiency or trauma. However, as of yet, there is insufficient evidence to implicate these factors as causes of ALS. Future research may show that many factors, including a genetic predisposition, are involved in the development of ALS.

How is ALS treated?

No cure has yet been found for ALS. However, the Food and Drug Administration (FDA) has approved the first drug treatment for the disease—riluzole (Rilutek). Riluzole is believed to reduce damage to motor neurons by decreasing the release of glutamate. Clinical trials with ALS patients showed that riluzole prolongs survival by several months, mainly in those with difficulty swallowing. The drug also extends the time before a patient needs ventilation support. Riluzole does not reverse the damage already done to motor neurons, and patients taking the drug must be monitored for liver damage and other possible side effects. However, this first disease-specific therapy offers hope that the progression of ALS may one day be slowed by new medications or combinations of drugs.

Other treatments for ALS are designed to relieve symptoms and improve the quality of life for patients. This supportive care is best provided by multidisciplinary teams of health care professionals such as physicians; pharmacists; physical, occupational, and speech therapists; nutritionists; social workers; and home care and hospice nurses. Working with patients and caregivers, these teams can design an individualized plan of medical and physical therapy and provide special equipment aimed at keeping patients as mobile and comfortable as possible.

Physicians can prescribe medications to help reduce fatigue, ease muscle cramps, control spasticity, and reduce excess saliva and phlegm. Drugs also are available to help patients with pain, depression, sleep disturbances, and constipation. Pharmacists can give advice on the proper use of medications and monitor a patient's prescriptions to avoid risks of drug interactions.

Physical therapy and special equipment can enhance patients' independence and safety throughout the course of ALS. Gentle, low-impact aerobic exercise such as walking, swimming, and stationary bicycling can strengthen unaffected muscles, improve cardiovascular health, and help patients fight fatigue and depression. Range of motion and stretching exercises can help prevent painful spasticity and shortening (contracture) of muscles. Physical therapists can recommend exercises that provide these benefits without overworking muscles. Occupational therapists can suggest devices such as ramps, braces, walkers, and wheelchairs that help patients conserve energy and remain mobile.

ALS patients who have difficulty speaking may benefit from working with a speech therapist. These health professionals can teach patients adaptive strategies such as techniques to help them speak louder and more clearly. As ALS progresses, speech therapists can help patients develop ways for responding to yes-or-no questions with their eyes or by other nonverbal means and can recommend aids such as speech synthesizers and computer-based communication systems. These methods and devices help patients communicate when they can no longer speak or produce vocal sounds.

Patients and caregivers can learn from speech therapists and nutritionists how to plan and prepare numerous small meals throughout the day that provide enough calories, fiber, and fluid and how to avoid foods that are difficult to swallow. Patients may begin using suction devices to remove excess fluids or saliva and prevent choking. When patients can no longer get enough nourishment from eating, doctors may advise inserting a feeding tube into the stomach. The use of a feeding tube also reduces the risk of choking and pneumonia that can result from inhaling liquids into the lungs. The tube is not painful and does not prevent patients from eating food orally if they wish.

When the muscles that assist in breathing weaken, use of nocturnal ventilatory assistance (intermittent positive pressure ventilation [IPPV] or bilevel positive airway pressure [BIPAP]) may be used to aid breathing during sleep. Such devices artificially inflate the patient's lungs from various external sources that are applied directly to the face or body. When muscles are no longer able to maintain oxygen and carbon dioxide levels, these devices may be used full-time.

Patients may eventually consider forms of mechanical ventilation (respirators) in which a machine inflates and deflates the lungs. To be effective, this may require a tube that passes from the nose or mouth to the windpipe (trachea) and for long-term use, an operation such as a tracheostomy, in which a plastic breathing tube is inserted directly in the patient's windpipe through an opening in the neck. Patients and their families should consider several factors when deciding whether and when to use one of these options. Ventilation devices differ in their effect on the patient's quality of life and in cost. Although ventilation support can ease problems with breathing and prolong survival, it does not affect the progression of ALS. Patients need to be fully informed about these considerations and the long-term effects of life without movement before they make decisions about ventilation support.

Social workers and home care and hospice nurses help patients, families, and caregivers with the medical, emotional, and financial challenges of coping with ALS, particularly during the final stages of the disease. Social workers provide support such as assistance in obtaining financial aid, arranging durable power of attorney, preparing a living will, and finding support groups for patients and caregivers. Respiratory therapists can help caregivers with tasks such as operating and maintaining respirators, and home care nurses are available not only to provide medical care but also to teach caregivers about giving tube feedings and moving patients to avoid painful skin problems and contractures. Home hospice nurses work in consultation with physicians to ensure proper medication, pain control, and other care affecting the quality of life of patients who wish to remain at home. The home hospice team can also counsel patients and caregivers about end-of-life issues.

What research is being done?

The National Institute of Neurological Disorders and Stroke, part of the National Institutes of Health, is the Federal Government's leading supporter of biomedical research on ALS. The goals of this research are to find the cause or causes of ALS, understand the mechanisms involved in the progression of the disease, and develop effective treatment.

Scientists are seeking to understand the mechanisms that trigger selective motor neurons to degenerate in ALS and to find effective approaches to halt the processes leading to cell death. This work includes studies in animals to identify the means by which SOD1 mutations lead to the destruction of neurons. The excessive accumulation of free radicals, which has been implicated in a number of neurodegenerative diseases including ALS, is also being closely studied. In addition, researchers are examining how the loss of neurotrophic factors may be involved in ALS. Neurotrophic factors are chemicals found in the brain and spinal cord that play a vital role in the development, specification, maintenance, and protection of neurons. Studying how these factors may be lost and how such a loss may contribute to motor neuron degeneration may lead to a greater understanding of ALS and the development of neuroprotective strategies. By exploring these and other possible factors, researchers hope to find the cause or causes of motor neuron degeneration in ALS and develop therapies to slow the progression of the disease.

Researchers are also conducting investigations to increase their understanding of the role of programmed cell death or apoptosis in ALS. In normal physiological processes, apoptosis acts as a means to rid the body of cells that are no longer needed by prompting the cells to commit "cell suicide." The critical balance between necessary cell death and the maintenance of essential cells is thought to be controlled by trophic factors. In addition to ALS, apoptosis is pervasive in other chronic neurodegenerative conditions such as Parkinson disease and Alzheimer disease and is thought to be a major cause of the secondary brain damage seen after stroke and trauma. Discovering what triggers apoptosis may eventually lead to therapeutic interventions for ALS and other neurological diseases.

Scientists have not yet identified a reliable biological marker for ALS—a biochemical abnormality shared by all patients with the disease. Once such a biomarker is discovered and tests are developed to detect the marker in patients, allowing early detection and diagnosis of ALS, physicians will have a valuable tool to help them follow the effects of new therapies and monitor disease progression.

NINDS-supported researchers are studying families with ALS who lack the SOD1 mutation to locate additional genes that cause the disease. Identification of additional ALS genes will allow genetic testing useful for diagnostic confirmation of ALS and prenatal screening for the disease. This work with familial ALS could lead to a greater understanding of sporadic ALS as well. Because familial ALS is virtually indistinguishable from sporadic ALS clinically, some researchers believe that familial ALS genes may also be involved in the manifestations of the more common sporadic form of ALS. Scientists also hope to identify genetic risk factors that predispose people to sporadic ALS.

Potential therapies for ALS are being investigated in animal models. Some of this work involves experimental treatments with normal SOD1 and other antioxidants. In addition, neurotrophic factors are being studied for their potential to protect motor neurons from pathological degeneration. Investigators are optimistic that these and other basic research studies will eventually lead to treatments for ALS.

Results of an NINDS-sponsored phase III randomized, placebo-controlled trial of the drug minocycline to treat ALS were reported in 2007. This study showed that people with ALS who received minocycline had a 25 percent greater rate of decline than those who received the placebo, according to the ALS functional rating scale (ALSFRS-R).

Chapter 22

Cerebellar or Spinocerebellar Degeneration

Chapter Contents

Section 22.1

Ataxia-Telangiectasia

Excerpted from "Ataxia Telangiectasia: Fact Sheet," by the National
Cancer Institute (NCI, www.cancer.gov), part of the National Institutes
of Health, January 26, 2006.

What is ataxia telangiectasia?

Ataxia telangiectasia (A-T) is a primary immunodeficiency disease
which affects a number of different organs in the body. An immunodeficiency disease is one that causes the immune system to break
down, making the body susceptible to diseases. It is a rare, recessive
genetic disorder of childhood that occurs in between 1 out of 40,000
and 1 out of 100,000 persons worldwide. The ailment is progressive.
Patients with A-T are frequently wheelchair-bound by their teens, and
the disease is generally fatal to patients by the time they reach their
twenties.

A-T is characterized by neurological problems, particularly abnormalities of balance, recurrent sinus and respiratory infections, and
dilated blood vessels in the eyes and on the surface of the skin. Patients usually have immune system abnormalities and are very sensitive to the effects of radiation treatments.

In the United States, where recurrent infections typical of the disorder are usually controlled by antibiotics, patients are at high risk
of developing and dying of cancer, particularly leukemias and lymphomas.

What are the signs of ataxia telangiectasia?

The first signs of the disease, which include delayed development
of motor skills, poor balance, and slurred speech, usually occur during the first decade of life. Telangiectasias (tiny, red "spider" veins),
which appear in the corners of the eyes or on the surface of the ears
and cheeks, are characteristic of the disease, but are not always present
and generally do not appear in the first years of life. About 20% of those
with A-T develop cancer, most frequently acute lymphocytic leukemia

or lymphoma. Many individuals with A-T have a weakened immune system, making them susceptible to recurrent respiratory infections. Other features of the disease may include mild diabetes mellitus, premature graying of the hair, difficulty swallowing, and delayed physical and sexual development. Children with A-T usually have normal or above normal intelligence.

Is the disorder curable?

There is no cure for A-T at this time. The cloning and sequencing of the gene (named ATM, for ataxia telangiectasia, mutated) has opened several avenues of research to develop better treatment, including: (1) gene therapy; (2) the design of drugs to correct the function of the altered protein; and (3) direct replacement of the functional protein. Physical, occupational, and speech therapy are used to help maintain flexibility, gamma-globulin injections help supplement the immune systems of A-T patients and high-dose vitamin regimens are being researched with some moderate results.

Research shows that a protein kinase called ATM reacts to DNA damage by chemically modifying and triggering accumulation of a molecular or tumor suppressor called p53. This tumor suppressor is defective in about half of all human cancers and is the master control switch for a process that normally prevents cells from dividing. In A-T patients, the ATM protein is missing or defective. This delays the accumulation of p53, allowing cells to replicate without repair of their DNA and thereby increasing the risk of cancer. This research was reported by two separate groups of researchers in the September 1998 issue of *Science*.

Section 22.2

Friedreich Ataxia

Excerpted from "Friedreich's Ataxia Fact Sheet," by the National Institute of Neurological Disorders and Stroke (NINDS, www.ninds.nih.gov), part of the National Institutes of Health, December 11, 2007.

What is Friedreich ataxia?

Friedreich ataxia is an inherited disease that causes progressive damage to the nervous system resulting in symptoms ranging from gait disturbance and speech problems to heart disease. It is named after the physician Nicholaus Friedreich, who first described the condition in the 1860s. "Ataxia," which refers to coordination problems such as clumsy or awkward movements and unsteadiness, occurs in many different diseases and conditions. The ataxia of Friedreich ataxia results from the degeneration of nerve tissue in the spinal cord and of nerves that control muscle movement in the arms and legs. The spinal cord becomes thinner and nerve cells lose some of their myelin sheath—the insular covering on all nerve cells that helps conduct nerve impulses.

Friedreich ataxia, although rare, is the most prevalent inherited ataxia, affecting about 1 in every 50,000 people in the United States. Males and females are affected equally.

What are the signs and symptoms?

Symptoms usually begin between the ages of 5 and 15 but can, on rare occasions, appear as early as 18 months or as late as 50 years of age. The first symptom to appear is usually difficulty in walking, or gait ataxia. The ataxia gradually worsens and slowly spreads to the arms and then the trunk. Foot deformities such as clubfoot, flexion (involuntary bending) of the toes, hammer toes, or foot inversion (turning inward) may be early signs. Over time, muscles begin to weaken and waste away, especially in the feet, lower legs, and hands, and deformities develop. Other symptoms include loss of tendon reflexes, especially in the knees and ankles. There is often a gradual loss of

198

sensation in the extremities, which may spread to other parts of the body. Dysarthria (slowness and slurring of speech) develops, and the person is easily fatigued. Rapid, rhythmic, involuntary movements of the eye (nystagmus) are common. Most people with Friedreich ataxia develop scoliosis (a curving of the spine to one side), which, if severe, may impair breathing.

Other symptoms that may occur include chest pain, shortness of breath, and heart palpitations. These symptoms are the result of various forms of heart disease that often accompany Friedreich ataxia, such as cardiomyopathy (enlargement of the heart), myocardial fibrosis (formation of fiber-like material in the muscles of the heart), and cardiac failure. Heart rhythm abnormalities such as tachycardia (fast heart rate) and heart block (impaired conduction of cardiac impulses within the heart) are also common. About 20 percent of people with Friedreich ataxia develop carbohydrate intolerance and 10 percent develop diabetes mellitus. Some people lose hearing or eyesight.

The rate of progression varies from person to person. Generally, within 10 to 20 years after the appearance of the first symptoms, the person is confined to a wheelchair, and in later stages of the disease individuals become completely incapacitated. Life expectancy may be affected, and many people with Friedreich ataxia die in adulthood from the associated heart disease, the most common cause of death. However, some people with less severe symptoms of Friedreich ataxia live much longer, sometimes into their sixties or seventies.

Can Friedreich ataxia be cured or treated?

As with many degenerative diseases of the nervous system, there is currently no cure or effective treatment for Friedreich ataxia. However, many of the symptoms and accompanying complications can be treated to help patients maintain optimal functioning as long as possible. Diabetes, if present, can be treated with diet and medications such as insulin, and some of the heart problems can be treated with medication as well. Orthopedic problems such as foot deformities and scoliosis can be treated with braces or surgery. Physical therapy may prolong use of the arms and legs. Scientists hope that recent advances in understanding the genetics of Friedreich ataxia may lead to breakthroughs in treatment.

Section 22.3

Machado-Joseph Disease

Excerpted from "Machado-Joseph Disease Fact Sheet," by the National Institute of Neurological Disorders and Stroke (NINDS, www.ninds.nih.gov), part of the National Institutes of Health, June 3, 2008.

What is Machado-Joseph disease?

Machado-Joseph disease (MJD)—also called spinocerebellar ataxia type 3—is a rare hereditary ataxia. (Ataxia is a general term meaning lack of muscle control.) The disease is characterized by clumsiness and weakness in the arms and legs, spasticity, a staggering lurching gait easily mistaken for drunkenness, difficulty with speech and swallowing, involuntary eye movements, double vision, and frequent urination. Some patients have dystonia (sustained muscle contractions that cause twisting of the body and limbs, repetitive movements, abnormal postures, and/or rigidity), or symptoms similar to those of Parkinson disease. Others have twitching of the face or tongue or peculiar bulging eyes.

The severity of the disease is related to the age of onset, with earlier onset associated with a more severe form of the disease. Symptoms can begin any time between early adolescence and about 70 years of age. MJD is also a progressive disease, meaning that symptoms get worse with time. Life expectancy ranges from the mid-thirties for those with severe forms of MJD to a normal life expectancy for those with mild forms. For those who die early from the disease, the cause of death is often aspiration pneumonia.

The name, Machado-Joseph, comes from two families of Portuguese/Azorean descent who were among the first families described with the unique symptoms of the disease in the 1970s. The prevalence of the disease is still highest among people of Portuguese/Azorean descent. For immigrants of Portuguese ancestry in New England, the prevalence is around one in 4,000. The highest prevalence in the world, about one in 140, occurs on the small Azorean island of Flores. Recently, researchers have identified MJD in several family groups not of obvious Portuguese descent, including an African-American family from

North Carolina, an Italian-American family, and several Japanese families. On a worldwide basis, MJD is the most prevalent autosomal dominant inherited form of ataxia, based on DNA studies.

What are the different types of Machado-Joseph disease?

The types of MJD are distinguished by the age of onset and range of symptoms. Type I is characterized by onset between 10 and 30 years of age, fast progression, and severe dystonia and rigidity. Type II MJD generally begins between the ages of 20 and 50 years, has an intermediate progression, and causes symptoms that include spasticity (continuous, uncontrollable muscle contractions), spastic gait, and exaggerated reflex responses. Type III MJD patients have an onset between 40 and 70 years of age, a relatively slow progression, and some muscle twitching, muscle atrophy, and unpleasant sensations such as numbness, tingling, cramps, and pain in the hands, feet, and limbs. Almost all MJD patients experience vision problems, including double vision (diplopia) or blurred vision, loss of ability to distinguish color and/or contrast, and inability to control eye movements. Some MJD patients also experience Parkinson-like symptoms, such as slowness of movement, rigidity or stiffness of the limbs and trunk, tremor or trembling in the hands, and impaired balance and coordination.

What causes Machado-Joseph disease?

MJD is classified as a disorder of movement, specifically a spinocerebellar ataxia. In these disorders, degeneration of cells in an area of the brain called the hindbrain leads to deficits in movement. The hindbrain includes the cerebellum (a bundle of tissue about the size of an apricot located at the back of the head), the brainstem, and the upper part of the spinal cord. MJD is an inherited, autosomal dominant disease, meaning that if a child inherits one copy of the defective gene from either parent, the child will develop symptoms of the disease. People with a defective gene have a 50 percent chance of passing the mutation on to their children.

MJD belongs to a class of genetic disorders called triplet repeat diseases. The genetic mutation in triplet repeat diseases involves the extensive abnormal repetition of three letters of the DNA genetic code. In the case of MJD the code "CAG" is repeated within a gene located on chromosome 14q. The MJD gene produces a mutated protein called ataxin-3. This protein accumulates in affected cells and forms intranuclear inclusion bodies, which are insoluble spheres located in the nucleus of the cell. These spheres interfere with the normal operation of the nucleus and cause the cell to degenerate and die.

One trait of MJD and other triplet repeat diseases is a phenomenon called anticipation, in which the children of affected parents tend to develop symptoms of the disease much earlier in life, have a faster progression of the disease, and experience more severe symptoms. This is due to the tendency of the triplet repeat mutation to expand with the passing of genetic material to offspring. A longer expansion is associated with an earlier age of onset and a more severe form of the disease. It is impossible to predict precisely the course of the disease for an individual based solely on the repeat length.

How is Machado-Joseph disease treated?

MJD is incurable, but some symptoms of the disease can be treated. For those patients who show parkinsonian features, levodopa therapy can help for many years. Treatment with antispasmodic drugs, such as baclofen, can help reduce spasticity. Botulinum toxin can also treat severe spasticity as well as some symptoms of dystonia. However, botulinum toxin should be used as a last resort due to the possibility of side effects, such as swallowing problems (dysphagia). Speech problems (dysarthria) and dysphagia can be treated with medication and speech therapy. Wearing prism glasses can reduce blurred or double vision, but eye surgery has only short-term benefits due to the progressive degeneration of eye muscles. Physiotherapy can help patients cope with disability associated with gait problems, and physical aids, such as walkers and wheelchairs, can assist the patient with everyday activities. Other problems, such as sleep disturbances, cramps, and urinary dysfunction, can be treated with medications and medical care.

Chapter 23

Cerebral Palsy

What is cerebral palsy?

Doctors use the term cerebral palsy to refer to any one of a number of neurological disorders that appear in infancy or early childhood and permanently affect body movement and muscle coordination but aren't progressive, in other words, they don't get worse over time. The term cerebral refers to the two halves or hemispheres of the brain, in this case to the motor area of the brain's outer layer (called the cerebral cortex), the part of the brain that directs muscle movement; palsy refers to the loss or impairment of motor function.

Even though cerebral palsy affects muscle movement, it isn't caused by problems in the muscles or nerves. It is caused by abnormalities inside the brain that disrupt the brain's ability to control movement and posture.

In some cases of cerebral palsy, the cerebral motor cortex hasn't developed normally during fetal growth. In others, the damage is a result of injury to the brain either before, during, or after birth. In either case, the damage is not repairable and the disabilities that result are permanent.

Children with cerebral palsy exhibit a wide variety of symptoms, including:

Excerpted from "Cerebral Palsy: Hope Through Research," by the National Institute of Neurological Disorders and Stroke (NINDS, www.ninds.nih.gov), part of the National Institutes of Health (NIH), February 7, 2008.

- lack of muscle coordination when performing voluntary movements (ataxia);

- stiff or tight muscles and exaggerated reflexes (spasticity);

- walking with one foot or leg dragging;

- walking on the toes, a crouched gait, or a "scissored" gait;

- variations in muscle tone, either too stiff or too floppy;

- excessive drooling or difficulties swallowing or speaking;

- shaking (tremor) or random involuntary movements; and

- difficulty with precise motions, such as writing or buttoning a shirt.

The symptoms of cerebral palsy differ in type and severity from one person to the next, and may even change in an individual over time. Some people with cerebral palsy also have other medical disorders, including mental retardation, seizures, impaired vision or hearing, and abnormal physical sensations or perceptions.

Cerebral palsy doesn't always cause profound disabilities. While one child with severe cerebral palsy might be unable to walk and need extensive, lifelong care, another with mild cerebral palsy might be only slightly awkward and require no special assistance.

Cerebral palsy isn't a disease. It isn't contagious and it can't be passed from one generation to the next. There is no cure for cerebral palsy, but supportive treatments, medications, and surgery can help many individuals improve their motor skills and ability to communicate with the world.

How many people have cerebral palsy?

The United Cerebral Palsy (UCP) Foundation estimates that nearly 800,000 children and adults in the United States are living with one or more of the symptoms of cerebral palsy. According to the federal government's Centers for Disease Control and Prevention, each year about 10,000 babies born in the United States will develop cerebral palsy.

Despite advances in preventing and treating certain causes of cerebral palsy, the percentage of babies who develop the condition has remained the same over the past 30 years. Improved care in neonatal intensive care units has resulted in higher survival rates for very low birthweight babies. Many of these infants will have developmental defects in their nervous systems or suffer brain damage that will cause the characteristic symptoms of cerebral palsy.

What are the early signs?

The early signs of cerebral palsy usually appear before a child reaches 3 years of age. Parents are often the first to suspect that their baby's motor skills aren't developing normally. Infants with cerebral palsy frequently have developmental delay, in which they are slow to reach developmental milestones such as learning to roll over, sit, crawl, smile, or walk. Some infants with cerebral palsy have abnormal muscle tone as infants. Decreased muscle tone (hypotonia) can make them appear relaxed, even floppy. Increased muscle tone (hypertonia) can make them seem stiff or rigid. In some cases, an early period of hypotonia will progress to hypertonia after the first 2 to 3 months of life. Children with cerebral palsy may also have unusual posture or favor one side of the body when they move.

Parents who are concerned about their baby's development for any reason should contact their pediatrician. A doctor can determine the difference between a normal lag in development and a delay that could indicate cerebral palsy.

What causes cerebral palsy?

The majority of children with cerebral palsy are born with it, although it may not be detected until months or years later. This is called congenital cerebral palsy. In the past, if doctors couldn't identify another cause, they attributed most cases of congenital cerebral palsy to problems or complications during labor that caused asphyxia (a lack of oxygen) during birth. However, extensive research by NINDS scientists and others has shown that few babies who experience asphyxia during birth grow up to have cerebral palsy or any other neurological disorder. Birth complications, including asphyxia, are now estimated to account for only 5 to 10 percent of the babies born with congenital cerebral palsy.

A small number of children have acquired cerebral palsy, which means the disorder begins after birth. In these cases, doctors can often pinpoint a specific reason for the problem, such as brain damage in the first few months or years of life, brain infections such as bacterial meningitis or viral encephalitis, or head injury from a motor vehicle accident, a fall, or child abuse.

What causes the remaining 90 to 95 percent? Research has given us a bigger and more accurate picture of the kinds of events that can happen during early fetal development, or just before, during, or after birth, that cause the particular types of brain damage that will result in congenital cerebral palsy. There are multiple reasons why cerebral palsy happens—as the result of genetic abnormalities, maternal infections or fevers, or fetal injury, for example. But in all cases the disorder is the result of four types of brain damage that cause its characteristic symptoms:

Damage to the white matter of the brain (periventricular leukomalacia [PVL]): The white matter of the brain is responsible for transmitting signals inside the brain and to the rest of the body. PVL describes a type of damage that looks like tiny holes in the white matter of an infant's brain. These gaps in brain tissue interfere with the normal transmission of signals. There are a number of events that can cause PVL, including maternal or fetal infection. Researchers have also identified a period of selective vulnerability in the developing fetal brain, a period of time between 26 and 34 weeks of gestation, in which periventricular white matter is particularly sensitive to insults and injury.

Abnormal development of the brain (cerebral dysgenesis): Any interruption of the normal process of brain growth during fetal development can cause brain malformations that interfere with the transmission of brain signals. The fetal brain is particularly vulnerable during the first 20 weeks of development. Mutations in the genes that control brain development during this early period can keep the brain from developing normally. Infections, fevers, trauma, or other conditions that cause unhealthy conditions in the womb also put an unborn baby's nervous system at risk.

Bleeding in the brain (intracranial hemorrhage): Intracranial hemorrhage describes bleeding inside the brain caused by blocked or broken blood vessels. A common cause of this kind of damage is fetal stroke. Some babies suffer a stroke while still in the womb because of blood clots in the placenta that block blood flow. Other types of fetal stroke are caused by malformed or weak blood vessels in the brain or by blood-clotting abnormalities. Maternal high blood pressure (hypertension) is a common medical disorder during pregnancy that has been known to cause fetal stroke. Maternal infection, especially pelvic inflammatory disease, has also been shown to increase the risk of fetal stroke.

Brain damage caused by a lack of oxygen in the brain (hypoxic-ischemic encephalopathy or intrapartum asphyxia): Asphyxia, a lack of oxygen in the brain caused by an interruption in breathing or poor oxygen supply, is common in babies due to the stress of labor and delivery. But even though a newborn's blood is equipped to compensate for short-term low levels of oxygen, if the supply of oxygen is cut off or reduced for lengthy periods, an infant can develop a type of brain damage called hypoxic-ischemic encephalopathy, which destroys tissue in the cerebral motor cortex and other areas of the brain. This kind of damage can also be caused by severe maternal low blood pressure, rupture of the uterus, detachment of the placenta, or problems involving the umbilical cord.

What are the different forms?

The specific forms of cerebral palsy are determined by the extent, type, and location of a child's abnormalities. Doctors classify cerebral palsy according to the type of movement disorder involved—spastic (stiff muscles), athetoid (writhing movements), or ataxic (poor balance and coordination)—plus any additional symptoms. Doctors will often describe the type of cerebral palsy a child has based on which limbs are affected. The names of the most common forms of cerebral palsy use Latin terms to describe the location or number of affected limbs, combined with the words for weakened (paresis) or paralyzed (plegia). For example, hemiparesis (hemi = half) indicates that only one side of the body is weakened. Quadriplegia (quad = four) means all four limbs are paralyzed.

Spastic hemiplegia/hemiparesis: This type of cerebral palsy typically affects the arm and hand on one side of the body, but it can also include the leg. Children with spastic hemiplegia generally walk later and on tip-toe because of tight heel tendons. The arm and leg of the affected side are frequently shorter and thinner. Some children will develop an abnormal curvature of the spine (scoliosis). Depending on the location of the brain damage, a child with spastic hemiplegia may also have seizures. Speech will be delayed and, at best, may be competent, but intelligence is usually normal.

Spastic diplegia/diparesis: In this type of cerebral palsy, muscle stiffness is predominantly in the legs and less severely affects the arms and face, although the hands may be clumsy. Tendon reflexes are hyperactive. Toes point up. Tightness in certain leg muscles makes the legs move like the arms of a scissor. Children with this kind of cerebral palsy may require a walker or leg braces. Intelligence and language skills are usually normal.

Spastic quadriplegia/quadriparesis: This is the most severe form of cerebral palsy, often associated with moderate-to-severe mental retardation. It is caused by widespread damage to the brain or significant brain malformations. Children will often have severe stiffness in their limbs but a floppy neck. They are rarely able to walk. Speaking and being understood are difficult. Seizures can be frequent and hard to control.

Dyskinetic cerebral palsy (also includes athetoid, choreoathetoid, and dystonic cerebral palsies): This type of cerebral palsy is characterized by slow and uncontrollable writhing movements of the hands, feet, arms, or legs. In some children, hyperactivity in the muscles of the face and tongue makes them grimace or drool. They find it difficult to sit straight or walk. Children may also have problems coordinating the muscle movements required for speaking. Intelligence is rarely affected in these forms of cerebral palsy.

Ataxic cerebral palsy: This rare type of cerebral palsy affects balance and depth perception. Children will often have poor coordination and walk unsteadily with a wide-based gait, placing their feet unusually far apart. They have difficulty with quick or precise movements, such as writing or buttoning a shirt. They may also have intention tremor, in which a voluntary movement, such as reaching for a book, is accompanied by trembling that gets worse the closer their hand gets to the object.

Mixed types: It is common for children to have symptoms that don't correspond to any single type of cerebral palsy. Their symptoms are a mix of types. For example, a child with mixed cerebral palsy may have some muscles that are too tight and others that are too relaxed, creating a mix of stiffness and floppiness.

What other conditions are associated with cerebral palsy?

Many individuals with cerebral palsy have no additional medical disorders. However, because cerebral palsy involves the brain and the brain controls so many of the body's functions, cerebral palsy can also cause seizures, impair intellectual development, and affect vision, hearing, and behavior. Coping with these disabilities may be even more of a challenge than coping with the motor impairments of cerebral palsy.

These additional medical conditions include:

Mental retardation: Two thirds of individuals with cerebral palsy will be intellectually impaired. Mental impairment is more common among those with spastic quadriplegia than in those with other types of cerebral palsy, and children who have epilepsy and an abnormal electroencephalogram (EEG) or MRI [magnetic resonance imaging test] are also more likely to have mental retardation.

Seizure disorder: As many as half of all children with cerebral palsy have seizures. Seizures can take the form of the classic convulsions of tonic-clonic seizures or the less obvious focal (partial) seizures, in which the only symptoms may be muscle twitches or mental confusion.

Delayed growth and development: A syndrome called failure to thrive is common in children with moderate-to-severe cerebral palsy, especially those with spastic quadriparesis. Failure to thrive is a general term doctors use to describe children who lag behind in growth and development. In babies this lag usually takes the form of too little weight gain. In young children it can appear as abnormal shortness, and in teenagers it may appear as a combination of shortness and lack of sexual development.

In addition, the muscles and limbs affected by cerebral palsy tend to be smaller than normal. This is especially noticeable in children with spastic hemiplegia because limbs on the affected side of the body may not grow as quickly or as long as those on the normal side.

Spinal deformities: Deformities of the spine—curvature (scoliosis), humpback (kyphosis), and saddle back (lordosis)—are associated with cerebral palsy. Spinal deformities can make sitting, standing, and walking difficult and cause chronic back pain.

Impaired vision, hearing, or speech: A large number of children with cerebral palsy have strabismus, commonly called "cross eyes," in which the eyes are misaligned because of differences between the left and right eye muscles. In an adult, strabismus causes double vision. In children, the brain adapts to the condition by ignoring signals from one of the misaligned eyes. Untreated, this can lead to poor vision in one eye and can interfere with the ability to judge distance. In some cases, doctors will recommend surgery to realign the muscles.

Children with hemiparesis may have hemianopia, which is defective vision or blindness that blurs the normal field of vision in one eye. In homonymous hemianopia, the impairment affects the same part of the visual field in both eyes.

Impaired hearing is also more frequent among those with cerebral palsy than in the general population. Speech and language disorders, such as difficulty forming words and speaking clearly, are present in more than a third of those with cerebral palsy.

Drooling: Some individuals with cerebral palsy drool because they have poor control of the muscles of the throat, mouth, and tongue. Drooling can cause severe skin irritation. Because it is socially unacceptable, drooling may also isolate children from their peers.

Incontinence: A common complication of cerebral palsy is incontinence, caused by poor control of the muscles that keep the bladder closed. Incontinence can take the form of bedwetting, uncontrolled urination during physical activities, or slow leaking of urine throughout the day.

Abnormal sensations and perceptions: Some children with cerebral palsy have difficulty feeling simple sensations, such as touch. They may have stereognosia, which makes it difficult to perceive and identify objects using only the sense of touch. A child with stereognosia, for example, would have trouble closing his eyes and sensing the difference between a hard ball or a sponge ball placed in his hand.

How is cerebral palsy managed?

Cerebral palsy can't be cured, but treatment will often improve a child's capabilities. Many children go on to enjoy near-normal adult lives if their disabilities are properly managed. In general, the earlier treatment begins, the better chance children have of overcoming developmental disabilities or learning new ways to accomplish the tasks that challenge them.

There is no standard therapy that works for every individual with cerebral palsy. Once the diagnosis is made, and the type of cerebral palsy is determined, a team of health care professionals will work with a child and his or her parents to identify specific impairments and needs, and then develop an appropriate plan to tackle the core disabilities that affect the child's quality of life.

A comprehensive management plan will pull in a combination of health professionals with expertise in the following:

- Physical therapy to improve walking and gait, stretch spastic muscles, and prevent deformities

- Occupational therapy to develop compensating tactics for every-day activities such as dressing, going to school, and participating in day-to-day activities

- Speech therapy to address swallowing disorders, speech impediments, and other obstacles to communication

- Counseling and behavioral therapy to address emotional and psychological needs and help children cope emotionally with their disabilities

- Drugs to control seizures, relax muscle spasms, and alleviate pain

- Surgery to correct anatomical abnormalities or release tight muscles

- Braces and other orthotic devices to compensate for muscle imbalance, improve posture and walking, and increase independent mobility

- Mechanical aids such as wheelchairs and rolling walkers for individuals who are not independently mobile

- Communication aids such as computers, voice synthesizers, or symbol boards to allow severely impaired individuals to communicate with others

Doctors use tests and evaluation scales to determine a child's level of disability, and then make decisions about the types of treatments and the best timing and strategy for interventions. Early intervention programs typically provide all the required therapies within a single treatment center. Centers also focus on parents' needs, often offering support groups, babysitting services, and respite care.

Regardless of age or the types of therapy that are used, treatment doesn't end when an individual with cerebral palsy leaves the treatment center. Most of the work is done at home. Members of the treatment team often act as coaches, giving parents and children techniques and strategies to practice at home. Studies have shown that family support and personal determination are two of the most important factors in helping individuals with cerebral palsy reach their long-term goals.

While mastering specific skills is an important focus of treatment on a day-to-day basis, the ultimate goal is to help children grow into adulthood with as much independence as possible.

As a child with cerebral palsy grows older, the need for therapy and the kinds of therapies required, as well as support services, will likely change. Counseling for emotional and psychological challenges may be needed at any age, but is often most critical during adolescence. Depending on their physical and intellectual abilities, adults may need help finding attendants to care for them, a place to live, a job, and a way to get to their place of employment.

Addressing the needs of parents and caregivers is also an important component of the treatment plan. The well-being of an individual with cerebral palsy depends upon the strength and well-being of his or her family. For parents to accept a child's disabilities and come to grips with the extent of their caregiving responsibilities will take time and support from health care professionals. Family-centered programs in hospitals and clinics and community-based organizations usually work together with families to help them make well-informed decisions about the services they need. They also coordinate services to get the most out of treatment.

A good program will encourage the open exchange of information, offer respectful and supportive care, encourage partnerships between parents and the health care professionals they work with, and acknowledge that although medical specialists may be the experts, it's parents who know their children best.

What specific treatments are available?

Physical therapy: Physical therapy, usually begun in the first few years of life or soon after the diagnosis is made, is a cornerstone of cerebral palsy treatment. Physical therapy programs use specific sets of exercises and activities to work toward two important goals: preventing weakening or deterioration in the muscles that aren't being used (disuse atrophy), and keeping muscles from becoming fixed in a rigid, abnormal position (contracture).

Resistive exercise programs (also called strength training) and other types of exercise are often used to increase muscle performance, especially in children and adolescents with mild cerebral palsy. Daily bouts of exercise keep muscles that aren't normally used moving and active and less prone to wasting away. Exercise also reduces the risk of contracture, one of the most common and serious complications of cerebral palsy.

Normally growing children stretch their muscles and tendons as they run, walk, and move through their daily activities. This insures that their muscles grow at the same rate as their bones. But in children with

212

cerebral palsy, spasticity prevents muscles from stretching. As a result, their muscles don't grow fast enough to keep up with their lengthening bones. The muscle contracture that results can set back the gains in function they've made. Physical therapy alone or in combination with special braces (called orthotic devices) helps prevent contracture by stretching spastic muscles.

Occupational therapy: This kind of therapy focuses on optimizing upper body function, improving posture, and making the most of a child's mobility. An occupational therapist helps a child master the basic activities of daily living, such as eating, dressing, and using the bathroom alone. Fostering this kind of independence boosts self-reliance and self-esteem, and also helps reduce demands on parents and caregivers.

Recreational therapies: Recreational therapies, such as therapeutic horseback riding (also called hippotherapy), are sometimes used with mildly impaired children to improve gross motor skills. Parents of children who participate in recreational therapies usually notice an improvement in their child's speech, self-esteem, and emotional well-being.

Controversial physical therapies: "Patterning" is a physical therapy based on the principle that children with cerebral palsy should be taught motor skills in the same sequence in which they develop in normal children. In this controversial approach, the therapist begins by teaching a child elementary movements such as crawling—regardless of age—before moving on to walking skills. Some experts and organizations, including the American Academy of Pediatrics, have expressed strong reservations about the patterning approach because studies have not documented its value.

Experts have similar reservations about the Bobath technique (which is also called "neurodevelopmental treatment"), named for a husband and wife team who pioneered the approach in England. In this form of physical therapy, instructors inhibit abnormal patterns of movement and encourage more normal movements.

The Bobath technique has had a widespread influence on the core physical therapies of cerebral palsy treatment, but there is no evidence that the technique improves motor control. The American Academy of Cerebral Palsy and Developmental Medicine reviewed studies that measured the impact of neurodevelopmental treatment and concluded that there was no strong evidence supporting its effectiveness for children with cerebral palsy.

Conductive education, developed in Hungary in the 1940s, is another physical therapy that at one time appeared to hold promise. Conductive education instructors attempt to improve a child's motor abilities by combining rhythmic activities, such as singing and clapping, with physical maneuvers on special equipment. The therapy, however, has not been able to produce consistent or significant improvements in study groups.

Speech and language therapy: About 20 percent of children with cerebral palsy are unable to produce intelligible speech. They also experience challenges in other areas of communication, such as hand gestures and facial expressions, and they have difficulty participating in the basic give and take of a normal conversation. These challenges will last throughout their lives.

Speech and language therapists (also known as speech therapists or speech-language pathologists) observe, diagnose, and treat the communication disorders associated with cerebral palsy. They use a program of exercises to teach children how to overcome specific communication difficulties.

For example, if a child has difficulty saying words that begin with "b," the therapist may suggest daily practice with a list of "b" words, increasing their difficulty as each list is mastered. Other kinds of exercises help children master the social skills involved in communicating by teaching them to keep their head up, maintain eye contact, and repeat themselves when they are misunderstood.

Speech therapists can also help children with severe disabilities learn how to use special communication devices, such as a computer with a voice synthesizer, or a special board covered with symbols of everyday objects and activities to which a child can point to indicate his or her wishes.

Speech interventions often use a child's family members and friends to reinforce the lessons learned in a therapeutic setting. This kind of indirect therapy encourages people who are in close daily contact with a child to create opportunities for him or her to use their new skills in conversation.

Treatments for problems with eating and drooling are often necessary when children with cerebral palsy have difficulty eating and drinking because they have little control over the muscles that move their mouth, jaw, and tongue. They are also at risk for breathing food or fluid into the lungs. Some children develop gastroesophageal reflux disease (GERD, commonly called heartburn) in which a weak diaphragm can't keep stomach acids from spilling into the esophagus. The irritation of the acid can cause bleeding and pain.

Individuals with cerebral palsy are also at risk for malnutrition, recurrent lung infections, and progressive lung disease. The individuals most at risk for these problems are those with spastic quadriplegia.

Initially, children should be evaluated for their swallowing ability, which is usually done with a modified barium swallow study. Recommendations regarding diet modifications will be derived from the results of this study.

In severe cases where swallowing problems are causing malnutrition, a doctor may recommend tube feeding, in which a tube delivers food and nutrients down the throat and into the stomach, or gastrostomy, in which a surgical opening allows a tube to be placed directly into the stomach.

Although numerous treatments for drooling have been tested over the years, there is no one treatment that helps reliably. Anticholinergic drugs—such as glycopyrrolate—can reduce the flow of saliva but may cause unpleasant side effects, such as dry mouth, constipation, and urinary retention. Surgery, while sometimes effective, carries the risk of complications. Some children benefit from biofeedback techniques that help them recognize more quickly when their mouths fall open and they begin to drool. Intraoral devices (devices that fit into the mouth) that encourage better tongue positioning and swallowing are still being evaluated, but appear to reduce drooling for some children.

What are the drug treatments for cerebral palsy?

Oral medications such as diazepam, baclofen, dantrolene sodium, and tizanidine are usually used as the first line of treatment to relax stiff, contracted, or overactive muscles. These drugs are easy to use, except that dosages high enough to be effective often have side effects, among them drowsiness, upset stomach, high blood pressure, and possible liver damage with long-term use. Oral medications are most appropriate for children who need only mild reduction in muscle tone or who have widespread spasticity.

Doctors also sometimes use alcohol "washes"—injections of alcohol into muscles—to reduce spasticity. The benefits last from a few months to 2 years or more, but the adverse effects include a significant risk of pain or numbness, and the procedure requires a high degree of skill to target the nerve.

The availability of new and more precise methods to deliver anti-spasmodic medications is moving treatment for spasticity toward chemodenervation, in which injected drugs are used to target and relax muscles.

Botulinum toxin (BT-A), injected locally, has become a standard treatment for overactive muscles in children with spastic movement disorders such as cerebral palsy. BT-A relaxes contracted muscles by keeping nerve cells from over-activating muscle. Although BT-A is not approved by the Food and Drug Administration (FDA) for treating cerebral palsy, since the 1990s doctors have been using it off-label to relax spastic muscles. A number of studies have shown that it reduces spasticity and increases the range of motion of the muscles it targets.

The relaxing effect of a BT-A injection lasts approximately 3 months. Undesirable side effects are mild and short-lived, consisting of pain upon injection and occasionally mild flu-like symptoms. BT-A injections are most effective when followed by a stretching program including physical therapy and splinting. BT-A injections work best for children who have some control over their motor movements and have a limited number of muscles to treat, none of which is fixed or rigid.

Because BT-A does not have FDA approval to treat spasticity in children, parents and caregivers should make sure that the doctor giving the injection is trained in the procedure and has experience using it in children.

Intrathecal baclofen therapy uses an implantable pump to deliver baclofen, a muscle relaxant, into the fluid surrounding the spinal cord. Baclofen works by decreasing the excitability of nerve cells in the spinal cord, which then reduces muscle spasticity throughout the body. Because it is delivered directly into the nervous system, the intrathecal dose of baclofen can be as low as one one-hundredth of the oral dose. Studies have shown it reduces spasticity and pain and improves sleep.

The pump is the size of a hockey puck and is implanted in the abdomen. It contains a refillable reservoir connected to an alarm that beeps when the reservoir is low. The pump is programmable with an electronic telemetry wand. The program can be adjusted if muscle tone is worse at certain times of the day or night.

The baclofen pump carries a small but significant risk of serious complications if it fails or is programmed incorrectly, if the catheter becomes twisted or kinked, or if the insertion site becomes infected. Undesirable, but infrequent, side effects include overrelaxation of the muscles, sleepiness, headache, nausea, vomiting, dizziness, and constipation.

As a muscle-relaxing therapy, the baclofen pump is most appropriate for individuals with chronic, severe stiffness or uncontrolled muscle movement throughout the body. Doctors have successfully implanted the pump in children as young as 3 years of age.

What surgeries are available for cerebral palsy?

Orthopedic surgery is often recommended when spasticity and stiffness are severe enough to make walking and moving about difficult or painful. For many people with cerebral palsy, improving the appearance of how they walk—their gait—is also important. A more upright gait with smoother transitions and foot placements is the primary goal for many children and young adults.

In the operating room, surgeons can lengthen muscles and tendons that are proportionately too short. But first, they have to determine the specific muscles responsible for the gait abnormalities. Finding these muscles can be difficult. It takes more than 30 major muscles working at the right time using the right amount of force to walk two strides with a normal gait. A problem with any of those muscles can cause an abnormal gait.

In addition, because the body makes natural adjustments to compensate for muscle imbalances, these adjustments could appear to be the problem, instead of a compensation. In the past, doctors relied on clinical examination, observation of the gait, and the measurement of motion and spasticity to determine the muscles involved. Now, doctors have a diagnostic technique known as gait analysis.

Gait analysis uses cameras that record how an individual walks, force plates that detect when and where feet touch the ground, a special recording technique that detects muscle activity (known as electromyography), and a computer program that gathers and analyzes the data to identify the problem muscles. Using gait analysis, doctors can precisely locate which muscles would benefit from surgery and how much improvement in gait can be expected.

The timing of orthopedic surgery has also changed in recent years. Previously, orthopedic surgeons preferred to perform all of the necessary surgeries a child needed at the same time, usually between the ages of 7 and 10. Because of the length of time spent in recovery, which was generally several months, doing them all at once shortened the amount of time a child spent in bed. Now most of the surgical procedures can be done on an outpatient basis or with a short inpatient stay. Children usually return to their normal lifestyle within a week.

Consequently, doctors think it is much better to stagger surgeries and perform them at times appropriate to a child's age and level of motor development. For example, spasticity in the upper leg muscles (the adductors), which causes a "scissor pattern" walk, is a major obstacle to normal gait. The optimal age to correct this spasticity with adduction release surgery is 2 to 4 years of age. On the other hand, the best time to perform surgery to lengthen the hamstrings or Achilles tendon is 7 to 8 years of age. If adduction release surgery is delayed so that it can be performed at the same time as hamstring lengthening, the child will have learned to compensate for spasticity in the adductors. By the time the hamstring surgery is performed, the child's abnormal gait pattern could be so ingrained that it might not be easily corrected.

With shorter recovery times and new, less invasive surgical techniques, doctors can schedule surgeries at times that take advantage of a child's age and developmental abilities for the best possible result.

Selective dorsal rhizotomy (SDR) is a surgical procedure recommended only for cases of severe spasticity when all of the more conservative treatments—physical therapy, oral medications, and intrathecal baclofen—have failed to reduce spasticity or chronic pain. In the procedure, a surgeon locates and selectively severs overactivated nerves at the base of the spinal column.

Because it reduces the amount of stimulation that reaches muscles via the nerves, SDR is most commonly used to relax muscles and decrease chronic pain in one or both of the lower or upper limbs. It is also sometimes used to correct an overactive bladder. Potential side effects include sensory loss, numbness, or uncomfortable sensations in limb areas once supplied by the severed nerve.

Even though the use of microsurgery techniques has refined the practice of SDR surgery, there is still controversy about how selective SDR actually is. Some doctors have concerns since it is invasive and irreversible and may only achieve small improvements in function. Although recent research has shown that combining SDR with physical therapy reduces spasticity in some children, particularly those with spastic diplegia, whether or not it improves gait or function has still not been proven. Ongoing research continues to look at this surgery's effectiveness.

Spinal cord stimulation was developed in the 1980s to treat spinal cord injury and other neurological conditions involving motor neurons. An implanted electrode selectively stimulates nerves at the base of the spinal cord to inhibit and decrease nerve activity. The effectiveness of spinal cord stimulation for the treatment of cerebral palsy has yet to be proven in clinical studies. It is considered a treatment alternative only when other conservative or surgical treatments have been unsuccessful at relaxing muscles or relieving pain.

What are some orthotic devices used to treat cerebral palsy?

Orthotic devices—such as braces and splints—use external force to correct muscle abnormalities. The technology of orthotics has advanced over the past 30 years from metal rods that hooked up to bulky orthopedic shoes, to appliances that are individually molded from high-temperature plastics for a precise fit.

Ankle-foot orthoses are frequently prescribed for children with spastic diplegia to prevent muscle contracture and to improve gait. Splints are also used to correct spasticity in the hand muscles.

What assistive technologies are available to treat cerebral palsy?

Devices that help individuals move about more easily and communicate successfully at home, at school, or in the workplace can help a child or adult with cerebral palsy overcome physical and communication limitations. There are a number of devices that help individuals stand straight and walk, such as postural support or seating systems, open-front walkers, quadrupedal canes (lightweight metal canes with four feet), and gait poles. Electric wheelchairs let more severely impaired adults and children move about successfully.

The computer is probably the most dramatic example of a communication device that can make a big difference in the lives of people with cerebral palsy. Equipped with a computer and voice synthesizer, a child or adult with cerebral palsy can communicate successfully with others. For example, a child who is unable to speak or write but can make head movements may be able to control a computer using a special light pointer that attaches to a headband.

What alternative therapies are available to treat cerebral palsy?

Therapeutic (subthreshold) electrical stimulation, also called neuromuscular electrical stimulation (NES), pulses electricity into the motor nerves to stimulate contraction in selective muscle groups.

Many studies have demonstrated that NES appears to increase range of motion and muscular strength.

Threshold electrical stimulation, which involves the application of electrical stimulation at an intensity too low to stimulate muscle contraction, is a controversial therapy. Studies have not been able to demonstrate its effectiveness or any significant improvement with its use.

Hyperbaric oxygen therapy: Some children have cerebral palsy as the result of brain damage from oxygen deprivation. Proponents of hyperbaric oxygen therapy propose that the brain tissue surrounding the damaged area can be "awakened" by forcing high concentrations of oxygen into the body under greater than atmospheric pressure.

A recent study compared a group of children who received no hyperbaric treatment to a group that received 40 treatments over 8 weeks. On every measure of function (gross motor, cognitive, communication, and memory) at the end of 2 months of treatment and after a further 3 months of follow up, the two groups were identical in outcome. There was no added benefit from hyperbaric oxygen therapy.

Chapter 24

Charcot-Marie-Tooth Disease

What is Charcot-Marie-Tooth disease?

Charcot-Marie-Tooth disease (CMT) is one of the most common inherited neurological disorders, affecting approximately 1 in 2,500 people in the United States. The disease is named for the three physicians who first identified it in 1886—Jean-Martin Charcot and Pierre Marie in Paris, France, and Howard Henry Tooth in Cambridge, England. CMT, also known as hereditary motor and sensory neuropathy (HMSN) or peroneal muscular atrophy, comprises a group of disorders that affect peripheral nerves. The peripheral nerves lie outside the brain and spinal cord and supply the muscles and sensory organs in the limbs. Disorders that affect the peripheral nerves are called peripheral neuropathies.

What are the symptoms of Charcot-Marie-Tooth disease?

The neuropathy of CMT affects both motor and sensory nerves. A typical feature includes weakness of the foot and lower leg muscles, which may result in foot drop and a high-stepped gait with frequent tripping or falls. Foot deformities, such as high arches and hammertoes (a condition in which the middle joint of a toe bends upwards) are also characteristic due to weakness of the small muscles in the

"Charcot-Marie-Tooth Disease Fact Sheet," is from the National Institute on Neurological Disorders and Stroke (NINDS, www.ninds.nih.gov), part of the National Institutes of Health, December 11, 2007.

feet. In addition, the lower legs may take on an "inverted champagne bottle" appearance due to the loss of muscle bulk. Later in the disease, weakness and muscle atrophy may occur in the hands, resulting in difficulty with fine motor skills.

Onset of symptoms is most often in adolescence or early adulthood, however presentation may be delayed until mid-adulthood. The severity of symptoms is quite variable in different patients and even among family members with the disease. Progression of symptoms is gradual. Pain can range from mild to severe, and some patients may need to rely on foot or leg braces or other orthopedic devices to maintain mobility. Although in rare cases patients may have respiratory muscle weakness, CMT is not considered a fatal disease and people with most forms of CMT have a normal life expectancy.

What causes Charcot-Marie-Tooth disease?

A nerve cell communicates information to distant targets by sending electrical signals down a long, thin part of the cell called the axon. In order to increase the speed at which these electrical signals travel, the axon is insulated by myelin, which is produced by another type of cell called the Schwann cell. Myelin twists around the axon like a jelly-roll cake and prevents dissipation of the electrical signals. Without an intact axon and myelin sheath, peripheral nerve cells are unable to activate target muscles or relay sensory information from the limbs back to the brain.

CMT is caused by mutations in genes that produce proteins involved in the structure and function of either the peripheral nerve axon or the myelin sheath. Although different proteins are abnormal in different forms of CMT disease, all of the mutations affect the normal function of the peripheral nerves. Consequently, these nerves slowly degenerate and lose the ability to communicate with their distant targets. The degeneration of motor nerves results in muscle weakness and atrophy in the extremities (arms, legs, hands, or feet), and in some cases the degeneration of sensory nerves results in a reduced ability to feel heat, cold, and pain.

The gene mutations in CMT disease are usually inherited. Each of us normally possesses two copies of every gene, one inherited from each parent. Some forms of CMT are inherited in an autosomal dominant fashion, which means that only one copy of the abnormal gene is needed to cause the disease. Other forms of CMT are inherited in an autosomal recessive fashion, which means that both copies of the abnormal gene must be present to cause the disease. Still other forms of CMT are inherited in an X-linked fashion, which means that the abnormal gene is located on the X chromosome. The X and Y chromosomes determine an individual's sex. Individuals with two X chromosomes are female and individuals with one X and one Y chromosome are male. In rare cases the gene mutation causing CMT disease is a new mutation which occurs spontaneously in the patient's genetic material and has not been passed down through the family.

How is Charcot-Marie-Tooth disease treated?

There is no cure for CMT, but physical therapy, occupational therapy, braces and other orthopedic devices, and even orthopedic surgery can help patients cope with the disabling symptoms of the disease. In addition, pain-killing drugs can be prescribed for patients who have severe pain.

Physical and occupational therapy, the preferred treatment for CMT, involves muscle strength training, muscle and ligament stretching, stamina training, and moderate aerobic exercise. Most therapists recommend a specialized treatment program designed with the approval of the patient's physician to fit individual abilities and needs. Therapists also suggest entering into a treatment program early; muscle strengthening may delay or reduce muscle atrophy, so strength training is most useful if it begins before nerve degeneration and muscle weakness progress to the point of disability.

Stretching may prevent or reduce joint deformities that result from uneven muscle pull on bones. Exercises to help build stamina or increase endurance will help prevent the fatigue that results from performing everyday activities that require strength and mobility. Moderate aerobic activity can help to maintain cardiovascular fitness and overall health. Most therapists recommend low-impact or no-impact exercises, such as biking or swimming, rather than activities such as walking or jogging, which may put stress on fragile muscles and joints.

Many CMT patients require ankle braces and other orthopedic devices to maintain everyday mobility and prevent injury. Ankle braces can help prevent ankle sprains by providing support and stability during activities such as walking or climbing stairs. High-top shoes or boots can also give the patient support for weak ankles. Thumb splints can help with hand weakness and loss of fine motor skills. Assistive devices should be used before disability sets in because the devices may prevent muscle strain and reduce muscle weakening. Some CMT patients may decide to have orthopedic surgery to reverse foot and joint deformities.

Chapter 25

Muscular Dystrophy

Muscular dystrophy (MD) is a genetic disorder that gradually weakens the body's muscles. It's caused by incorrect or missing genetic information that prevents the body from making the proteins it needs to build and maintain healthy muscles.

A child who is diagnosed with MD gradually loses the ability to do things like walk, sit upright, breathe easily, and move the arms and hands. This increasing weakness can lead to other health problems.

There are several major forms of muscular dystrophy, which can affect a child's muscles in different levels of severity. In some cases, MD starts causing muscle problems in infancy, while in others, symptoms don't appear until adulthood.

There is no cure for MD, but researchers are quickly learning more about how to prevent and treat the condition. Doctors are also working on improving muscle and joint function, and slowing muscle deterioration so that kids, teens, and adults with MD can live as actively and independently as possible.

What Are the First Symptoms of Muscular Dystrophy?

Many kids with muscular dystrophy follow a normal pattern of development during their first few years of life.

"Muscular Dystrophy," August 2005, reprinted with permission from www .kidshealth.org. Copyright © 2005 The Nemours Foundation. This information was provided by KidsHealth, one of the largest resources online for medically reviewed health information written for parents, kids, and teens. For more articles like this one, visit www.KidsHealth.org, or www.TeensHealth.org.

But in time common symptoms begin to appear. A child who has MD may start to stumble, waddle, have difficulty going up stairs, and toe walk (walk on the toes without the heels hitting the floor). A child may start to struggle to get up from a sitting position or have a hard time pushing things, like a wagon or a tricycle. It is also common for a young child with MD to develop enlarged calf muscles, a condition called calf pseudohypertrophy, as muscle tissue is destroyed and re-placed by fat.

How Is Muscular Dystrophy Diagnosed?

When a doctor first suspects that a child has muscular dystrophy, he or she probably will do a physical exam, take a family history, and ask about any problems—particularly those affecting the muscles—that the child might be experiencing.

In addition, the doctor may perform a series of tests to determine what type of MD a child may have and to rule out any other diseases that may be causing a problem. This might include a blood test to mea-sure levels of serum creatine kinase, an enzyme that's released into the bloodstream when muscle fibers are deteriorating. Elevated lev-els of this enzyme indicate that something is causing muscle damage.

The doctor also may do a blood test to check a child's DNA for gene abnormalities, or a muscle biopsy to examine a muscle tissue sample for patterns of deterioration and abnormal levels of dystrophin, a pro-tein that helps muscle cells keep their shape and length. Without dystrophin, the muscles break down.

Types of Muscular Dystrophy

The different types of muscular dystrophy affect different sets of muscles and result in different degrees of muscle weakness.

Duchenne muscular dystrophy is the most common and the most severe form of the disease. It affects about 1 out of every 3,500 boys. (Girls can carry the gene that causes the disease, but they usually have no symptoms.) This form of MD occurs because of a problem with the gene that makes dystrophin. Without this protein, the muscles break down and a child becomes weaker.

In cases of Duchenne muscular dystrophy, symptoms usually be-gin to appear around age 5, as the pelvic muscles begin to weaken. Most kids with this form of MD need to use a wheelchair by age 12. Over time, their muscles weaken in the shoulders, back, arms, and legs. Eventually, the respiratory muscles are affected, and a ventilator is required to assist breathing. Kids who have Duchenne muscular dystrophy typically have a life span of about 20 years.

Although most kids with Duchenne muscular dystrophy have average intelligence, about one-third of them experience learning disabilities and a small number of them have mental retardation.

While the incidence of Duchenne is known, it's unclear how common other forms of MD are because the symptoms can vary so widely between individuals. In fact, in some people the symptoms are so mild that the disease goes undiagnosed.

Becker muscular dystrophy is similar to Duchenne, but it is less common and progresses more slowly. This form of MD affects approximately 1 in 30,000 boys. It too is caused by insufficient production of dystrophin.

With this form of MD, symptoms typically begin during the teen years, then follow a pattern similar to Duchenne muscular dystrophy. Muscle weakness first begins in the pelvic muscles, then moves into the shoulders and back. Many children with Becker have a normal life span and can lead long, active lives without the use of a wheelchair.

Myotonic dystrophy, also known as Steinert's disease, is the most common adult form of muscular dystrophy, although half of all cases are diagnosed in people who are younger than 20 years old. It is caused by a portion of a particular gene that is larger than it should be. The symptoms can appear at any time during a child's life.

The main symptoms include muscle weakness, myotonia (in which the muscles have trouble relaxing once they contract), and muscle wasting, where the muscles shrink over time. Kids with myotonic dystrophy also can experience cataracts and heart problems.

Limb-girdle muscular dystrophy affects boys and girls equally. Typically, symptoms begin when kids are between 8 and 15 years old. This form of MD progresses slowly, affecting the pelvic, shoulder, and back muscles. The severity of muscle weakness varies from person to person. Some kids develop only mild weakness while others develop severe disabilities and as adults need a wheelchair to get around.

Facioscapulohumeral muscular dystrophy can affect both boys and girls, and the symptoms usually first appear during the teen years. This form of muscular dystrophy tends to progress slowly.

Muscle weakness first develops in the face, making it difficult for a child to close the eyes, whistle, or puff out the cheeks. The shoulder and back muscles gradually become weak, and kids who are affected have difficulty lifting objects or raising their hands overhead. Over time, the legs and pelvic muscles also may lose strength.

Other types of muscular dystrophy, which are rare, include distal, ocular, oculopharyngeal, and Emery-Dreifuss.

Caring for a Child with Muscular Dystrophy

Though there's no cure for MD yet, doctors are working to improve muscle and joint function, and slow muscle deterioration in kids who are living with the condition.

If your child is diagnosed with muscular dystrophy, a team of medical specialists will work with you and your family. That team will likely include: a neurologist, orthopedist, pulmonologist, physical and occupational therapist, nurse practitioner, cardiologist, registered dietitian, and a social worker.

Muscular dystrophy is often degenerative, so kids may pass through different stages as the disease progresses and require different kinds of treatment. During the early stages, physical therapy, joint bracing, and the medication prednisone are often used. During the later stages, doctors may use assistive devices such as:

- physical therapy and bracing to improve your child's flexibility;
- power wheelchairs and scooters to improve your child's mobility;
- a ventilator to support your child's breathing;
- robotics to help your child perform routine daily tasks.

Physical Therapy and Bracing

Physical therapy can help a child to maintain muscle tone and reduce the severity of joint contractures with exercises that keep the muscles strong and the joints flexible.

A physical therapist also uses bracing to help prevent joint contractures, a stiffening of the muscles near the joints that can make it harder to move and can lock the joints in painful positions. By providing extra support in just the right places, bracing can extend the time that a child with MD can walk independently.

Prednisone

If a child has Duchenne muscular dystrophy, the doctor may prescribe the steroid prednisone to help slow the rate of muscle deterioration. By doing so, a child with muscular dystrophy may be able to walk longer and live a more active life.

There is some debate over the best time to begin treating a child with prednisone, but most doctors prescribe it when a child with MD is 5 or 6 years old, or when the child's strength begins to show a significant decline. Prednisone does have side effects, though. It can cause weight gain, which can put even greater strain on a child's already-weak muscles. It also can cause a loss of bone density and, possibly, lead to fractures. If your doctor prescribes prednisone, he or she will closely monitor your child.

Spinal Fusion

Many children who have the Duchenne and Becker forms of muscular dystrophy develop severe scoliosis—an S- or C-shaped curvature of the spine that develops when the back muscles are too weak to hold the spine erect. Some kids who have severe cases of scoliosis undergo spinal fusion, a surgery that can reduce pain, lessen the severity of the spine curvature so that a child can sit upright and comfortably in a chair, and ensure that the spine curvature doesn't have an effect on the child's breathing. Typically, spinal fusion surgery only requires a short hospital stay.

Respiratory Care

Many kids with muscular dystrophy also have weakened heart and respiratory muscles. As a result, they can't cough out phlegm and sometimes develop respiratory infections that can quickly become serious. Good general health care and regular vaccinations are especially important for children with muscular dystrophy to help prevent these infections.

Assistive Devices

A variety of new technologies are available to create independence and mobility for kids with muscular dystrophy.

Some kids with Duchenne muscular dystrophy may use a manual wheelchair once it becomes difficult to walk. Others go directly to a motorized wheelchair, which can be equipped to meet their needs as muscle deterioration advances.

Robotic technologies also are under development to help kids move their arms and perform activities of daily living.

If your child would benefit from an assistive technological device, it's a good idea to contact your local chapter of the Muscular Dystrophy

Association to ask about financial assistance that might be available. In some cases, health insurers cover the cost of these devices.

The Search for a Cure

Researchers are quickly learning more about what causes the genetic disorder that leads to muscular dystrophy, and about possible treatments for the disease. If you'd like to know more about the most current research on muscular dystrophy, contact the local chapter of the Muscular Dystrophy Association, or talk to your child's doctor.

Chapter 26

Multiple Sclerosis

What is multiple sclerosis?

During an MS attack, inflammation occurs in areas of the white matter of the central nervous system in random patches called plaques. This process is followed by destruction of myelin, the fatty covering that insulates nerve cell fibers in the brain and spinal cord. Myelin facilitates the smooth, high-speed transmission of electrochemical messages between the brain, the spinal cord, and the rest of the body; when it is damaged, neurological transmission of messages may be slowed or blocked completely, leading to diminished or lost function. The name "multiple sclerosis" signifies both the number (multiple) and condition (sclerosis, from the Greek term for scarring or hardening) of the demyelinated areas in the central nervous system.

How many people have MS?

No one knows exactly how many people have MS. It is believed that, currently, there are approximately 250,000 to 350,000 people in the United States with MS diagnosed by a physician. This estimate suggests that approximately 200 new cases are diagnosed each week.

Excerpted from "Multiple Sclerosis: Hope Through Research," by the National Institute of Neurological Disorders and Stroke (NINDS, www.ninds.nih.gov), part of the National Institutes of Health, April 8, 2008.

Who gets MS?

Most people experience their first symptoms of MS between the ages of 20 and 40, but a diagnosis is often delayed. This is due to both the transitory nature of the disease and the lack of a specific diagnostic test—specific symptoms and changes in the brain must develop before the diagnosis is confirmed.

Although scientists have documented cases of MS in young children and elderly adults, symptoms rarely begin before age 15 or after age 60. Whites are more than twice as likely as other races to develop MS. In general, women are affected at almost twice the rate of men; however, among patients who develop the symptoms of MS at a later age, the gender ratio is more balanced.

MS is five times more prevalent in temperate climates—such as those found in the northern United States, Canada, and Europe—than in tropical regions. Furthermore, the age of 15 seems to be significant in terms of risk for developing the disease: some studies indicate that a person moving from a high-risk (temperate) to a low-risk (tropical) area before the age of 15 tends to adopt the risk (in this case, low) of the new area and vice versa. Other studies suggest that people moving after age 15 maintain the risk of the area where they grew up.

These findings indicate a strong role for an environmental factor in the cause of MS. It is possible that, at the time of or immediately following puberty, patients acquire an infection with a long latency period. Or, conversely, people in some areas may come in contact with an unknown protective agent during the time before puberty. Other studies suggest that the unknown geographic or climatic element may actually be simply a matter of genetic predilection and reflect racial and ethnic susceptibility factors.

Periodically, scientists receive reports of MS "clusters." The most famous of these MS "epidemics" took place in the Faeroe Islands north of Scotland in the years following the arrival of British troops during World War II. Despite intense study of this and other clusters, no direct environmental factor has been identified. Nor has any definitive evidence been found to link daily stress to MS attacks, although there is evidence that the risk of worsening is greater after acute viral illnesses.

What causes MS?

Scientists have learned a great deal about MS in recent years; still, its cause remains elusive. Many investigators believe MS to be an autoimmune disease—one in which the body, through its immune system, launches a defensive attack against its own tissues. In the case of MS, it is the nerve-insulating myelin that comes under assault. Such assaults may be linked to an unknown environmental trigger, perhaps a virus.

What is the course of MS?

Each case of MS displays one of several patterns of presentation and subsequent course. Most commonly, MS first manifests itself as a series of attacks followed by complete or partial remissions as symptoms mysteriously lessen, only to return later after a period of stability. This is called relapsing-remitting (RR) MS. Primary-progressive (PP) MS is characterized by a gradual clinical decline with no distinct remissions, although there may be temporary plateaus or minor relief from symptoms. Secondary-progressive (SP) MS begins with a relapsing-remitting course followed by a later primary-progressive course. Rarely, patients may have a progressive-relapsing (PR) course in which the disease takes a progressive path punctuated by acute attacks. PP, SP, and PR are sometimes lumped together and called chronic progressive MS.

In addition, 20 percent of the MS population has a benign form of the disease in which symptoms show little or no progression after the initial attack; these patients remain fully functional. A few patients experience malignant MS, defined as a swift and relentless decline resulting in significant disability or even death shortly after disease onset. However, MS is very rarely fatal and most people with MS have a fairly normal life expectancy.

Studies throughout the world are causing investigators to redefine the natural course of the disease. These studies use a technique called magnetic resonance imaging (MRI) to visualize the evolution of MS lesions in the white matter of the brain. Bright spots on a T2 MRI scan indicate the presence of lesions, but do not provide information about when they developed.

Because investigators speculate that the breakdown of the blood/brain barrier is the first step in the development of MS lesions, it is important to distinguish new lesions from old. To do this, physicians give patients injections of gadolinium, a chemical contrast agent that normally does not cross the blood/brain barrier, before performing a scan. On this type of scan, called T1, the appearance of bright areas indicates periods of recent disease activity (when gadolinium is able to cross the barrier). The ability to estimate the age of lesions through

MRI has allowed investigators to show that, in some patients, lesions occur frequently throughout the course of the disease even when no symptoms are present.

What are the symptoms of MS?

Symptoms of MS may be mild or severe, of long duration or short, and may appear in various combinations, depending on the area of the nervous system affected. Complete or partial remission of symptoms, especially in the early stages of the disease, occurs in approximately 70 percent of MS patients.

The initial symptom of MS is often blurred or double vision, red-green color distortion, or even blindness in one eye. Inexplicably, visual problems tend to clear up in the later stages of MS. Inflammatory problems of the optic nerve may be diagnosed as retrobulbar optic neuritis. Fifty-five percent of MS patients will have an attack of optic neuritis at some time or other and it will be the first symptom of MS in approximately 15 percent. This has led to general recognition of optic neuritis as an early sign of MS, especially if tests also reveal abnormalities in the patient's spinal fluid.

Most MS patients experience muscle weakness in their extremities and difficulty with coordination and balance at some time during the course of the disease. These symptoms may be severe enough to impair walking or even standing. In the worst cases, MS can produce partial or complete paralysis. Spasticity—the involuntary increased tone of muscles leading to stiffness and spasms—is common, as is fatigue. Fatigue may be triggered by physical exertion and improve with rest, or it may take the form of a constant and persistent tiredness.

Most people with MS also exhibit paresthesias, transitory abnormal sensory feelings such as numbness, prickling, or "pins and needles" sensations; uncommonly, some may also experience pain. Loss of sensation sometimes occurs. Speech impediments, tremors, and dizziness are other frequent complaints. Occasionally, people with MS have hearing loss.

Approximately half of all people with MS experience cognitive impairments such as difficulties with concentration, attention, memory, and poor judgment, but such symptoms are usually mild and are frequently overlooked. In fact, they are often detectable only through comprehensive testing. Patients themselves may be unaware of their cognitive loss; it is often a family member or friend who first notices a deficit. Such impairments are usually mild, rarely disabling, and intellectual and language abilities are generally spared.

Cognitive symptoms occur when lesions develop in brain areas responsible for information processing. These deficits tend to become more apparent as the information to be processed becomes more complex. Fatigue may also add to processing difficulties. Scientists do not yet know whether altered cognition in MS reflects problems with information acquisition, retrieval, or a combination of both. Types of memory problems may differ depending on the individual's disease course (relapsing-remitting, primary-progressive, etc.), but there does not appear to be any direct correlation between duration of illness and severity of cognitive dysfunction.

Depression, which is unrelated to cognitive problems, is another common feature of MS. In addition, about 10 percent of patients suffer from more severe psychotic disorders such as manic-depression and paranoia. Five percent may experience episodes of inappropriate euphoria and despair—unrelated to the patient's actual emotional state—known as "laughing/weeping syndrome." This syndrome is thought to be due to demyelination in the brainstem, the area of the brain that controls facial expression and emotions, and is usually seen only in severe cases.

As the disease progresses, sexual dysfunction may become a problem. Bowel and bladder control may also be lost.

In about 60 percent of MS patients, heat—whether generated by temperatures outside the body or by exercise—may cause temporary worsening of many MS symptoms. In these cases, eradicating the heat eliminates the problem. Some temperature-sensitive patients find that a cold bath may temporarily relieve their symptoms. For the same reason, swimming is often a good exercise choice for people with MS.

The erratic symptoms of MS can affect the entire family as patients may become unable to work at the same time they are facing high medical bills and additional expenses for housekeeping assistance and modifications to homes and vehicles. The emotional drain on both patient and family is immeasurable. Support groups and counseling may help MS patients, their families, and friends find ways to cope with the many problems the disease can cause.

Can MS be treated?

There is as yet no cure for MS. Many patients do well with no therapy at all, especially since many medications have serious side effects and some carry significant risks. Naturally occurring or spontaneous remissions make it difficult to determine therapeutic effects of experimental treatments; however, the emerging evidence that MRIs can chart the development of lesions is already helping scientists evaluate new therapies.

In the past, the principal medications physicians used to treat MS were steroids possessing anti-inflammatory properties; these include adrenocorticotropic hormone (better known as ACTH), prednisone, prednisolone, methylprednisolone, betamethasone, and dexamethasone. Studies suggest that intravenous methylprednisolone may be superior to the more traditional intravenous ACTH for patients experiencing acute relapses; no strong evidence exists to support the use of these drugs to treat progressive forms of MS. Also, there is some indication that steroids may be more appropriate for people with movement, rather than sensory, symptoms.

While steroids do not affect the course of MS over time, they can reduce the duration and severity of attacks in some patients. The mechanism behind this effect is not known; one study suggests the medications work by restoring the effectiveness of the blood/brain barrier. Because steroids can produce numerous adverse side effects (acne, weight gain, seizures, psychosis), they are not recommended for long-term use.

One of the most promising MS research areas involves naturally occurring antiviral proteins known as interferons. Three forms of beta interferon (Avonex, Betaseron, and Rebif) have now been approved by the U.S. Food and Drug Administration (FDA) for treatment of relapsing-remitting MS. Beta interferon has been shown to reduce the number of exacerbations and may slow the progression of physical disability. When attacks do occur, they tend to be shorter and less severe. In addition, MRI scans suggest that beta interferon can decrease myelin destruction.

Investigators speculate that the effects of beta interferon may be due to the drug's ability to correct an MS-related deficiency of certain white blood cells that suppress the immune system and/or its ability to inhibit gamma interferon, a substance believed to be involved in MS attacks. Alpha interferon is also being studied as a possible treatment for MS. Common side effects of interferons include fever, chills, sweating, muscle aches, fatigue, depression, and injection site reactions.

Scientists continue their extensive efforts to create new and better therapies for MS. Goals of therapy are threefold: to improve recovery from attacks, to prevent or lessen the number of relapses, and to halt disease progression. Some therapies currently under investigation are discussed in the following text.

Immunotherapy: As evidence of immune system involvement in the development of MS has grown, trials of various new treatments to alter or suppress immune response are being conducted. Most of these therapies are, at this time, still considered experimental.

Results of recent clinical trials have shown that immunosuppressive agents and techniques can positively (if temporarily) affect the course of MS; however, toxic side effects often preclude their widespread use. In addition, generalized immunosuppression leaves the patient open to a variety of viral, bacterial, and fungal infections.

Over the years, MS investigators have studied a number of immunosuppressant treatments. One such treatment, Novantrone (mitoxantrone), was approved by the FDA for the treatment of advanced or chronic MS. Other therapies being studied are cyclosporine (Sandimmune), cyclophosphamide (Cytoxan), methotrexate, azathioprine (Imuran), and total lymphoid irradiation (a process whereby the MS patient's lymph nodes are irradiated with x-rays in small doses over a few weeks to destroy lymphoid tissue, which is actively involved in tissue destruction in autoimmune diseases). Inconclusive and/or contradictory results of these trials, combined with the therapies' potentially dangerous side effects, dictate that further research is necessary to determine what, if any, role they should play in the management of MS. Studies are also being conducted with the immune system modulating drug cladribine (Leustatin).

Another potential treatment for MS is monoclonal antibodies, which are identical, laboratory-produced antibodies that are highly specific for a single antigen. They are injected into the patient in the hope that they will alter the patient's immune response. One monoclonal antibody, natalizumab (Tysabri), was shown in clinical trials to significantly reduce the frequency of attacks in people with relapsing forms of MS and was approved for marketing by the U.S. Food and Drug Administration (FDA) in 2004. However, in 2005 the drug's manufacturer voluntarily suspended marketing of the drug after several reports of significant adverse events. In 2006, the FDA again approved sale of the drug for MS but under strict treatment guidelines involving infusion centers where patients can be monitored by specially trained physicians.

Another experimental treatment for MS is plasma exchange, or plasmapheresis. Plasmapheresis is a procedure in which blood is removed from the patient and the blood plasma is separated from other blood substances that may contain antibodies and other immunologically active products. These other blood substances are discarded and the plasma is then transfused back into the patient. Because its worth as a treatment for MS has not yet been proven, this experimental treatment remains at the stage of clinical testing.

Bone marrow transplantation (a procedure in which bone marrow from a healthy donor is infused into patients who have undergone drug or radiation therapy to suppress their immune system so they will not reject the donated marrow) and injections of venom from honey bees are also being studied. Each of these therapies carries the risk of potentially severe side effects.

Therapy to improve nerve impulse conduction: Because the transmission of electrochemical messages between the brain and body is disrupted in MS, medications to improve the conduction of nerve impulses are being investigated. Since demyelinated nerves show abnormalities of potassium activity, scientists are studying drugs that block the channels through which potassium moves, thereby restoring conduction of the nerve impulse. In several small experimental trials, derivatives of a drug called aminopyridine temporarily improved vision, coordination, and strength when given to MS patients who suffered from both visual symptoms and heightened sensitivity to temperature. Possible side effects of these therapies include paresthesias (tingling sensations), dizziness, and seizures.

Therapies targeting an antigen: Trials of a synthetic form of myelin basic protein, called copolymer I (Copaxone), were successful, leading the FDA to approve the agent for the treatment of relapsing-remitting MS. Copolymer I, unlike so many drugs tested for the treatment of MS, has few side effects, and studies indicate that the agent can reduce the relapse rate by almost one third. In addition, patients given copolymer I are more likely to show neurologic improvement than those given a placebo.

Investigators are also looking at the possibility of developing an MS vaccine. Myelin-attacking T cells were removed, inactivated, and injected back into animals with experimental allergic encephalomyelitis (EAE). This procedure results in destruction of the immune system cells that were attacking myelin basic protein. In a couple of small trials scientists have tested a similar vaccine in humans. The product was well-tolerated and had no side effects, but the studies were too small to establish efficacy. Patients with progressive forms of MS did not appear to benefit, although relapsing-remitting patients showed some neurologic improvement and had fewer relapses and reduced numbers of lesions in one study. Unfortunately, the benefits did not last beyond 2 years.

A similar approach, known as peptide therapy, is based on evidence that the body can mount an immune response against the T cells that destroy myelin, but this response is not strong enough to overcome the disease. To induce this response, the investigator scans the myelin-attacking T cells for the myelin-recognizing receptors on the cells' surface. A fragment, or peptide, of those receptors is then injected into the body. The immune system "sees" the injected peptide as a foreign invader and launches an attack on any myelin-destroying T cells that carry the peptide. The injection of portions of T cell receptors may heighten the immune system reaction against the errant T cells much the same way a booster shot heightens immunity to tetanus. Or, peptide therapy may jam the errant cells' receptors, preventing the cells from attacking myelin.

Despite these promising early results, there are some major obstacles to developing vaccine and peptide therapies. Individual patients' T cells vary so much that it may not be possible to develop a standard vaccine or peptide therapy beneficial to all, or even most, MS patients. At this time, each treatment involves extracting cells from each individual patient, purifying the cells, and then growing them in culture before inactivating and chemically altering them. This makes the production of quantities sufficient for therapy extremely time consuming, labor intensive, and expensive. Further studies are necessary to determine whether universal inoculations can be developed to induce suppression of MS patients' overactive immune systems.

Protein antigen feeding is similar to peptide therapy, but is a potentially simpler means to the same end. Whenever we eat, the digestive system breaks each food or substance into its primary "non-antigenic" building blocks, thereby averting a potentially harmful immune attack. So, strange as it may seem, antigens that trigger an immune response when they are injected can encourage immune system tolerance when taken orally. Furthermore, this reaction is directed solely at the specific antigen being fed; wholesale immunosuppression, which can leave the body open to a variety of infections, does not occur. Studies have shown that when rodents with EAE are fed myelin protein antigens, they experience fewer relapses. Data from a small, preliminary trial of antigen feeding in humans found limited suggestion of improvement, but the results were not statistically significant. A multi-center trial is being conducted to determine whether protein antigen feeding is effective.

Cytokines: As our growing insight into the workings of the immune system gives us new knowledge about the function of cytokines,

239

the powerful chemicals produced by T cells, the possibility of using them to manipulate the immune system becomes more attractive. Scientists are studying a variety of substances that may block harmful cytokines, such as those involved in inflammation, or that encourage the production of protective cytokines.

A drug that has been tested as a depression treatment, rolipram, has been shown to reduce levels of several destructive cytokines in animal models of MS. Its potential as a therapy for MS is not known at this time, but side effects seem modest. Protein antigen feeding, discussed earlier, may release transforming growth factor beta (TGF), a protective cytokine that inhibits or regulates the activity of certain immune cells. Preliminary tests indicate that it may reduce the number of immune cells commonly found in MS patients' spinal fluid. Side effects include anemia and altered kidney function.

Interleukin 4 (IL-4) is able to diminish demyelination and improve the clinical course of mice with EAE, apparently by influencing developing T cells to become protective rather than harmful. This also appears to be true of a group of chemicals called retinoids. When fed to rodents with EAE, retinoids increase levels of TGF and IL-4, which encourage protective T cells, while decreasing numbers of harmful T cells. This results in improvement of the animals' clinical symptoms.

Remyelination: Some studies focus on strategies to reverse the damage to myelin and oligodendrocytes (the cells that make and maintain myelin in the central nervous system), both of which are destroyed during MS attacks. Scientists now know that oligodendrocytes may proliferate and form new myelin after an attack. Therefore, there is a great deal of interest in agents that may stimulate this reaction. To learn more about the process, investigators are looking at how drugs used in MS trials affect remyelination. Studies of animal models indicate that monoclonal antibodies and two immunosuppressant drugs, cyclophosphamide and azathioprine, may accelerate remyelination, while steroids may inhibit it. The ability of intravenous immunoglobulin (IVIg) to restore visual acuity and/or muscle strength is also being investigated.

Diet: Over the years, many people have tried to implicate diet as a cause of or treatment for MS. Some physicians have advocated a diet low in saturated fats; others have suggested increasing the patient's intake of linoleic acid, a polyunsaturated fat, via supplements of sunflower seed, safflower, or evening primrose oils. Other proposed dietary "remedies" include megavitamin therapy, including increased intake of vitamins B12 or C; various liquid diets; and sucrose-, tobacco-, or gluten-free diets. To date, clinical studies have not been able to confirm benefits from dietary changes; in the absence of any evidence that diet therapy is effective, patients are best advised to eat a balanced, wholesome diet.

Unproven therapies: MS is a disease with a natural tendency to remit spontaneously, and for which there is no universally effective treatment and no known cause. These factors open the door for an array of unsubstantiated claims of cures. At one time or another, many ineffective and even potentially dangerous therapies have been promoted as treatments for MS. A partial list of these "therapies" includes: injections of snake venom, electrical stimulation of the spinal cord's dorsal column, removal of the thymus gland, breathing pressurized (hyperbaric) oxygen in a special chamber, injections of beef heart and hog pancreas extracts, intravenous or oral calcium orotate (calcium EAP), hysterectomy, removal of dental fillings containing silver or mercury amalgams, and surgical implantation of pig brain into the patient's abdomen. None of these treatments is an effective therapy for MS or any of its symptoms.

Table 26.1. Drugs Used to Treat Symptoms of Multiple Sclerosis

Symptom	Drug
Spasticity	Baclofen (Lioresal)
	Tizanidine (Zanaflex)
	Diazepam (Valium)
	Clonazepam (Klonopin)
	Dantrolene (Dantrium)
Optic neuritis	Methylprednisolone (Solu-Medrol)
	Oral steroids
Fatigue	Antidepressants
	Amantadine (Symmetrel)
	Pemoline (Cylert)
Pain	Aspirin or acetaminophen
	Antidepressants
	Codeine
Trigeminal neuralgia	Carbamazepine, other anticonvulsant
Sexual dysfunction	Papaverine injections (in men)

Chapter 27

Myasthenia

Chapter Contents

Section 27.1

Myasthenia Gravis

From "Myasthenia Gravis Fact Sheet," from the National Institute
of Neurological Disorders and Stroke (NINDS, www.ninds.nih.gov),
part of the National Institutes of Health, April 9, 2008.

What is myasthenia gravis?

Myasthenia gravis is a chronic autoimmune neuromuscular disease characterized by varying degrees of weakness of the skeletal (voluntary) muscles of the body. The name myasthenia gravis, which is Latin and Greek in origin, literally means "grave muscle weakness." With current therapies, however, most cases of myasthenia gravis are not as "grave" as the name implies. In fact, for the majority of individuals with myasthenia gravis, life expectancy is not lessened by the disorder.

The hallmark of myasthenia gravis is muscle weakness that increases during periods of activity and improves after periods of rest. Certain muscles such as those that control eye and eyelid movement, facial expression, chewing, talking, and swallowing are often, but not always, involved in the disorder. The muscles that control breathing and neck and limb movements may also be affected.

What causes myasthenia gravis?

Myasthenia gravis is caused by a defect in the transmission of nerve impulses to muscles. It occurs when normal communication between the nerve and muscle is interrupted at the neuromuscular junction—the place where nerve cells connect with the muscles they control. Normally when impulses travel down the nerve, the nerve endings release a neurotransmitter substance called acetylcholine. Acetylcholine travels through the neuromuscular junction and binds to acetylcholine receptors which are activated and generate a muscle contraction.

In myasthenia gravis, antibodies block, alter, or destroy the receptors for acetylcholine at the neuromuscular junction which prevents the muscle contraction from occurring. Individuals with seronegative myasthenia gravis have no antibodies at all to receptors for acetylcholine and muscle-specific kinase, which is involved in cell signaling and the formation of the neuromuscular junction. These antibodies are produced by the body's own immune system. Thus, myasthenia gravis is an autoimmune disease because the immune system—which normally protects the body from foreign organisms—mistakenly attacks itself.

What is the role of the thymus gland in myasthenia gravis?

The thymus gland, which lies in the upper chest area beneath the breastbone, plays an important role in the development of the immune system in early life. Its cells form a part of the body's normal immune system. The gland is somewhat large in infants, grows gradually until puberty, and then gets smaller and is replaced by fat with age. In adults with myasthenia gravis, the thymus gland is abnormal. It contains certain clusters of immune cells indicative of lymphoid hyperplasia—a condition usually found only in the spleen and lymph nodes during an active immune response. Some individuals with myasthenia gravis develop thymomas or tumors of the thymus gland. Generally thymomas are benign, but they can become malignant.

The relationship between the thymus gland and myasthenia gravis is not yet fully understood. Scientists believe the thymus gland may give incorrect instructions to developing immune cells, ultimately resulting in autoimmunity and the production of the acetylcholine receptor antibodies, thereby setting the stage for the attack on neuromuscular transmission.

What are the symptoms of myasthenia gravis?

Although myasthenia gravis may affect any voluntary muscle, muscles that control eye and eyelid movement, facial expression, and swallowing are most frequently affected. The onset of the disorder may be sudden. Symptoms often are not immediately recognized as myasthenia gravis.

In most cases, the first noticeable symptom is weakness of the eye muscles. In others, difficulty in swallowing and slurred speech may be the first signs. The degree of muscle weakness involved in myasthenia gravis varies greatly among patients, ranging from a localized form, limited to eye muscles (ocular myasthenia), to a severe or generalized form in which many muscles—sometimes including those that control breathing—are affected. Symptoms, which vary in type and severity, may include a drooping of one or both eyelids (ptosis), blurred or double vision (diplopia) due to weakness of the muscles that control eye movements, unstable or waddling gait, weakness in arms, hands, fingers, legs, and neck, a change in facial expression, difficulty in swallowing and shortness of breath, and impaired speech (dysarthria).

Who gets myasthenia gravis?

Myasthenia gravis occurs in all ethnic groups and both genders. It most commonly affects young adult women (under 40) and older men (over 60), but it can occur at any age.

In neonatal myasthenia, the fetus may acquire immune proteins (antibodies) from a mother affected with myasthenia gravis. Generally, cases of neonatal myasthenia gravis are transient (temporary) and the child's symptoms usually disappear within 2-3 months after birth. Other children develop myasthenia gravis indistinguishable from adults. Myasthenia gravis in juveniles is common.

Myasthenia gravis is not directly inherited nor is it contagious. Occasionally, the disease may occur in more than one member of the same family.

Rarely, children may show signs of congenital myasthenia or congenital myasthenic syndrome. These are not autoimmune disorders, but are caused by defective genes that produce proteins in the acetylcholine receptor or in acetylcholinesterase.

How is myasthenia gravis diagnosed?

Unfortunately, a delay in diagnosis of one or two years is not unusual in cases of myasthenia gravis. Because weakness is a common symptom of many other disorders, the diagnosis is often missed in people who experience mild weakness or in those individuals whose weakness is restricted to only a few muscles.

The first steps of diagnosing myasthenia gravis include a review of the individual's medical history, and physical and neurological examinations. The signs a physician must look for are impairment of eye movements or muscle weakness without any changes in the individual's ability to feel things. If the doctor suspects myasthenia gravis, several tests are available to confirm the diagnosis.

A special blood test can detect the presence of immune molecules or acetylcholine receptor antibodies. Most patients with myasthenia gravis have abnormally elevated levels of these antibodies. However, antibodies may not be detected in patients with only ocular forms of the disease.

Another test is called the edrophonium test. This approach requires the intravenous administration of edrophonium chloride or Tensilon®, a drug that blocks the degradation (breakdown) of acetylcholine and temporarily increases the levels of acetylcholine at the neuromuscular junction. In people with myasthenia gravis involving the eye muscles, edrophonium chloride will briefly relieve weakness. Other methods to confirm the diagnosis include a version of nerve conduction study which tests for specific muscle "fatigue" by repetitive nerve stimulation. This test records weakening muscle responses when the nerves are repetitively stimulated. Repetitive stimulation of a nerve during a nerve conduction study may demonstrate decrements of the muscle action potential due to impaired nerve-to-muscle transmission.

A different test called single fiber electromyography (EMG), in which single muscle fibers are stimulated by electrical impulses, can also detect impaired nerve-to-muscle transmission. EMG measures the electrical potential of muscle cells. Muscle fibers in myasthenia gravis, as well as other neuromuscular disorders, do not respond as well to repeated electrical stimulation compared to muscles from normal individuals. Computed tomography (CT) may be used to identify an abnormal thymus gland or the presence of a thymoma.

A special examination called pulmonary function testing—which measures breathing strength—helps to predict whether respiration may fail and lead to a myasthenic crisis.

How is myasthenia gravis treated?

Today, myasthenia gravis can be controlled. There are several therapies available to help reduce and improve muscle weakness. Medications used to treat the disorder include anticholinesterase agents such as neostigmine and pyridostigmine, which help improve neuromuscular transmission and increase muscle strength. Immunosuppressive drugs such as prednisone, cyclosporine, and azathioprine may also be used. These medications improve muscle strength by suppressing the production of abnormal antibodies. They must be used with careful medical follow up because they may cause major side effects.

Thymectomy, the surgical removal of the thymus gland (which often is abnormal in myasthenia gravis patients), reduces symptoms in more than 70 percent of patients without thymoma and may cure some individuals, possibly by rebalancing the immune system. Other therapies used to treat myasthenia gravis include plasmapheresis, a procedure in which abnormal antibodies are removed from the blood, and high-dose intravenous immune globulin, which temporarily modifies the immune system and provides the body with normal antibodies from donated blood. These therapies may be used to help individuals during especially difficult periods of weakness. A neurologist will determine which treatment option is best for each individual depending on the severity of the weakness, which muscles are affected, and the individual's age and other associated medical problems.

What are myasthenic crises?

A myasthenic crisis occurs when the muscles that control breathing weaken to the point that ventilation is inadequate, creating a medical emergency and requiring a respirator for assisted ventilation. In patients whose respiratory muscles are weak, crises—which generally call for immediate medical attention—may be triggered by infection, fever, or an adverse reaction to medication.

What is the prognosis?

With treatment, the outlook for most patients with myasthenia gravis is bright: they will have significant improvement of their muscle weakness and they can expect to lead normal or nearly normal lives. Some cases of myasthenia gravis may go into remission temporarily and muscle weakness may disappear completely so that medications can be discontinued. Stable, long-lasting complete remissions are the goal of thymectomy. In a few cases, the severe weakness of myasthenia gravis may cause a crisis (respiratory failure), which requires immediate emergency medical care.

What research is being done?

Within the federal government, the National Institute of Neurological Disorders and Stroke (NINDS), one of the federal government's National Institutes of Health (NIH), has primary responsibility for conducting and supporting research on myasthenia gravis.

Much has been learned about myasthenia gravis in recent years. Technological advances have led to more timely and accurate diagnosis, and new and enhanced therapies have improved management of the disorder. Much knowledge has been gained about the structure and function of the neuromuscular junction, the fundamental aspects of the thymus gland and of autoimmunity, and the disorder itself.

Despite these advances, however, there is still much to learn. The ultimate goal of myasthenia gravis research is to increase scientific understanding of the disorder. Researchers are seeking to learn what causes the autoimmune response in myasthenia gravis, and to better define the relationship between the thymus gland and myasthenia gravis.

Today's myasthenia gravis research includes a broad spectrum of studies conducted and supported by NINDS. NINDS scientists are evaluating new and improving current treatments for the disorder. One such study is testing the efficacy of intravenous immune globulin in patients with myasthenia gravis. The goal of the study is to determine whether this treatment safely improves muscle strength. Another study seeks further understanding of the molecular basis of synaptic transmission in the nervous system. The objective of this study is to expand current knowledge of the function of receptors and to apply this knowledge to the treatment of myasthenia gravis.

Section 27.2

Congenital Myasthenia

What is congenital myasthenia?

Congenital myasthenia is the term used for a group of uncommon hereditary disorders of the neuromuscular junction. Patients with congenital myasthenia tend to have lifelong or relatively stable symptoms of generalized fatigable weakness. These disorders are non-immunologic in nature and patients do not have acetylcholine receptor antibodies; therefore, patients do not typically respond to immune therapy often used in patients with autoimmune myasthenia gravis (steroids, thymectomy, plasma exchange). Most patients with congenital myasthenia develop symptoms in infancy or childhood with variable degrees of fluctuating weakness.

Are there different types of congenital myasthenia?

Yes. Not all forms of congenital myasthenia are the same. A number of different types of congenital myasthenia have been identified with a variety of different structural and functional abnormalities of the neuromuscular junction. Patterns of inheritance, clinical symptoms, electrophysiology, and response to therapy vary depending on the type. Some of the subtypes that one may encounter include familial infantile myasthenia, a congenital absence of acetylcholinesterase presenting in infancy or childhood with generalized weakness and reduced muscle tone; the slow channel syndrome, which often follows an autosomal dominant pattern of inheritance with a variable age of onset and severity of symptoms; and a collection of disorders characterized by defective acetylcholine receptors.

Is there any reason to try to determine the exact type of congenital myasthenia?

A thorough diagnostic evaluation is worthwhile in patients with suspected congenital myasthenia because of the different types, and somewhat different treatment options. Patients with some subtypes may respond best to Mestinon® (pyridostigmine), while patients with other subtypes may respond best to other therapies (some types respond to ephedrine, some to 3, 4 DAP, as well as a variety of other drugs depending on the type of congenital myasthenia).

In general, what is the long-term prognosis for patients with congenital myasthenia?

Most patients remain fairly stable throughout their lifetime and tend not to have wide fluctuations of symptoms or function nor myasthenic crises. Overall, patients tend to stay about the same on a long-term basis.

What is the difference between congenital myasthenia and transient neonatal myasthenia?

Transient neonatal myasthenia occurs in 10–15% of babies born to mothers with autoimmune myasthenia gravis. Within the first few days after delivery, the infant has a weak cry or suck, appears generally weak, and, on occasion, requires mechanical ventilation. Maternal antibodies that cross the placenta late in pregnancy cause the condition. As these maternal antibodies are replaced by the infant's own antibodies, the symptoms gradually disappear, usually within a few weeks, and the baby is normal thereafter. Infants with severe weakness from transient neonatal myasthenia may be treated with oral pyridostigmine and whatever degree of general support (mechanical respiratory ventilation, for example) is necessary until the condition clears. Infants with transient neonatal myasthenia gravis do not have an increased risk for the long-term or future development of myasthenia gravis.

Should patients with congenital myasthenia avoid the same medications that may aggravate autoimmune myasthenia gravis?

Yes. It is advisable to be cautious when starting newly prescribed or even some over-the-counter medications. Patients should check with their myasthenia physician prior to taking any new medications.

Chapter 28

Myoclonus

What is myoclonus?

Myoclonus describes a symptom and generally is not a diagnosis of a disease. It refers to sudden, involuntary jerking of a muscle or group of muscles. Myoclonic twitches or jerks usually are caused by sudden muscle contractions, called positive myoclonus, or by muscle relaxation, called negative myoclonus. Myoclonic jerks may occur alone or in sequence, in a pattern or without pattern. They may occur infrequently or many times each minute. Myoclonus sometimes occurs in response to an external event or when a person attempts to make a movement. The twitching cannot be controlled by the person experiencing it.

In its simplest form, myoclonus consists of a muscle twitch followed by relaxation. A hiccup is an example of this type of myoclonus. Other familiar examples of myoclonus are the jerks or "sleep starts" that some people experience while drifting off to sleep. These simple forms of myoclonus occur in normal, healthy persons and cause no difficulties. When more widespread, myoclonus may involve persistent, shock-like contractions in a group of muscles. In some cases, myoclonus begins in one region of the body and spreads to muscles in other areas. More severe cases of myoclonus can distort movement and severely limit a

Excerpted from "Myoclonus Fact Sheet," from the National Institute of Neurological Disorders and Stroke (NINDS, www.ninds.nih.gov), part of the National Institutes of Health, December 11, 2007.

person's ability to eat, talk, or walk. These types of myoclonus may indicate an underlying disorder in the brain or nerves.

What are the types of myoclonus?

Classifying the many different forms of myoclonus is difficult because the causes, effects, and responses to therapy vary widely. Listed below are the types most commonly described.

- **Action myoclonus** is characterized by muscular jerking triggered or intensified by voluntary movement or even the intention to move. It may be made worse by attempts at precise, coordinated movements. Action myoclonus is the most disabling form of myoclonus and can affect the arms, legs, face, and even the voice. This type of myoclonus often is caused by brain damage that results from a lack of oxygen and blood flow to the brain when breathing or heartbeat is temporarily stopped.

- **Cortical reflex myoclonus** is thought to be a type of epilepsy that originates in the cerebral cortex—the outer layer, or "gray matter," of the brain, responsible for much of the information processing that takes place in the brain. In this type of myoclonus, jerks usually involve only a few muscles in one part of the body, but jerks involving many muscles also may occur. Cortical reflex myoclonus can be intensified when patients attempt to move in a certain way or perceive a particular sensation.

- **Essential myoclonus** occurs in the absence of epilepsy or other apparent abnormalities in the brain or nerves. It can occur randomly in people with no family history, but it also can appear among members of the same family, indicating that it sometimes may be an inherited disorder. Essential myoclonus tends to be stable without increasing in severity over time. Some scientists speculate that some forms of essential myoclonus may be a type of epilepsy with no known cause.

- **Palatal myoclonus** is a regular, rhythmic contraction of one or both sides of the rear of the roof of the mouth, called the soft palate. These contractions may be accompanied by myoclonus in other muscles, including those in the face, tongue, throat, and diaphragm. The contractions are very rapid, occurring as often as 150 times a minute, and may persist during sleep. The condition usually appears in adults and can last indefinitely. People with palatal myoclonus usually regard it as a minor problem, although some occasionally complain of a "clicking" sound in the ear, a noise made as the muscles in the soft palate contract.

- **Progressive myoclonus epilepsy (PME)** is a group of diseases characterized by myoclonus, epileptic seizures, and other serious symptoms such as trouble walking or speaking. These rare disorders often get worse over time and sometimes are fatal. Studies have identified at least three forms of PME. Lafora body disease is inherited as an autosomal recessive disorder, meaning that the disease occurs only when a child inherits two copies of a defective gene, one from each parent. Lafora body disease is characterized by myoclonus, epileptic seizures, and dementia (progressive loss of memory and other intellectual functions). A second group of PME diseases belonging to the class of cerebral storage diseases usually involves myoclonus, visual problems, dementia, and dystonia (sustained muscle contractions that cause twisting movements or abnormal postures). Another group of PME disorders in the class of system degenerations often is accompanied by action myoclonus, seizures, and problems with balance and walking. Many of these PME diseases begin in childhood or adolescence.

- **Reticular reflex myoclonus** is thought to be a type of generalized epilepsy that originates in the brainstem, the part of the brain that connects to the spinal cord and controls vital functions such as breathing and heartbeat. Myoclonic jerks usually affect the whole body, with muscles on both sides of the body affected simultaneously. In some people, myoclonic jerks occur in only a part of the body, such as the legs, with all the muscles in that part being involved in each jerk. Reticular reflex myoclonus can be triggered by either a voluntary movement or an external stimulus.

- **Stimulus-sensitive myoclonus** is triggered by a variety of external events, including noise, movement, and light. Surprise may increase the sensitivity of the patient.

- **Sleep myoclonus** occurs during the initial phases of sleep, especially at the moment of dropping off to sleep. Some forms appear to be stimulus-sensitive. Some persons with sleep myoclonus are rarely troubled by, or need treatment for, the condition. However, myoclonus may be a symptom in more complex and disturbing sleep disorders, such as restless legs syndrome, and may require treatment by a doctor.

How is myoclonus treated?

Treatment of myoclonus focuses on medications that may help reduce symptoms. The drug of first choice to treat myoclonus, especially certain types of action myoclonus, is clonazepam, a type of tranquilizer. Dosages of clonazepam usually are increased gradually until the patient improves or side effects become harmful. Drowsiness and loss of coordination are common side effects. The beneficial effects of clonazepam may diminish over time if the patient develops a tolerance for the drug.

Many of the drugs used for myoclonus, such as barbiturates, phenytoin, and primidone, are also used to treat epilepsy. Barbiturates slow down the central nervous system and cause tranquilizing or antiseizure effects. Phenytoin and primidone are effective antiepileptic drugs, although phenytoin can cause liver failure or have other harmful long-term effects in patients with PME. Sodium valproate is an alternative therapy for myoclonus and can be used either alone or in combination with clonazepam. Although clonazepam and/or sodium valproate are effective in the majority of patients with myoclonus, some people have adverse reactions to these drugs.

Some studies have shown that doses of 5-hydroxytryptophan (5-HTP), a building block of serotonin, leads to improvement in patients with some types of action myoclonus and PME. However, other studies indicate that 5-HTP therapy is not effective in all people with myoclonus, and, in fact, may worsen the condition in some patients. These differences in the effect of 5-HTP on patients with myoclonus have not yet been explained, but they may offer important clues to underlying abnormalities in serotonin receptors.

The complex origins of myoclonus may require the use of multiple drugs for effective treatment. Although some drugs have a limited effect when used individually, they may have a greater effect when used with drugs that act on different pathways or mechanisms in the brain. By combining several of these drugs, scientists hope to achieve greater control of myoclonic symptoms. Some drugs currently being studied in different combinations include clonazepam, sodium valproate, piracetam, and primidone. Hormonal therapy also may improve responses to antimyoclonic drugs in some people.

Chapter 29

Progressive Supranuclear Palsy (PSP)

It is unlikely that any of the approximately 4,500 people in the United States who have been diagnosed as having progressive supranuclear palsy had ever heard of that disease before. In fact, most of my patients with PSP report that their family doctors knew nothing about PSP until a neurologist made the diagnosis. Moreover, the neurologist probably thought the diagnosis was Parkinson's disease until several years into the illness. For every person with a diagnosis of PSP, there are three with PSP who could be diagnosed if their doctor suspected it and performed the appropriate examination. Recently, more and more has appeared in medical journals to help doctors remedy their unfamiliarity with PSP. This information was written to help patients and their families do the same.

Why has no one heard of PSP?

PSP is poorly known because it is rare—only about one percent as common as Parkinson's disease—and because even when it does occur, it is often misdiagnosed. This is gradually changing. As more doctors become familiar with PSP, it will be diagnosed more readily. No one even realized it existed until 1964, when several patients were first described at a national neurology research convention and the disease received its name. In retrospect, at least 12 cases of PSP had

"PSP: Some Answers," by Lawrence L. Golbe, M.D. Excerpted from *A Guide for People Living with PSP*, © 2007 Society for Progressive Supranuclear Palsy (www.psp.org). Reprinted with permission.

appeared in the medical literature since 1909, but because of its resemblance to Parkinson's disease, no one had recognized it as a distinct disease until the 1960s.

What are the common early symptoms of PSP?

The most common first symptom, occurring on average in the 60s, is loss of balance while walking. This may take the form of unexplained falls or of a stiffness and awkwardness in the walk that can resemble Parkinson's disease. Sometimes the falls are described by the person experiencing them as attacks of dizziness. This often prompts the doctor to suspect an inner ear problem or hardening of the arteries supplying the brain. Other common early symptoms are forgetfulness and changes in personality. The latter can take the form of a loss of interest in ordinary pleasurable activities or increased irritability and cantankerousness. These mental changes are misinterpreted as depression or even as senility. Less common early symptoms include trouble with eyesight, slurring of speech, and mild shaking of the hands. Difficulty driving a car, with several accidents or near misses, is common early in the course of PSP. The exact reason for this problem is not clear.

What happens next?

The term "progressive" was included in the name of the disease because, unfortunately, the early symptoms get worse, and new symptoms develop sooner or later. After 5 to 6 years, on average, the imbalance and stiffness worsen to make walking very difficult or impossible. If trouble with eyesight was not present early on, it eventually develops in almost all cases and can sometimes be as disabling as the movement difficulty. Difficulty with speech and swallowing are additional important features of PSP that occur eventually in most patients.

What does the name "supranuclear palsy" mean?

In general, a "palsy" is a weakness or paralysis of a part of the body. The term "supranuclear" refers to the nature of the eye problem in PSP. Although some patients with PSP describe their symptom as "blurring," the actual problem is an inability to aim the eyes properly because of weakness or paralysis (palsy) of the muscles that move the eyeballs. These muscles are controlled by nerve cells residing in clusters or "nuclei" near the base of the brain in the brainstem. Most other brain problems that affect eye movements originate in those nuclei, but in PSP, the problem lies in parts of the brain that control those eye-movement nuclei themselves. These "higher" control areas are what the prefix "supra" in "supranuclear" refers to. Sometimes, complicated disease names are avoided by the use of the name of the physician who discovered the disease. However, for PSP, there were three such physicians and the string of names—Steele, Richardson, and Olszewski—is even less convenient than the descriptive name. Steele-Richardson-Olszewski syndrome is rarely used these days as a synonym for PSP. Incidentally, although Drs. John Clifford Richardson and Jerzy Olszewski are deceased, Dr. John C. Steele, who was a neurology resident (i.e., a trainee) when he collaborated in the original description of PSP, still does neurological research and serves as Honorary Chairman of the Society for PSP.

Is the visual problem the most important part of PSP?

In most cases, the visual problem is at least as important as the walking difficulty, though it does not appear, on average, until 3 to 5 years after the walking problem. Because the main difficulty with the eyes is in aiming them properly, reading often becomes difficult. The patient finds it hard to shift down to the beginning of the next line automatically after reaching the end of the first line. This is very different from just needing reading glasses. An eye doctor unfamiliar with PSP may be baffled by the patient's complaint of being unable to read a newspaper despite normal ability to read the individual letters on an eye chart. Some patients have their mild cataracts extracted in a vain effort to relieve such a visual problem.

Another common visual problem is an inability to maintain eye contact during conversation. This can give the mistaken impression that the patient is senile, hostile, or uninterested. The same eye movement problem can create the symptom of "tunnel vision" and can interfere with driving a car.

The most common eye movement problem in PSP is an impaired ability to move the eyes up or down. This can interfere with eating or with descending a flight of stairs, among other things. This problem is not usually as vexing for the patient and family as the inability to maintain eye contact or to coordinate eye movements while reading, but is much easier for the doctor to detect. This reduction in vertical eye movement is usually the first clue to the doctor that the diagnosis is PSP. Other conditions, particularly Parkinson's disease and normal aging, can sometimes cause difficulty moving the eyes up. However, PSP is nearly unique in also causing problems moving the eyes down.

Yet another eye problem in PSP can be abnormal eyelid movement—either too much or too little. A few patients experience forceful involuntary closing of the eyes for a few seconds or minutes at a time, called blepharospasm. Others have difficulty opening the eyes, even though the lids seem to be relaxed, and will try to use the muscles of the forehead, or even the fingers, in an effort to open the eyelids (apraxia of lid opening). About 20 percent of patients with PSP eventually develop one of these problems. Others, on the contrary, have trouble closing the eyes and blink very little. While about 15 to 25 blinks per minute are normal, people with PSP blink, on average, only about three or four times per minute. This can allow the eyes to become irritated. They often react by producing extra tears, which, in itself, can become annoying.

What sort of speech problems occur?

The same general area of the brain that controls eye movement also controls movements of the mouth, tongue, and throat, and these movements also weaken in PSP. Speech becomes slurred in most patients after 3 or 4 years, on average, although it is the first symptom in a few patients. In Parkinson's disease, the speech problem is characterized by soft volume and rapid succession of words. In PSP, however, the speech may have an irregular, explosive quality (called spastic speech, a drunken quality (ataxic speech) or may have the features of speech in Parkinson's disease. Most commonly, there is a combination of at least two of these three features in the speech of PSP.

An erroneous impression of senility or dementia can be created by the PSP patient's combination of speech difficulty, slight forgetfulness, slow (albeit accurate) mental responses, personality change, apathy and poor eye contact during conversation. Dementia of a sort does occur in many people with PSP, however, and is discussed below.

What about the swallowing problems?

Swallowing tough foods or thin liquids can become difficult because of throat muscle weakness or incoordination. This tends to occur later than the walking, visual, and speech problems, but can become very troublesome if the patient tends to choke on food. Unlike the other difficulties in PSP, this one can sometimes pose a danger for the patient—the danger of food going down the wrong pipe into the breathing passages, termed aspiration. Usually, difficulty managing thin liquids precedes difficulty with solid food. This is because in PSP, the swallowing muscles have difficulty creating a watertight seal separating the path to the stomach from the path to the lungs. The same is true for the swallowing difficulty of many neurological diseases. For non-neurologic conditions such as stricture of the esophagus, however, the difficulties start with solid foods.

Repeated, minor, often unnoticed episodes of small amounts of food and drink dripping into the lungs can cause pneumonia. Often, it is not apparent to the physician or family that the PSP patient's pneumonia is in fact the result of subtle aspiration. But aspiration pneumonia is the most common cause of death in PSP.

Does PSP lead to dementia like that in Alzheimer's disease?

Although mental confusion in patients with PSP is more apparent than real, most patients do eventually develop some degree of mental impairment. Some are mislabeled as having Alzheimer's disease. This is not very different from the situation in Parkinson's disease. In PSP, the dementia, if it does occur, does not feature the memory problem that is so apparent in Alzheimer's disease. Rather, the dementia of PSP is characterized by slowed thought and difficulty synthesizing several different ideas into a new idea or plan. These mental functions are performed mostly by the front part of the brain (the frontal lobes). In Alzheimer's, on the other hand, the problem is mostly in the part of the brain just above the ears (the temporal lobes), where memory functions are concentrated.

Alzheimer's disease also includes either difficulty with language (such as trouble recalling correct names of common objects) or difficulty finding one's way around a previously familiar environment. Fortunately, these symptoms almost never occur in PSP. Nevertheless, the "frontal" problems of PSP can interfere to a major degree with the ability to function independently, and the patient's irritability in some cases can make it difficult for caregivers to help.

Slowing of thought can cause major problems for people with PSP by making it difficult to partake in conversation. A question may be answered with great accuracy and detail, but with a delay of several minutes. Probably the most important aspect of the dementia of PSP is apathy. People with PSP seem to lose interest in their surroundings, again creating the impression of loss of thinking ability and interfering with family interactions.

How is PSP different from Parkinson's disease?

Both PSP and Parkinson's disease cause stiffness, slowness, and clumsiness, a combination called parkinsonism. This is why early on, PSP may be difficult to distinguish from Parkinson's disease. However, shaking (tremor), while prominent in about two thirds of people with Parkinson's disease, occurs in only about one in 20 people with PSP. A more common type of tremor occurring in PSP is irregular, mild, and present only when the hand is in use, not at rest as in Parkinson's disease.

Patients with PSP usually stand up straight or occasionally even tilt the head backward and tend to fall backward, while those with Parkinson's usually are bent forward. The problems with vision, speech, and swallowing are much more common and severe in PSP than in Parkinson's. Parkinson's causes more difficulty using the hands and more stiffness in the limbs than does PSP. Finally, the medications that are so effective for Parkinson's disease are of much less benefit in PSP.

The mainstay of drugs for Parkinson's disease are those that enhance, replace, or mimic a brain chemical called dopamine. Parkinson's responds better to such drugs than does PSP because in PD, deficiency of dopamine is by far the most important abnormality, while in PSP, deficiencies of several other brain chemicals are at least as severe as the dopamine deficiency, and no good way exists to replace those. Also, in PSP, there is damage to the brain cells that receive the dopamine-encoded messages, while these remain intact in Parkinson's.

What about treatment with medication?

Several medications, all available only by prescription, can help PSP in some cases.

Sinemet: This is the brand name for a combination of levodopa and carbidopa. Levodopa is the component that helps the disease symptoms. Carbidopa simply helps prevent the nausea that levodopa alone can cause. When levodopa came along in the late 1960s, it was a revolutionary advance for Parkinson's but, unfortunately, it is of only modest benefit in PSP. It can help the slowness, stiffness, and balance problems of PSP to a degree, but usually not the mental, speech, visual, or swallowing difficulties. It usually loses its benefit after 2 or 3 years, but a few patients with PSP never fully lose their responsiveness to Sinemet.

Some patients with PSP require large dosages, up to 1,500 milligrams (mg) of levodopa as Sinemet per day to see an improvement, so the dosage should be pushed to at least that level, under the close supervision of a physician, unless a benefit or intolerable side effects occur sooner. The most common side effects of Sinemet in patients with PSP are confusion, hallucinations, and dizziness. These generally disappear after the drug is stopped. The most common side effect in patients with Parkinson's disease, involuntary writhing movements (chorea or dyskinesias) occur very rarely in PSP, even at high Sinemet dosages.

Patients with PSP should generally receive the standard Sinemet (or generic levodopa/ carbidopa) preparation rather than the controlled-release (Sinemet CR or generic levodopa/carbidopa ER) form. The CR form is absorbed from the intestine into the blood slowly and can be useful for people with Parkinson's disease who respond well to Sinemet but need to prolong the number of hours of benefit from each dose. In PSP, however, such response fluctuations almost never occur. Because Sinemet CR is sometimes absorbed very little or erratically, a poor CR response in a patient with PSP might be incorrectly blamed on the fact that the disease is usually unresponsive to the drug. Such a patient might actually respond to the standard form, which reaches the brain in a more predictable way.

A new formulation of levodopa-carbidopa is Parcopa, which dissolves under the tongue. For people with PSP who cannot swallow medication safely, this could be useful. Another approach for such patients is to crush a regular levodopa-carbidopa tablet into a food or beverage that is easily swallowed. Another new formulation of levodopa-carbidopa (called Stalevo) combines those two drugs with a third drug, entacapone, in the same tablet. The entacapone slows the rate at which dopamine is broken down. It is useful for patients with Parkinson's whose levodopa-carbidopa works well but only for a few hours per dose. This situation rarely, if ever, occurs in PSP.

Dopamine receptor agonists: There are four such drugs on the market—Parlodel (generic name, bromocriptine), Permax (pergolide), Mirapex (pramipexole) and Requip (ropinirole). These are helpful in most people with Parkinson's disease, but in PSP, they rarely give any benefit beyond that provided by carbidopa/levodopa. One careful trial of Mirapex showed no benefit at all in PSP. The main possible side effects of the dopamine receptor agonists are hallucinations and confusion, which can be more troublesome for PSP than for Parkinson's. They can also cause excessive involuntary movements, dizziness, and nausea.

Antidepressants: Another group of drugs that has been of some modest success in PSP are the antidepressant drugs. The anti-PSP benefit of these drugs is not related to their ability to relieve depression. The best antidepressant drug for the movement problems of PSP is probably Elavil (generic name, amitriptyline). It has been used against depression since the early 1960s. The dosage should start at 10 mg once daily, preferably at bedtime. It can be increased slowly and taken divided into at least two doses per day. Past 40 mg per day, the likelihood of side effects increases to an unacceptable level for most patients. Elavil is also a good sleep medication for some elderly people and may provide this benefit in PSP if taken at bedtime. One important side effect in some people is constipation. Others are dry mouth, confusion, and difficulty urinating (in men). Unfortunately, some patients with PSP find that their balance difficulty worsens on Elavil.

Symmetrel: This drug (generic name, amantadine) has been used for Parkinson's since the 1960s. Because it affects more than just the dopamine system, it can be effective in PSP even if Sinemet is not. It seems to help the gait disorder more than anything else. Its benefit generally lasts only a few months, however. Its principal potential side effects are dry mouth, constipation, confusion, and swelling of the ankles.

Experimental drugs: In the past 15 years, research trials have been completed with the drugs physostigmine, idazoxan, and methysergide. While each showed initial promise and prompted an optimistic article or two in a prestigious neurological journal, none has proven effective enough to justify use in patients. The most recent trial was of efaroxan, a drug similar to idazoxan, but it, too, proved ineffective. Cognex (tacrine), Aricept (donepezil), and Reminyl (galantamine) are drugs that enhance the activity of the brain chemical acetylcholine and are modestly useful against the dementia of Alzheimer's disease. But, they do not help the mental difficulties of PSP. A fourth anti-Alzheimer drug, Namenda (memantine), acts on a different brain chemical, glutamate. It works no better for PSP than the others and, in addition, can cause confusion and agitation in those patients.

Botox: A different sort of drug that can be useful for people whose PSP is complicated by blepharospasm is Botox or Myobloc (two types of botulinum toxin). This substance is produced by certain bacteria that can contaminate food. Its poisonous action occurs because it weakens muscles. A very diluted solution of the toxin can be carefully injected by a neurologist into the eyelid muscles as a temporary remedy for abnormal involuntary eyelid closure. Botox can also be used for involuntary turning or bending of the head that occurs in PSP, but injection of Botox into the neck muscles can sometimes cause slight weakness of the swallowing muscles, which are nearby. In PSP, where swallowing is already impaired in many patients, caution should be used when considering use of Botox in neck muscles.

Is tube feeding advisable for advanced patients?

An operation that may be advised for extreme cases of poor swallowing where choking is a definite risk is the placement of a tube through the skin of the abdomen into the stomach (gastrostomy or percutaneous endoscopic gastrostomy or PEG) for feeding purposes. PEG feeding may allow patients to regain lost weight, avoid hunger, and receive the nourishment they need to fight off other potential complications of PSP. A patient who is receiving the necessary nutrients and fluids is much happier and stronger overall and will probably find general movement, speech, and thinking easier.

PEG placement may be considered when any of the following occur: aspiration pneumonia; small amounts of aspiration with each swallow; significant weight loss from insufficient feeding; or when a meal requires so much time that the functioning of the household is disrupted.

The PEG tube can be inserted with the patient awake but sedated, often as an outpatient procedure. The tube is clamped shut and hidden under the clothes when not in use. The feeding can easily be managed at home by pureeing the family's regular food in a blender and injecting it into the tube with what looks like a basting syringe. The skin site where the tube enters requires only a little care that can easily be provided by a family member or even by the patient. If the need for tube feeding abates (as through a new medication, for example), normal oral feeding can be resumed and the tube can be kept as a backup or removed.

The potential downside of tube feedings for some patients is a loss of the feeling of "wholeness" or humanity. The issue of how much additional quality will be introduced into the patient's life is one that must be considered carefully. The family, physician, and if possible, the patient must all voice their opinions. Some patients who are in the advanced stages of PSP may feel that their quality of life is so poor that prolonging that life by having a PEG installed is not what they want.

It may be useful to note that some nursing homes will advise PEG placement because it reduces the personnel time needed to feed the patients and because third-party payers often will pay an additional fee for tube feeding, but not for the time-consuming task of hand feeding a patient by mouth.

Do any of the new brain operations for Parkinson's work for PSP?

Not so far, unfortunately. The operations for Parkinson's disease fall into two categories. One is based on the theory that the output of the basal ganglia (the group of nuclei that control movement) to the rest of the brain is overactive in Parkinson's. The operations dampen this overactivity. The main operations for this purpose are pallidotomy, which is rarely performed nowadays, and subthalamic nucleus stimulation, which is the most common Parkinson's operation at present. In PSP, the area of the basal ganglia from which the output comes is itself damaged, so its activity is already dampened down. The operations would only make things worse.

The other category of operation for Parkinson's attempts to replace the lost dopamine-producing brain cells. The reason this is unlikely to work for PSP is that while in Parkinson's, most of the movement problem is caused by loss of the main dopamine-producing nucleus, the substantia nigra, in PSP, the movement problems caused by loss of many other nuclei in addition. Many of those other nuclei receive their input from the substantia nigra, so replacing only the first "link in the chain" will not help much. It would be impractical to replace cells in all of the nuclei involved in PSP and would require too much trauma to the brain.

What about other non-drug treatment?

Probably the most important part of dealing with PSP is for the patient's family to understand that the problems with visual inattention and personality changes are part of the illness. The patient is not lacking willpower, nor "faking." Furthermore, many of the problems in PSP are intermittent and can be aggravated by the patient's mental or emotional state. For example, walking, writing and eating may be poor one hour and better the next. The family should understand that these fluctuations are not under the patient's conscious control and that nagging and shouting usually just make matters worse. A wise policy is to be prepared to take advantage of the "good" periods to have an outing, a relaxing shower, or some other activity that would be more difficult during the "bad" times.

Walking aids are often important for patients with PSP. Because of the tendency to fall backward, if a walker is required, it should be weighted in front with sandbags over the lower rung. A better but more expensive solution is a large, heavy walker resembling a small shopping cart with three or four fat, soft rubber wheels and a hand brake. The tendency to fall backward can also be countered by the use of built-up heels. Leg braces are not helpful because the problem in PSP is coordination and balance rather than actual muscle weakness.

Shoes with smooth soles are often better than rubber-soled athletic shoes. In many people with PSP, the gait disorder includes some element of freezing, a phenomenon that makes it difficult to lift a foot from the ground to initiate gait. Such people can fall if they move their body forward before the foot moves. In these cases, a smooth sole could make it easier to slide the first foot forward.

Hand rails installed in the home, especially in the bathroom, may also be helpful. The difficulty in looking down dictates that low objects such as throw rugs and low coffee tables, be removed from the patient's living space.

To remedy the difficulty of looking down, bifocals or special glasses called prisms are sometimes prescribed for people with PSP. These are sometimes worth trying, but are usually of limited value because there is not only a problem moving the eyes in PSP, but also a problem directing the person's attention (the "mind's eye") to objects located below the eyes. If this additional problem exists, special glasses would not help.

Formal physical therapy is of no proven benefit in PSP, but certain exercises done in the home by oneself on a regular schedule can keep the joints limber. Exercise also has a clear psychological benefit that improves the sense of well-being of anyone with a chronic illness. The special balance problems in PSP dictate caution in performing any exercises while standing. Many useful exercises can be performed seated in a chair or lying on a mat. Using a stationary bicycle is usually feasible as long as there is help in mounting and dismounting safely.

What is the cause of PSP?

The symptoms of PSP are caused by a gradual deterioration of brain cells in a few tiny but important places in the base of the brain. The most important such place, the substantia nigra is also affected

267

in Parkinson's disease and damage to it accounts for the symptoms that PSP and Parkinson's have in common. However, several important areas are affected in PSP that are normal in Parkinson's (and vice versa). Moreover, under the microscope, the appearance of the damaged brain cells in PSP is quite different from those in Parkinson's and resembles, rather, the degeneration in Alzheimer's disease. However, the location of the damaged cells is quite different in PSP and Alzheimer's. Furthermore, in PSP there are no amyloid plaques, deposits of waxy protein that are a hallmark of brain cells in Alzheimer's.

But what causes the brain cells to degenerate in the first place?

No one knows yet, but we have some clues. In the brain cells that are degenerating in PSP, there is an abnormal accumulation of a normal protein called tau. These clumps of tau are called neurofibrillary tangles. The normal function of tau is to help support the internal "skeleton" of the brain cells whose long extensions make contact with other brain cells. We do not know whether the problem is that the tau is defective from the time of its manufacture or whether it becomes damaged later. We also do not know if the problem is that the brain cells are deprived of the normal function of tau or if tau aggregates into clumps that are themselves toxic.

A clue to what is going wrong with tau protein is that most tau in the neurofibrillary tangles of PSP are of one type called "four-repeat" tau. In the normal brain cells, there are equal amounts of four-repeat and three-repeat tau. The "repeat" number refers to the number of copies of the part of the protein that binds it to another component of the cell's internal skeleton, the microtubules. So in PSP, the problem may be that too much four-repeat tau is made, or that too little three-repeat tau is made, the result being clumps of four-repeat tau.

Is PSP genetic?

PSP very rarely runs in families. Fewer than one in 100 people with PSP knows of even one other family member with PSP. However, a variant in the gene on chromosome 17 that encodes the tau protein is more common in PSP than in the rest of the population. The variant is called the H1 haplotype. About 95% of people with PSP have this variant on both of their copies of chromosome 17, while this is true for only about 60% of the rest of us. Clearly, the H1 haplotype is (nearly) necessary, but far from sufficient to cause the disease. There is evidence that this variant is directing the brain cells to produce too much tau protein. The theory is that the excess tau forms neurofibrillary tangles and that these, or an early, embryonic form of them, damages the cells.

One very large family where PSP is present in multiple members has a variant in a gene other than the tau gene. The specific gene has not yet been identified. Similarly, two other genetic variant that are ordinarily associated with hereditary Parkinson's disease—the parkin gene (PARK2) and the dardarin gene (PARK8) can in some cases, cause changes in the brain very similar to what happens in PSP. This means that there may be many different genetic contributors to PSP with no single one laying claim to the title of "the PSP gene." It also means that PSP, Parkinson's, and perhaps other neurodegenerative disorders may share come causative factors.

Chapter 30

Rett Syndrome

What is Rett syndrome?

Rett syndrome is a childhood neurodevelopmental disorder characterized by normal early development followed by loss of purposeful use of the hands, distinctive hand movements, slowed brain and head growth, gait abnormalities, seizures, and mental retardation. It affects females almost exclusively.

The disorder was identified by Dr. Andreas Rett, an Austrian physician who first described it in a journal article in 1966. It was not until after a second article about the disorder was published in 1983 that the disorder was generally recognized.

The course of Rett syndrome, including the age of onset and the severity of symptoms, varies from child to child. Before the symptoms begin, however, the child appears to grow and develop normally. Then, gradually, mental and physical symptoms appear. Hypotonia (loss of muscle tone) is usually the first symptom. As the syndrome progresses, the child loses purposeful use of her hands and the ability to speak. Other early symptoms may include problems crawling or walking and diminished eye contact. The loss of functional use of the hands is followed by compulsive hand movements such as wringing and washing. The onset of this period of regression is sometimes sudden.

"Rett Syndrome Fact Sheet," is from the National Institute of Neurological Disorders and Stroke (NINDS, www.ninds.nih.gov), part of the National Institutes of Health, February 7, 2008.

271

Another symptom, apraxia—the inability to perform motor functions—is perhaps the most severely disabling feature of Rett syndrome, interfering with every body movement, including eye gaze and speech.

Individuals with Rett syndrome often exhibit autistic-like behaviors in the early stages. Other symptoms may include toe walking; sleep problems; wide-based gait; teeth grinding and difficulty chewing; slowed growth; seizures; cognitive disabilities; and breathing difficulties while awake such as hyperventilation, apnea (breath holding), and air swallowing.

What causes Rett syndrome?

Rett syndrome is caused by mutations (structural alterations or defects) in the MECP2 gene, which is found on the X chromosome. Scientists identified the gene—which is believed to control the functions of several other genes—in 1999. The MECP2 gene contains instructions for the synthesis of a protein called methyl cytosine binding protein 2 (MeCP2), which acts as one of the many biochemical switches that tell other genes when to turn off and stop producing their own unique proteins. Because the MECP2 gene does not function properly in those with Rett syndrome, insufficient amounts or structurally abnormal forms of the protein are formed. The absence or malfunction of the protein is thought to cause other genes to be abnormally expressed, but this hypothesis has not yet been confirmed.

Seventy to 80 percent of girls given a diagnosis of Rett syndrome have the MECP2 genetic mutation detected by current diagnostic techniques. Scientists believe the remaining 20 to 30 percent of cases may be caused by partial gene deletions, by mutations in other parts of the gene, or by genes that have not yet been identified; thus, they continue to search for other mutations.

Is Rett syndrome inherited?

Although Rett syndrome is a genetic disorder—resulting from a faulty gene or genes—less than 1 percent of recorded cases are inherited or passed from one generation to the next. Most cases are sporadic, which means the mutation occurs randomly, mostly during spermatogenesis, and is not inherited.

Who gets Rett syndrome?

Rett syndrome affects one in every 10,000 to 15,000 live female births. It occurs in all racial and ethnic groups worldwide. Prenatal testing is available for families with an affected daughter who has an identified MECP2 mutation. Since the disorder occurs spontaneously in most affected individuals, however, the risk of a family having a second child with the disorder is less than 1 percent.

Genetic testing is also available for sisters of girls with Rett syndrome and an identified MECP2 mutation to determine if they are asymptomatic carriers of the disorder, which is an extremely rare possibility.

Girls have two X chromosomes, but only one is active in any given cell. This means that in a child with Rett syndrome only about half the cells in the nervous system will use the defective gene. Some of the child's brain cells use the healthy gene and express normal amounts of the proteins.

The story is different for boys who have an MECP2 mutation known to cause Rett syndrome in girls. Because boys have only one X chromosome they lack a back-up copy that could compensate for the defective one, and they have no protection from the harmful effects of the disorder. Boys with such a defect die shortly after birth.

Different types of mutations in the MECP2 gene can cause mental retardation in boys.

Is treatment available?

There is no cure for Rett syndrome. Treatment for the disorder is symptomatic—focusing on the management of symptoms—and supportive, requiring a multidisciplinary approach. Medication may be needed for breathing irregularities and motor difficulties, and antiepileptic drugs may be used to control seizures. There should be regular monitoring for scoliosis and possible heart abnormalities. Occupational therapy (in which therapists help children develop skills needed for performing self-directed activities—occupations—such as dressing, feeding, and practicing arts and crafts), physiotherapy, and hydrotherapy may prolong mobility. Some children may require special equipment and aids such as braces to arrest scoliosis, splints to modify hand movements, and nutritional programs to help them maintain adequate weight. Special academic, social, vocational, and support services may also be required in some cases.

What is the outlook for those with Rett syndrome?

Despite the difficulties with symptoms, most individuals with Rett syndrome continue to live well into middle age and beyond. Because the disorder is rare, very little is known about long-term prognosis and life expectancy. While it is estimated that there are many middle-aged women (in their 40s and 50s) with the disorder, not enough women have been studied to make reliable estimates about life expectancy beyond age 40.

Chapter 31

Spina Bifida

The human nervous system develops from a small, specialized plate of cells along the back of an embryo. Early in development, the edges of this plate begin to curl up toward each other, creating the neural tube—a narrow sheath that closes to form the brain and spinal cord of the embryo. As development progresses, the top of the tube becomes the brain and the remainder becomes the spinal cord. This process is usually complete by the 28th day of pregnancy. But if problems occur during this process, the result can be brain disorders called neural tube defects, including spina bifida.

What is spina bifida?

Spina bifida, which literally means "cleft spine," is characterized by the incomplete development of the brain, spinal cord, and/or meninges (the protective covering around the brain and spinal cord). It is the most common neural tube defect in the United States—affecting 1,500 to 2,000 of the more than 4 million babies born in the country each year.

What are the different types of spina bifida?

There are four types of spina bifida: occulta, closed neural tube defects, meningocele, and myelomeningocele.

Excerpted from "Spina Bifida Fact Sheet," by the National Institute of Neurological Disorders and Stroke (NINDS, www.ninds.nih.gov), part of the National Institutes of Health, December 11, 2007.

275

Occulta is the mildest and most common form in which one or more vertebrae are malformed. The name "occulta," which means "hidden," indicates that the malformation, or opening in the spine, is covered by a layer of skin. This form of spina bifida rarely causes disability or symptoms.

Closed neural tube defects make up the second type of spina bifida. This form consists of a diverse group of spinal defects in which the spinal cord is marked by a malformation of fat, bone, or membranes. In some patients there are few or no symptoms; in others the malformation causes incomplete paralysis with urinary and bowel dysfunction.

In the third type, meningocele, the meninges protrude from the spinal opening, and the malformation may or may not be covered by a layer of skin. Some patients with meningocele may have few or no symptoms while others may experience symptoms similar to closed neural tube defects.

Myelomeningocele, the fourth form, is the most severe and occurs when the spinal cord is exposed through the opening in the spine, resulting in partial or complete paralysis of the parts of the body below the spinal opening. The paralysis may be so severe that the affected individual is unable to walk and may have urinary and bowel dysfunction.

What causes spina bifida?

The exact cause of spina bifida remains a mystery. No one knows what disrupts complete closure of the neural tube, causing a malformation to develop. Scientists suspect genetic, nutritional, and environmental factors play a role. Research studies indicate that insufficient intake of folic acid—a common B vitamin—in the mother's diet is a key factor in causing spina bifida and other neural tube defects. Prenatal vitamins that are prescribed for the pregnant mother typically contain folic acid as well as other vitamins.

What are the signs and symptoms of spina bifida?

The symptoms of spina bifida vary from person to person, depending on the type. Often, individuals with occulta have no outward signs of the disorder. Closed neural tube defects are often recognized early in life due to an abnormal tuft or clump of hair or a small dimple or birthmark on the skin at the site of the spinal malformation.

Meningocele and myelomeningocele generally involve a fluid-filled sac—visible on the back—protruding from the spinal cord. In meningocele, the sac may be covered by a thin layer of skin, whereas in most cases of myelomeningocele, there is no layer of skin covering the sac and a section of spinal cord tissue usually is exposed.

What are the complications of spina bifida?

Complications of spina bifida can range from minor physical problems to severe physical and mental disabilities. It is important to note, however, that most people with spina bifida are of normal intelligence. Severity is determined by the size and location of the malformation, whether or not skin covers it, whether or not spinal nerves protrude from it, and which spinal nerves are involved. Generally all nerves located below the malformation are affected. Therefore, the higher the malformation occurs on the back, the greater the amount of nerve damage and loss of muscle function and sensation.

In addition to loss of sensation and paralysis, another neurological complication associated with spina bifida is Chiari II malformation—a rare condition (but common in children with myelomeningocele) in which the brainstem and the cerebellum, or rear portion of the brain, protrude downward into the spinal canal or neck area. This condition can lead to compression of the spinal cord and cause a variety of symptoms including difficulties with feeding, swallowing, and breathing; choking; and arm stiffness.

Chiari II malformation may also result in a blockage of cerebrospinal fluid, causing a condition called hydrocephalus, which is an abnormal buildup of cerebrospinal fluid in the brain. Cerebrospinal fluid is a clear liquid that surrounds the brain and spinal cord. The buildup of fluid puts damaging pressure on the brain. Hydrocephalus is commonly treated by surgically implanting a shunt—a hollow tube—in the brain to drain the excess fluid into the abdomen.

Some newborns with myelomeningocele may develop meningitis, an infection in the meninges. Meningitis may cause brain injury and can be life-threatening.

Children with both myelomeningocele and hydrocephalus may have learning disabilities, including difficulty paying attention, problems with language and reading comprehension, and trouble learning math.

Additional problems such as latex allergies, skin problems, gastrointestinal conditions, and depression may occur as children with spina bifida get older.

How is spina bifida treated?

There is no cure for spina bifida. The nerve tissue that is damaged or lost cannot be repaired or replaced, nor can function be restored to the damaged nerves. Treatment depends on the type and severity of the disorder. Generally, children with the mild form need no treatment, although some may require surgery as they grow.

The key priorities for treating myelomeningocele are to prevent infection from developing through the exposed nerves and tissue of the defect on the spine, and to protect the exposed nerves and structures from additional trauma. Typically, a child born with spina bifida will have surgery to close the defect and prevent infection or further trauma within the first few days of life.

Doctors have recently begun performing fetal surgery for treatment of myelomeningocele. Fetal surgery—which is performed in utero (within the uterus)—involves opening the mother's abdomen and uterus and sewing shut the opening over the developing baby's spinal cord. Some doctors believe the earlier the defect is corrected, the better the outcome is for the baby. Although the procedure cannot restore lost neurological function, it may prevent additional loss from occurring. However, the surgery is considered experimental and there are risks to the fetus as well as to the mother.

The major risks to the fetus are those that might occur if the surgery stimulates premature delivery such as organ immaturity, brain hemorrhage, and death. Risks to the mother include infection, blood loss leading to the need for transfusion, gestational diabetes, and weight gain due to bed rest.

Still, the benefits of fetal surgery are promising, and include less exposure of the vulnerable spinal nerve tissue and bones to the intrauterine environment, in particular the amniotic fluid, which is considered toxic. As an added benefit, doctors have discovered that the procedure affects the way the brain develops in the uterus, allowing certain complications—such as Chiari II with associated hydrocephalus—to correct themselves, thus, reducing or, in some cases, eliminating the need for surgery to implant a shunt.

Many children with myelomeningocele develop a condition called progressive tethering, or tethered cord syndrome, in which their spinal cords become fastened to an immovable structure—such as overlying membranes and vertebrae—causing the spinal cord to become abnormally stretched and the vertebrae elongated with growth and movement. This condition can cause loss of muscle function to the legs, bowel, and bladder. Early surgery on the spinal cord may allow the child to regain a normal level of functioning and prevent further neurological deterioration.

Some children will need subsequent surgeries to manage problems with the feet, hips, or spine. Individuals with hydrocephalus generally will require additional surgeries to replace the shunt, which can be outgrown or become clogged.

Some individuals with spina bifida require assistive devices such as braces, crutches, or wheelchairs. The location of the malformation on the spine often indicates the type of assistive devices needed. Children with a defect high on the spine and more extensive paralysis will often require a wheelchair, while those with a defect lower on the spine may be able to use crutches, bladder catheterizations, leg braces, or walkers.

Treatment for paralysis and bladder and bowel problems typically begins soon after birth, and may include special exercises for the legs and feet to help prepare the child for walking with braces or crutches when he or she is older.

Can the disorder be prevented?

Folic acid, also called folate, is an important vitamin in the development of a healthy fetus. Although taking this vitamin cannot guarantee having a healthy baby, it can help. Recent studies have shown that by adding folic acid to their diets, women of childbearing age significantly reduce the risk of having a child with a neural tube defect, such as spina bifida. Therefore, it is recommended that all women of childbearing age consume 400 micrograms of folic acid daily. Foods high in folic acid include dark green vegetables, egg yolks, and some fruits. Many foods—such as some breakfast cereals, enriched breads, flours, pastas, rice, and other grain products—are now fortified with folic acid. A lot of multivitamins contain the recommended dosage of folic acid as well.

Women who have a child with spina bifida, have spina bifida themselves, or have already had a pregnancy affected by any neural tube defect are at greater risk of having a child with spina bifida or another neural tube defect. These women may require more folic acid before they become pregnant.

What is the prognosis?

Children with spina bifida can lead relatively active lives. Prognosis depends on the number and severity of abnormalities and associated complications. Most children with the disorder have normal intelligence and can walk, usually with assistive devices. If learning problems develop, early educational intervention is helpful.

Chapter 32

Spinal Cord Injury and Disease

What is a spinal cord injury?

Although the hard bones of the spinal column protect the soft tissues of the spinal cord, vertebrae can still be broken or dislocated in a variety of ways and cause traumatic injury to the spinal cord. Injuries can occur at any level of the spinal cord. The segment of the cord that is injured, and the severity of the injury, will determine which body functions are compromised or lost. Because the spinal cord acts as the main information pathway between the brain and the rest of the body, a spinal cord injury can have significant physiological consequences.

Catastrophic falls, being thrown from a horse or through a windshield, or any kind of physical trauma that crushes and compresses the vertebrae in the neck can cause irreversible damage at the cervical level of the spinal cord and below. Paralysis of most of the body including the arms and legs, called quadriplegia, is the likely result. Automobile accidents are often responsible for spinal cord damage in the middle back (the thoracic or lumbar area), which can cause paralysis of the lower trunk and lower extremities, called paraplegia.

Other kinds of injuries that directly penetrate the spinal cord, such as gunshot or knife wounds, can either completely or partially sever the spinal cord and create lifelong disabilities.

Excerpted from "Spinal Cord Injury: Hope through Research," by the National Institute of Neurological Disorders and Stroke (NINDS, www.ninds.nih.gov), part of the National Institutes of Health, May 7, 2008.

Most injuries to the spinal cord don't completely sever it. Instead, an injury is more likely to cause fractures and compression of the vertebrae, which then crush and destroy the axons, extensions of nerve cells that carry signals up and down the spinal cord between the brain and the rest of the body. An injury to the spinal cord can damage a few, many, or almost all of these axons. Some injuries will allow almost complete recovery. Others will result in complete paralysis.

Until World War II, a serious spinal cord injury usually meant certain death, or at best a lifetime confined to a wheelchair and an ongoing struggle to survive secondary complications such as breathing problems or blood clots. But today, improved emergency care for people with spinal cord injuries and aggressive treatment and rehabilitation can minimize damage to the nervous system and even restore limited abilities.

Advances in research are giving doctors and patients hope that all spinal cord injuries will eventually be repairable. With new surgical techniques and exciting developments in spinal nerve regeneration, the future for spinal cord injury survivors looks brighter every day.

This text has been written to explain what happens to the spinal cord when it is injured, the current treatments for spinal cord injury patients, and the most promising avenues of research currently under investigation.

What happens when the spinal cord is injured?

A spinal cord injury usually begins with a sudden, traumatic blow to the spine that fractures or dislocates vertebrae. The damage begins at the moment of injury when displaced bone fragments, disk material, or ligaments bruise or tear into spinal cord tissue. Axons are cut off or damaged beyond repair, and neural cell membranes are broken. Blood vessels may rupture and cause heavy bleeding in the central grey matter, which can spread to other areas of the spinal cord over the next few hours.

Within minutes, the spinal cord swells to fill the entire cavity of the spinal canal at the injury level. This swelling cuts off blood flow, which also cuts off oxygen to spinal cord tissue. Blood pressure drops, sometimes dramatically, as the body loses its ability to self-regulate. As blood pressure lowers even further, it interferes with the electrical activity of neurons and axons. All these changes can cause a condition known as spinal shock that can last from several hours to several days.

Although there is some controversy among neurologists about the extent and impact of spinal shock, and even its definition in terms of physiological characteristics, it appears to occur in approximately half the cases of spinal cord injury, and it is usually directly related to the size and severity of the injury. During spinal shock, even undamaged portions of the spinal cord become temporarily disabled and can't communicate normally with the brain. Complete paralysis may develop, with loss of reflexes and sensation in the limbs.

The crushing and tearing of axons is just the beginning of the devastation that occurs in the injured spinal cord and continues for days. The initial physical trauma sets off a cascade of biochemical and cellular events that kills neurons, strips axons of their myelin insulation, and triggers an inflammatory immune system response. Days or sometimes even weeks later, after this second wave of damage has passed, the area of destruction has increased—sometimes to several segments above and below the original injury—and so has the extent of disability.

Changes in blood flow cause ongoing damage: Changes in blood flow in and around the spinal cord begin at the injured area, spread out to adjacent, uninjured areas, and then set off problems throughout the body.

Immediately after the injury, there is a major reduction in blood flow to the site, which can last for as long as 24 hours and becomes progressively worse if untreated. Because of differences in tissue composition, the impact is greater on the interior grey matter of the spinal cord than on the outlying white matter.

Blood vessels in the grey matter also begin to leak, sometimes as early as 5 minutes after injury. Cells that line the still-intact blood vessels in the spinal cord begin to swell, for reasons that aren't yet clearly understood, and this continues to reduce blood flow to the injured area. The combination of leaking, swelling, and sluggish blood flow prevents the normal delivery of oxygen and nutrients to neurons, causing many of them to die.

The body continues to regulate blood pressure and heart rate during the first hour to hour-and-a-half after the injury, but as the reduction in the rate of blood flow becomes more widespread, self-regulation begins to turn off. Blood pressure and heart rate drop.

Excessive release of neurotransmitters kills nerve cells: After the injury, an excessive release of neurotransmitters (chemicals that allow neurons to signal each other) can cause additional damage by overexciting nerve cells.

Glutamate is an excitatory neurotransmitter, commonly used by nerve cells in the spinal cord to stimulate activity in neurons. But when spinal cells are injured, neurons flood the area with glutamate for reasons that are not yet well understood. Excessive glutamate triggers a destructive process called excitotoxicity, which disrupts normal processes and kills neurons and other cells called oligodendrocytes that surround and protect axons.

An invasion of immune system cells creates inflammation: Under normal conditions, the blood-brain barrier (which tightly controls the passage of cells and large molecules between the circulatory and central nervous systems) keeps immune system cells from entering the brain or spinal cord. But when the blood-brain barrier is broken by blood vessels bursting and leaking into spinal cord tissue, immune system cells that normally circulate in the blood—primarily white blood cells—can invade the surrounding tissue and trigger an inflammatory response. This inflammation is characterized by fluid accumulation and the influx of immune cells—neutrophils, T-cells, macrophages, and monocytes.

Neutrophils are the first to enter, within about 12 hours of injury, and they remain for about a day. Three days after the injury, T-cells arrive. Their function in the injured spinal cord is not clearly understood, but in the healthy spinal cord they kill infected cells and regulate the immune response. Macrophages and monocytes enter after the T-cells and scavenge cellular debris.

The up side of this immune system response is that it helps fight infection and cleans up debris. But the down side is that it sets off the release of cytokines—a group of immune system messenger molecules that exert a malign influence on the activities of nerve cells.

For example, microglial cells, which normally function as a kind of on-site immune cell in the spinal cord, begin to respond to signals from these cytokines. They transform into macrophage-like cells, engulf cell debris, and start to produce their own pro-inflammatory cytokines, which then stimulate and recruit other microglia to respond.

Injury also stimulates resting astrocytes to express cytokines. These "reactive" astrocytes may ultimately participate in the formation of scar tissue within the spinal cord.

Whether or not the immune response is protective or destructive is controversial among researchers. Some speculate that certain types of injury might evoke a protective immune response that actually reduces the loss of neurons.

Free radicals attack nerve cells: Another consequence of the immune system's entry into the CNS is that inflammation accelerates the production of highly reactive forms of oxygen molecules called free radicals.

Free radicals are produced as a by-product of normal cell metabolism. In the healthy spinal cord their numbers are small enough that they cause no harm. But injury to the spinal cord, and the subsequent wave of inflammation that sweeps through spinal cord tissue, signals particular cells to overproduce free radicals.

Free radicals then attack and disable molecules that are crucial for cell function—for example, those found in cell membranes—by modifying their chemical structure. Free radicals can also change how cells respond to natural growth and survival factors, and turn these protective factors into agents of destruction.

Nerve cells self-destruct: Researchers used to think that the only way in which cells died during spinal cord injury was as a direct result of trauma. But recent findings have revealed that cells in the injured spinal cord also die from a kind of programmed cell death called apoptosis, often described as cellular suicide, that happens days or weeks after the injury.

Apoptosis is a normal cellular event that occurs in a variety of tissues and cellular systems. It helps the body get rid of old and unhealthy cells by causing them to shrink and implode. Nearby scavenger cells then gobble up the debris. Apoptosis seems to be regulated by specific molecules that have the ability to either start or stop the process.

For reasons that are still unclear, spinal cord injury sets off apoptosis, which kills oligodendrocytes in damaged areas of the spinal cord days to weeks after the injury. The death of oligodendrocytes is another blow to the damaged spinal cord, since these are the cells that form the myelin that wraps around axons and speeds the conduction of nerve impulses. Apoptosis strips myelin from intact axons in adjacent ascending and descending pathways, which further impairs the spinal cord's ability to communicate with the brain.

Secondary damage takes a cumulative toll: All of these mechanisms of secondary damage—restricted blood flow, excitotoxicity, inflammation, free radical release, and apoptosis—increase the area of damage in the injured spinal cord. Damaged axons become dysfunctional, either because they are stripped of their myelin or because they are disconnected from the brain. Glial cells cluster to form a scar, which creates a barrier to any axons that could potentially regenerate and reconnect. A few whole axons may remain, but not enough to convey any meaningful information to the brain.

Researchers are especially interested in studying the mechanisms of this wave of secondary damage because finding ways to stop it could save axons and reduce disabilities. This could make a big difference in the potential for recovery.

What are the immediate treatments for spinal cord injury?

The outcome of any injury to the spinal cord depends upon the number of axons that survive: the higher the number of normally functioning axons, the less the amount of disability. Consequently, the most important consideration when moving people to a hospital or trauma center is preventing further injury to the spine and spinal cord.

Spinal cord injury isn't always obvious. Any injury that involves the head (especially with trauma to the front of the face), pelvic fractures, penetrating injuries in the area of the spine, or injuries that result from falling from heights should be suspect for spinal cord damage.

Until imaging of the spine is done at an emergency or trauma center, people who might have spinal cord injury should be cared for as if any significant movement of the spine could cause further damage. They are usually transported in a recumbent (lying down) position, with a rigid collar and backboard immobilizing the spine.

Respiratory complications are often an indication of the severity of spinal cord injury. About one third of those with injury to the neck area will need help with breathing and require respiratory support via intubation, which involves inserting a tube connected to an oxygen tank through the nose or throat and into the airway.

Methylprednisolone, a steroid drug, became standard treatment for acute spinal cord injury in 1990 when a large-scale clinical trial supported by the National Institute of Neurological Disorders and Stroke showed significantly better recovery in patients who were given the drug within the first 8 hours after their injury. Methylprednisolone appears to reduce the damage to nerve cells and decreases inflammation near the injury site by suppressing activities of immune cells.

Realignment of the spine using a rigid brace or axial traction is usually done as soon as possible to stabilize the spine and prevent additional damage.

On about the third day after the injury, doctors give patients a complete neurological examination to diagnose the severity of the injury and predict the likely extent of recovery. X-rays, MRIs, or more advanced imaging techniques are used to visualize the entire length of the spine.

Spinal cord injuries are classified as either complete or incomplete, depending on how much cord width is injured. An incomplete injury means that the ability of the spinal cord to convey messages to or from the brain is not completely lost. People with incomplete injuries retain some motor or sensory function below the injury.

A complete injury is indicated by a total lack of sensory and motor function below the level of injury.

How does rehabilitation help people recover from spinal cord injuries?

No two people will experience the same emotions after surviving a spinal cord injury, but almost everyone will feel frightened, anxious, or confused about what has happened. It's common for people to have very mixed feelings: relief that they are still alive, but disbelief at the nature of their disabilities.

Rehabilitation programs combine physical therapies with skill-building activities and counseling to provide social and emotional support. The education and active involvement of the newly injured person and his or her family and friends is crucial.

A rehabilitation team is usually led by a doctor specializing in physical medicine and rehabilitation (called a physiatrist), and often includes social workers, physical and occupational therapists, recreational therapists, rehabilitation nurses, rehabilitation psychologists, vocational counselors, nutritionists, and other specialists. A caseworker or program manager coordinates care.

In the initial phase of rehabilitation, therapists emphasize regaining leg and arm strength since mobility and communication are the two most important areas of function. For some, mobility will only be possible with the assistance of devices such as a walker, leg braces, or a wheelchair. Communication skills, such as writing, typing, and using the telephone, may also require adaptive devices.

Physical therapy includes exercise programs geared toward muscle strengthening. Occupational therapy helps redevelop fine motor skills. Bladder and bowel management programs teach basic toileting routines, and patients also learn techniques for self-grooming. People acquire coping strategies for recurring episodes of spasticity, autonomic dysreflexia, and neurogenic pain.

Vocational rehabilitation begins with an assessment of basic work skills, current dexterity, and physical and cognitive capabilities to determine the likelihood for employment. A vocational rehabilitation specialist then identifies potential work places, determines the type of assistive equipment that will be needed, and helps arrange for a user-friendly workplace. For those whose disabilities prevent them from returning to the workplace, therapists focus on encouraging productivity through participation in activities that provide a sense of satisfaction and self-esteem. This could include educational classes, hobbies, memberships in special interest groups, and participation in family and community events.

Recreation therapy encourages patients to build on their abilities so that they can participate in recreational or athletic activities at their level of mobility. Engaging in recreational outlets and athletics helps those with spinal cord injuries achieve a more balanced and normal lifestyle and also provides opportunities for socialization and self-expression.

Chapter 33

Spinal Muscular Atrophy

What is spinal muscular atrophy?

Spinal muscular atrophy (SMA) Types I, II, and III belong to a group of hereditary diseases that cause weakness and wasting of the voluntary muscles in the arms and legs of infants and children.

The disorders are caused by an abnormal or missing gene known as the survival motor neuron gene (SMN1), which is responsible for the production of a protein essential to motor neurons. Without this protein, lower motor neurons in the spinal cord degenerate and die.

The type of SMA (I, II, or III) is determined by the age of onset and the severity of symptoms. Type I has the earliest onset, usually at birth, and the most severe symptoms. Type II usually happens in early childhood and is less severe but still disabling. Type III can happen as late as adolescence and may be only moderately disabling.

There are other types of SMA disorders with similar symptoms, but different causes. Infantile SMA disorders, such as X-linked infantile SMA, SMA with cerebellar hypoplasia, diaphragmatic SMA, and SMA with congenital bone fractures are linked to genes other than SMN1. Kennedy syndrome (X-linked spinal and bulbar muscular atrophy, SMAX1), a disease of adult males, has symptoms similar to the childhood SMAs, but is caused by a different gene and genetic mutation.

Excerpted from "Spinal Muscular Atrophy Fact Sheet," by the National Institute of Neurological Disorders and Stroke (NINDS, www.ninds.nih.gov), part of the National Institutes of Health, July 9, 2008.

What are the symptoms of SMA in children?

SMA Type I, also known as Werdnig-Hoffman disease, or infantile-onset SMA, is evident at birth or within the first few months. Symptoms include floppy limbs and trunk, feeble movements of the arms and legs, swallowing difficulties, a weak sucking reflex, and impaired breathing. A baby with SMA Type I will not be able to sit without support. The majority of babies with SMA Type I die of respiratory failure within the first two years.

SMA Type II, also known as juvenile SMA, intermediate SMA, or chronic SMA, has an onset between 6 and 18 months. Legs tend to be more impaired than arms. The first indication that a baby may have the disease is when he or she fails to crawl or walk. Children with Type II are usually able to sit without support if placed in position. Some may be able to stand or walk with help. Although children with SMA II may not need artificial assistance to breathe, they are still at an increased risk for respiratory infections. These children often survive into adulthood, but with significant motor disability.

SMA Type III, also called Wolhlfart-Kugelberg-Welander disease, or mild SMA, can begin as early as the toddler years or as late as adolescence. Children can stand alone and walk, but may have difficulty getting up from a sitting position. Their fingers may tremble. Children with SMA Type III usually remain mobile well into adulthood. Like children with Type II, they are at an increased risk for respiratory infections.

How is SMA diagnosed in children?

A blood test is available that can indicate whether there are deletions or mutations of the SMN1 gene. This test identifies at least 95 percent of SMA Types I, II, and III. Other diagnostic tests may include electrodiagnosis with nerve conduction velocities (EMG), and muscle biopsy.

Are there treatments for SMA?

There is no cure for SMA. Treatment consists of managing the symptoms and preventing complications. Treatment for specific symptoms and common complications are described below.

Breathing issues: Babies with SMA (especially those with Type I) may need help breathing, especially at night, using non-invasive methods that include negative pressure ventilators and bi-level positive airway pressure support, which direct air through the nostrils via a small, gently fitted mask. Children who survive their first two years are at risk for complications involving the lungs, which may not be fully developed. A regular program of respiratory therapy and breathing exercises is helpful. Parents should be instructed in chest physiotherapy (CPT), a series of physical maneuvers that clear the lungs and airway.

Failure to thrive: Infants with SMA I may have difficulties getting adequate nutrition because they have a weak sucking reflex and tendency to tire easily. Their unprotected air passage makes it difficult for older babies to chew and swallow; they may inhale and choke on their food. Some babies may require feeding with nasogastric or gastric tubes.

Weak arms and legs: Children with SMA Types I and II are not likely to stand or walk on their own. They can be taught to operate a power wheelchair at two to three years of age. Less handicapped children may benefit from a standing frame, vertical stander, or standing wheelchair. Physical therapy and exercise may also help improve mobility and joint movement, brighten mood, and improve sleep patterns. Stretching exercises can preserve and increase flexibility.

Orthopedic complications: Scoliosis (curvature of the spine) occurs at some point in the majority of children with SMA Types I and II, and some with Type III. Custom seating systems, seating aids, and a body jacket can be used to prevent severe scoliosis. Spinal fusion surgery may be necessary for some children.

What is the prognosis?

The prognosis is poor for babies with SMA Type I. Most die within the first two years. For children with SMA Type II, the prognosis for life expectancy or for independent standing or walking roughly correlates with how old they are when they first begin to experience symptoms—older children tend to have less severe symptoms. Some children may have a normal life expectancy and learn to walk with the aid of a brace. Others may die from respiratory infections, such as pneumonia. Children with onset after 18 months are often able to walk and are fully functional for years before they need assistance. They may have a normal life expectancy.

Chapter 34

Other Types of Hypokinetic Movement Disorders

Chapter Contents

Section 34.1

Corticobasal Degeneration

From "Corticobasal Degeneration Information Page," by the National Institute of Neurological Disorders and Stroke (NINDS, www.ninds.nih .gov), part of the National Institutes of Health, April 25, 2008.

What is corticobasal degeneration?

Corticobasal degeneration is a progressive neurological disorder characterized by nerve cell loss and atrophy (shrinkage) of multiple areas of the brain including the cerebral cortex and the basal ganglia. Corticobasal degeneration progresses gradually. Initial symptoms, which typically begin at or around age 60, may first appear on one side of the body (unilateral), but eventually affect both sides as the disease progresses. Symptoms are similar to those found in Parkinson disease, such as poor coordination, akinesia (an absence of movements), rigidity (a resistance to imposed movement), disequilibrium (impaired balance); and limb dystonia (abnormal muscle postures). Other symptoms such as cognitive and visual-spatial impairments, apraxia (loss of the ability to make familiar, purposeful movements), hesitant and halting speech, myoclonus (muscular jerks), and dysphagia (difficulty swallowing) may also occur. An individual with corticobasal degeneration eventually becomes unable to walk.

Is there any treatment?

There is no treatment available to slow the course of corticobasal degeneration, and the symptoms of the disease are generally resistant to therapy. Drugs used to treat Parkinson disease-type symptoms do not produce any significant or sustained improvement. Clonazepam may help the myoclonus. Occupational, physical, and speech therapy can help in managing disability.

What is the prognosis?

Corticobasal degeneration usually progresses slowly over the course of 6 to 8 years. Death is generally caused by pneumonia or other complications of severe debility such as sepsis or pulmonary embolism.

Section 34.2

Multiple System Atrophy

From "Multiple System Atrophy Information Page," by the National Institute of Neurological Disorders and Stroke (NINDS, www.ninds.nih .gov), part of the National Institutes of Health, February 13, 2007.

What is multiple system atrophy?

Multiple system atrophy (MSA) is the current name for disorders once known individually as striatonigral degeneration, sporadic olivopontocerebellar atrophy, and the Shy-Drager syndrome. MSA is a progressive neurodegenerative disorder characterized by symptoms of autonomic nervous system failure (such as lightheadedness or fainting spells, constipation, erectile failure in men, and urinary retention) combined with tremor and rigidity, slurred speech, or loss of muscle coordination. MSA affects both men and women, primarily in their 50s. It can progress swiftly or slowly, but people with MSA generally survive for 9 years after the appearance of symptoms. There is no remission from the disease.

Is there any treatment?

There is no specific treatment for nerve degeneration in MSA. Levodopa, used to treat rigidity and tremor in Parkinson disease, may offer some help. However, striatonigral degeneration does not respond well to levodopa. Dopamine and anticholinergic drugs may be prescribed to treat spasms. Orthostatic hypotension may be treated with fludrocortisone and other drugs that raise blood pressure. Increased dietary fiber intake or use of laxatives may relieve constipation, and drugs or a penile implant may help with male impotence. A routine of stretching and exercise can help retain muscle strength and range of movement. An artificial feeding tube or breathing tube may be surgically inserted for management of swallowing and breathing difficulties.

What is the prognosis?

MSA is a progressive disorder and most patients have a life expectancy after diagnosis of about 10 years or less.

What research is being done?

The NINDS carries out and funds studies of basal ganglia and cerebellar degeneration and autonomic nerve system dysfunction, including multiple system atrophy. This research is aimed at obtaining a better understanding of these diseases and finding ways to treat, cure, and ultimately, prevent them.

Section 34.3

Postpolio Syndrome

From "Post-Polio Syndrome," by the National Institute of
Neurological Disorders and Stroke (NINDS, www.ninds.nih.gov),
part of the National Institutes of Health, April 9, 2008.

What is postpolio syndrome?

Postpolio syndrome (PPS) is a condition that affects polio survivors anywhere from 10 to 40 years after recovery from an initial paralytic attack of the poliomyelitis virus. PPS is characterized by a further weakening of muscles that were previously affected by the polio infection. Symptoms include fatigue, slowly progressive muscle weakness and, at times, muscular atrophy. Joint pain and increasing skeletal deformities such as scoliosis are common. Some patients experience only minor symptoms, while others develop spinal muscular atrophy, and very rarely, what appears to be, but is not, a form of amyotrophic lateral sclerosis (ALS), also called Lou Gehrig disease. PPS is rarely life-threatening.

Is there any treatment?

Presently, no prevention has been found. Doctors recommend that polio survivors follow standard healthy lifestyle practices: consuming a well-balanced diet, exercising in moderation, and visiting a doctor regularly. There has been much debate about whether to encourage or discourage exercise for polio survivors or individuals who already have PPS. A commonsense approach, in which people use individual tolerance as their limit, is currently recommended.

What is the prognosis?

PPS is a very slowly progressing condition marked by long periods of stability. The severity of PPS depends on the degree of the residual weakness and disability an individual has after the original polio attack. People who had only minimal symptoms from the original attack and subsequently develop PPS will most likely experience only mild PPS symptoms. People originally hit hard by the polio virus, who were left with severe residual weakness, may develop a more severe case of PPS with a greater loss of muscle function, difficulty in swallowing, and more periods of fatigue.

Section 34.4

Stiff Person Syndrome

From "Stiff Person Syndrome Information Page," is from the National Institute of Neurological Disorders and Stroke (NINDS, www.ninds.nih .gov), part of the National Institutes of Health, February 14, 2007.

What is stiff person syndrome?

Stiff person syndrome (SPS) is a rare neurological disorder with features of an autoimmune disease. SPS is characterized by fluctuating muscle rigidity in the trunk and limbs and a heightened sensitivity to stimuli such as noise, touch, and emotional distress, which can set off muscle spasms. Abnormal postures, often hunched over and stiffened, are characteristic of the disorder. People with SPS can be too disabled to walk or move, or they are afraid to leave the house because street noises, such as the sound of a horn, can trigger spasms and falls. SPS affects twice as many women as men. It is frequently associated with other autoimmune diseases such as diabetes, thyroiditis, vitiligo, and pernicious anemia. Scientists don't yet understand what causes SPS, but research indicates that it is the result of an autoimmune response gone awry in the brain and spinal cord. The disorder is often misdiagnosed as Parkinson disease, multiple sclerosis, fibromyalgia, psychosomatic illness, or anxiety and phobia. A definitive diagnosis can be made with a blood test that measures the level of glutamic acid decarboxylase (GAD) antibodies in the blood. People with SPS have elevated levels of GAD, an antibody that works against an enzyme involved in the synthesis of an important neurotransmitter in the brain.

Is there any treatment?

People with SPS respond to high doses of diazepam and several anticonvulsants, gabapentin, and tiagabine. A recent study funded by the NINDS demonstrated the effectiveness of intravenous immunoglobulin (IVIg) treatment in reducing stiffness and lowering sensitivity to noise, touch, and stress in people with SPS.

What is the prognosis?

Treatment with IVIg, antianxiety drugs, muscle relaxants, anticonvulsants, and pain relievers will improve the symptoms of SPS, but will not cure the disorder. Most individuals with SPS have frequent falls and because they lack the normal defensive reflexes; injuries can be severe. With appropriate treatment, the symptoms are usually well controlled.

What research is being done?

The National Institute of Neurological Disorders and Stroke (NINDS) conducts research related to SPS in its laboratories at the National Institutes of Health (NIH), and also supports additional research through grants to major medical institutions across the country. Current research is focused on understanding the cause of the disease and the role of the anti-GAD antibodies. A study using a new drug, Rituximab, is underway in patient trials at the NIH clinical center.

Part Four

Hyperkinetic Movement Disorders: Excessive or Unwanted Movements

Chapter 35

Dystonia

Chapter Contents

Section 35.1

Facts about Dystonias

From "Dystonias Fact Sheet," by the National Institute of
Neurological Disorders and Stroke (NINDS, www.ninds.nih.gov),
part of the National Institutes of Health, December 11, 2007.

What are the dystonias?

The dystonias are movement disorders in which sustained muscle contractions cause twisting and repetitive movements or abnormal postures. The movements, which are involuntary and sometimes painful, may affect a single muscle; a group of muscles such as those in the arms, legs, or neck; or the entire body. Those with dystonia usually have normal intelligence and no associated psychiatric disorders.

What are the symptoms?

Dystonia can affect many different parts of the body. Early symptoms may include a deterioration in handwriting after writing several lines, foot cramps, and/or a tendency of one foot to pull up or drag; this may occur "out of the blue" or may occur after running or walking some distance. The neck may turn or pull involuntarily, especially when the patient is tired or stressed. Sometimes both eyes will blink rapidly and uncontrollably, rendering a person functionally blind. Other possible symptoms are tremor and voice or speech difficulties. The initial symptoms can be very mild and may be noticeable only after prolonged exertion, stress, or fatigue. Over a period of time, the symptoms may become more noticeable and widespread and be unrelenting; sometimes, however, there is little or no progression.

How are the dystonias classified?

One way to classify the dystonias is according to the parts of the body they affect:

- Generalized dystonia affects most or all of the body.
- Focal dystonia is localized to a specific part of the body.

- Multifocal dystonia involves two or more unrelated body parts.

- Segmental dystonia affects two or more adjacent parts of the body.

- Hemidystonia involves the arm and leg on the same side of the body.

Some patterns of dystonia are defined as specific syndromes.

Torsion dystonia, previously called dystonia musculorum deformans or DMD, is a rare, generalized dystonia that may be inherited, usually begins in childhood, and becomes progressively worse. It can leave individuals seriously disabled and confined to a wheelchair. Genetic studies have revealed an underlying cause in many patients— a mutation in a gene named DYT1. And it has been discovered that this gene is related not only to generalized dystonia, but also to some forms of focal dystonia. Note, however, that most dystonia, of any type, is not due to this gene and has an unknown cause.

Cervical dystonia, also called spasmodic torticollis, or torticollis, is the most common of the focal dystonias. In torticollis, the muscles in the neck that control the position of the head are affected, causing the head to twist and turn to one side. In addition, the head may be pulled forward or backward. Torticollis can occur at any age, although most individuals first experience symptoms in middle age. It often begins slowly and usually reaches a plateau. About 10 to 20 percent of those with torticollis experience a spontaneous remission, but unfortunately the remission may not be lasting.

Blepharospasm, the second most common focal dystonia, is the involuntary, forcible closure of the eyelids. The first symptoms may be uncontrollable blinking. Only one eye may be affected initially, but eventually both eyes are usually involved. The spasms may leave the eyelids completely closed causing functional blindness even though the eyes and vision are normal.

Cranial dystonia is a term used to describe dystonia that affects the muscles of the head, face, and neck. Oromandibular dystonia affects the muscles of the jaw, lips, and tongue. The jaw may be pulled either open or shut, and speech and swallowing can be difficult. Spasmodic dysphonia involves the muscles of the throat that control speech. Also called spastic dysphonia or laryngeal dystonia, it causes strained and difficult speaking or breathy and effortful speech. Meige syndrome is the combination of blepharospasm and oromandibular dystonia and sometimes spasmodic dysphonia. Spasmodic torticollis can be classified as a type of cranial dystonia.

Writer's cramp is a dystonia that affects the muscles of the hand and sometimes the forearm, and only occurs during handwriting. Similar focal dystonias have also been called typist's cramp, pianist's cramp, and musician's cramp.

Dopa-responsive dystonia (DRD), of which Segawa dystonia is an important variant, is a condition successfully treated with drugs. Typically, DRD begins in childhood or adolescence with progressive difficulty in walking and, in some cases, spasticity. In Segawa dystonia, the symptoms fluctuate during the day from relative mobility in the morning to increasingly worse disability in the afternoon and evening as well as after exercise. The diagnosis of DRD may be missed since it mimics many of the symptoms of cerebral palsy.

What do scientists know about the dystonias?

Investigators believe that the dystonias result from an abnormality in an area of the brain called the basal ganglia where some of the messages that initiate muscle contractions are processed. Scientists suspect a defect in the body's ability to process a group of chemicals called neurotransmitters that help cells in the brain communicate with each other. Some of these neurotransmitters include:

- GABA (gamma-aminobutyric acid), an inhibitory substance that helps the brain maintain muscle control.

- Dopamine, an inhibitory chemical that influences the brain's control of movement.

- Acetylcholine, an excitatory chemical that helps regulate dopamine in the brain. In the body, acetylcholine released at nerve endings causes muscle contraction.

- Norepinephrine and serotonin, inhibitory chemicals that help the brain regulate acetylcholine.

Acquired dystonia, also called secondary dystonia, results from environmental or disease-related damage to the basal ganglia. Birth injury (particularly due to lack of oxygen), certain infections, reactions to certain drugs, heavy-metal or carbon monoxide poisoning, trauma, or stroke can cause dystonic symptoms. Dystonias can also be symptoms of other diseases, some of which may be hereditary.

About half the cases of dystonia have no connection to disease or injury and are called primary or idiopathic dystonia. Of the primary dystonias, many cases appear to be inherited in a dominant manner;

i.e., only one carrier parent need contribute the dystonia gene for the disease to occur, each child having a 50/50 chance of being a carrier. In dystonia, however, a carrier may or may not develop a dystonia and the symptoms may vary widely even among members of the same family. The product of one defective gene appears to be sufficient to cause the chemical imbalances that may lead to dystonia; but the possibility exists that another gene or genes and environmental factors may play a role.

Some cases of primary dystonia may have different types of hereditary patterns. Knowing the pattern of inheritance can help families understand the risk of passing dystonia along to future generations.

When do symptoms occur?

In some individuals, symptoms of a dystonia appear in childhood, approximately between the ages of 5 and 16, usually in the foot or in the hand. In generalized dystonia, the involuntary dystonic movements may progress quickly to involve all limbs and the torso, but the rate of progression usually slows noticeably after adolescence.

For other individuals, the symptoms emerge in late adolescence or early adulthood. In these cases, the dystonia often begins in upper body parts, with symptoms progressing slowly. A dystonia that begins in adulthood is more likely to remain as a focal or segmental dystonia.

Dystonias often progress through various stages. Initially, dystonic movements are intermittent and appear only during voluntary movements or stress. Later, individuals may show dystonic postures and movements while walking and ultimately even while they are relaxed. Dystonic motions may lead to permanent physical deformities by causing tendons to shorten.

In secondary dystonias due to injury or stroke, people often have abnormal movements of just one side of the body, which may begin at the time of the brain injury or sometime afterward. Symptoms generally plateau and do not usually spread to other parts of the body.

Are there any treatments?

No one treatment has been found universally effective. Instead, physicians use a variety of therapies aimed at reducing or eliminating muscle spasms and pain.

Medication: Several classes of drugs that may help correct imbalances in neurotransmitters have been found useful. But response to drugs varies among patients and even in the same person over time. The most effective therapy is often individualized, with physicians prescribing several types of drugs at different doses to treat symptoms and produce the fewest side effects. Note that not all of the medications mentioned in the following text are currently available for patients in the United States.

Frequently, the first drug administered belongs to a group that reduces the level of the neurotransmitter acetylcholine. Drugs in this group include trihexyphenidyl, benztropine, and procyclidine HCl. Sometimes these medications can be sedating, especially at higher doses, and this can limit their usefulness.

Drugs that regulate the neurotransmitter GABA may be used in combination with these drugs or alone in patients with mild symptoms. GABA-regulating drugs include the muscle relaxants diazepam, lorazepam, clonazepam, and baclofen. Other drugs act on dopamine, a neurotransmitter that helps the brain fine-tune muscle movement. Some drugs which increase dopamine effects include levodopa/carbidopa and bromocriptine. DRD has been remarkably responsive to small doses of this dopamine-boosting treatment. On the other hand, patients have occasionally benefited from drugs that decrease dopamine, such as reserpine or the investigational drug tetrabenazine. Once again, side effects can restrict the use of these medications.

Anticonvulsants including carbamazepine, usually prescribed to control epilepsy, have occasionally helped individuals with dystonia.

Botulinum toxin: Minute amounts of this familiar toxin can be injected into affected muscles to provide temporary relief of focal dystonias. First used to treat blepharospasm, such injections have gained wider acceptance among physicians for treating other focal dystonias. The toxin stops muscle spasms by blocking release of the excitatory neurotransmitter acetylcholine. The effect lasts for up to several months before the injections have to be repeated.

Surgery and other treatments: Surgery may be recommended for some patients when medication is unsuccessful or the side effects are too severe. In selected cases, advanced generalized dystonias have been helped, at least temporarily, by surgical destruction of parts of the thalamus, a structure deep in the brain that helps control movement. Speech disturbance is a special risk accompanying this procedure, since the thalamus lies near brain structures that help control speech. Surgically cutting or removing the nerves to the affected muscles has helped some

306

focal dystonias, including blepharospasm, spasmodic dysphonia and torticollis. The benefits of these operations, however, can be short-lived. They also carry the risk of disfigurement, can be unpredictable, and are irreversible.

Some patients with spasmodic dysphonia may benefit from treatment by a speech-language pathologist. Physical therapy, splinting, stress management, and biofeedback may also help individuals with certain forms of dystonia.

What research is being done?

The ultimate goals of research are to find the cause(s) of the dystonias so that they can be prevented, and to find ways to cure or more effectively treat people now affected. The National Institute of Neurological Disorders and Stroke (NINDS), a unit of the federal government's National Institutes of Health (NIH), is the agency with primary responsibility for brain and neuromuscular research. NINDS sponsors research on dystonia both in its facilities at the NIH and through grants to medical centers throughout the country. Scientists at the National Institute on Deafness and Other Communication Disorders (NIDCD), also part of the NIH, are studying improved treatments for speech and voice disorders associated with dystonias. The National Eye Institute (NEI) supports work on the study of blepharospasm and related problems and the National Institute of Child Health and Human Development (NICHD) supports work on dystonia, including the rehabilitation aspects of the disorder.

Scientists at the NINDS laboratories have conducted detailed investigations of the pattern of muscle activity in persons with focal dystonias. One of the most important characteristics is the failure of reciprocal inhibition, a normal process in which muscles with opposite actions work without opposing each other. In dystonia, the tightening of muscles is associated with an abnormal pattern of muscles fighting each other. Other studies at the NINDS have probed the spinal reflex function and found abnormalities consistent with the defect in reciprocal inhibition. Other studies using EEG analysis and neuroimaging are probing brain activity and its relation to these observations.

The search for the gene or genes responsible for some forms of dominantly inherited dystonias continues. In 1989 a team of researchers mapped a gene for early-onset torsion dystonia to chromosome 9; the gene was subsequently named DYT1. In 1997 the team sequenced the DYT1 gene and found that it codes for a previously unknown protein now called "torsin A." The discovery of the DYT1 gene and the torsin A protein provides the opportunity for prenatal testing, allows doctors to make a specific diagnosis in some cases of dystonia, and permits the investigation of molecular and cellular mechanisms that lead to disease.

The gene for Segawa dystonia has been found. It codes for an enzyme important in the brain's manufacture of dopamine.

Section 35.2

Blepharospasm

"Facts About Blepharospasm," is from the National Eye Institute (NEI, www.nei.nih.gov), part of the National Institutes of Health, March 2008.

What is blepharospasm?

Blepharospasm is an abnormal, involuntary blinking or spasm of the eyelids.

What causes blepharospasm?

Blepharospasm is associated with an abnormal function of the basal ganglion from an unknown cause. The basal ganglion is the part of the brain responsible for controlling the muscles. In rare cases, heredity may play a role in the development of blepharospasm.

What are the symptoms of blepharospasm?

Most people develop blepharospasm without any warning symptoms. It may begin with a gradual increase in blinking or eye irritation. Some people may also experience fatigue, emotional tension, or sensitivity to bright light. As the condition progresses, the symptoms become more frequent, and facial spasms may develop. Blepharospasm may decrease or cease while a person is sleeping or concentrating on a specific task.

How is blepharospasm treated?

To date, there is no successful cure for blepharospasm, although several treatment options can reduce its severity.

In the United States and Canada, the injection of Oculinum (botulinum toxin, or Botox) into the muscles of the eyelids is an approved treatment for blepharospasm. Botulinum toxin, produced by the bacterium *Clostridium botulinum*, paralyzes the muscles of the eyelids.

Medications taken by mouth for blepharospasm are available but usually produce unpredictable results. Any symptom relief is usually short term and tends to be helpful in only 15 percent of the cases.

Myectomy, a surgical procedure to remove some of the muscles and nerves of the eyelids, is also a possible treatment option. This surgery has improved symptoms in 75 to 85 percent of people with blepharospasm.

Alternative treatments may include biofeedback, acupuncture, hypnosis, chiropractic, and nutritional therapy. The benefits of these alternative therapies have not been proven.

Section 35.3

Cervical Dystonia (Spasmodic Torticollis)

What is cervical dystonia?

Cervical dystonia, sometimes known as spasmodic torticollis, is a focal dystonia of the neck and typically occurs in people over the age of 40. By causing neck muscles to contract involuntarily, it produces abnormal movements and postures of the neck and head.

The movements can lead to the head and neck twisting (torticollis) or being pulled forward (antecollis), backward (retrocollis), or sideways (laterocollis). Symptoms may vary from mild to severe and the muscular spasms may result in pain and discomfort. Sometimes, the condition may be partially relieved by touching the chin, other parts of the face, or the back of the head.

Though cervical dystonia may progress, it is not life-threatening and does not affect other brain functions. Cervical dystonia is unlikely to become generalized, although occasionally another part of the body may be affected.

The condition varies from one individual to another. In some cases it may progress for about 5 years and then gets no worse. In other cases it hardly progresses at all.

Occasionally, it may go into remission as symptoms disappear, but may return at a later date. Because every case of cervical dystonia is different from every other, it is difficult to predict accurately how it may change in the future.

What causes cervical dystonia?

Cervical dystonia is believed to be the result of abnormal functioning of the basal ganglia, an area deep within the brain that is involved in the control of movement. Much research is currently being undertaken and progress made toward a better understanding of this abnormality.

How is the condition treated?

To date, no cure has been found. Many drugs have been tried in the treatment of cervical dystonia, but while some of these may provide benefit for some individuals, none is universally effective. These drugs may also produce side effects in some people.

Botulinum toxin injections, which weaken the muscles affected by spasm, are the most effective treatment. Injections need to be repeated every 3 months or so. In cases where little improvement results from the injections, it may be because they have not been accurately targeted, or the dose needs adjusting, or a different type of botulinum toxin is required.

Sometimes electromyography (EMG) is used to identify the appropriate muscles to inject.

How do I live with cervical dystonia?

Cervical dystonia can be a challenging condition to live with. Engaging socially or carrying out certain activities, such as driving or walking, can sometimes become more difficult. Sensory tricks (e.g., touching a part of the head with a finger), relaxation techniques, and pacing yourself where possible may be among a number of coping strategies you may wish to pursue.

Learning about cervical dystonia and talking to others who have the condition may help you come to terms with it and find the best way to manage your condition. A brief explanation of cervical dystonia to others may not only help them to understand your condition, but also, in turn, help you to cope with it.

Section 35.4

Hemifacial Spasm

From "Hemifacial Spasm Information Page," by the National Institute of Neurological Disorders and Stroke (NINDS, www.ninds.nih.gov), part of the National Institutes of Health, February 13, 2007.

What is hemifacial spasm?

Hemifacial spasm is a neuromuscular disorder characterized by frequent involuntary contractions (spasms) of the muscles on one side (hemi-) of the face (facial). The disorder occurs in both men and women, although it more frequently affects middle-aged or elderly women. The first symptom is usually an intermittent twitching of the eyelid muscle that can lead to forced closure of the eye. The spasm may then gradually spread to involve the muscles of the lower face, which may cause the mouth to be pulled to one side. Eventually the spasms involve all of the muscles on one side of the face almost continuously. The condition may be caused by a facial nerve injury, or a tumor, or it may have no apparent cause. Rarely, doctors see individuals with spasm on both sides of the face. Most often hemifacial spasm is caused by a blood vessel pressing on the facial nerve at the place where it exits the brainstem.

Is there any treatment?

Surgical treatment in the form of microvascular decompression, which relieves pressure on the facial nerve, will relieve hemifacial spasm in many cases. Other treatments include injections of botulinum toxin (commonly called Botox) into the affected areas and drug therapy with medications such as clonazepam, diazepam, and levodopa, which are used to relax the muscles.

What is the prognosis?

The prognosis for an individual with hemifacial spasm depends on the treatment and their response. Some individuals will be relatively free from symptoms. Some may require additional surgery. Others may only be treatable with Botox or drugs and will have to live with a greater or lesser degree of facial spasms in their day-to-day life.

Section 35.5

Laryngeal Spasm

In laryngeal dystonia the vocal cords are affected by involuntary spasms. These involuntary spasms of the vocal cords cause the voice to change in quality.

When the vocal cords are pulled together (adductor laryngeal dystonia), the voice tends to have a strangled quality. If the vocal cords are pulled apart (abductor laryngeal dystonia) the voice can be breathy and very quiet. Like most types of dystonia, laryngeal dystonia can be made worse when people are anxious or tired.

In most people the condition has no known cause and usually starts in mid-life, but does not affect the mind or the senses. Sometimes the vocal cords are the only part of the body affected, but in some cases other muscles nearby can be affected, such as the neck, mouth, and the muscles around the eyes.

How can laryngeal dystonia be treated?

To date, no cure exists for laryngeal dystonia, although a great deal of research is being undertaken around the world, with significant progress. Whilst treatment for this condition is not essential since it is neither life-threatening nor life-shortening, those who depend on their voices for their work will usually need to be treated if they are to continue in work.

Treatment of laryngeal dystonia can be difficult, and results of treatment vary greatly between different people. The principal treatment involves the injection of botulinum toxin to weaken the muscles affected by spasm. Injections have to be repeated every 3 months or so. Injections into the vocal cords are technically quite difficult, and a very precise dose needs to be given to avoid weakening the muscle too much. Any excessive weakness of the injected muscles is usually temporary.

Because of these difficulties, muscles are usually injected using electromyography (EMG)—a tool that helps identify which muscles are affected most by the dystonia, and is only usually performed by ear, nose, and throat (ENT) doctors with special training.

Some people with laryngeal dystonia can gain benefit from speech therapy. In other people, tablet treatment can be tried, although the results can be quite variable from person to person and side effects can occur.

How do I live with laryngeal dystonia?

Laryngeal dystonia can be a challenging condition to live with. The poor quality of your voice can make it difficult for you to make yourself understood and it can make you feel embarrassed and self-conscious in company.

Giving a brief explanation to new folk you meet can ease their concerns that you might strain your voice by speaking, for example: "I have a neurological condition which affects my speech but it's not painful and I won't do any damage by talking to you."

As with all forms of dystonia, a positive attitude is important. Learning about laryngeal dystonia and communicating with others with the condition may help you come to terms with it and to find the best ways of coping with your specific symptoms.

Section 35.6

Oromandibular Dystonia

In oromandibular dystonia the muscles that move the mouth and jaw are affected by involuntary spasm. This unwanted muscle contraction can pull the mouth into different positions. This often happens when people are using their mouths (e.g., talking or eating), but can happen at rest as well. Like most types of dystonia it can be made worse when people are anxious or tired.

In most people the condition has no known cause and usually starts in mid-life. Typically the mouth is the only part of the body affected, although some people can experience dystonia around the eyes (blepharospasm) and/or neck (cervical dystonia, or torticollis) in association with oromandibular dystonia.

An old name for the condition when eyes, neck, and mouth are affected together by dystonia is Meige syndrome. Usually if the condition comes on in mid-life with no obvious cause, it does not spread further, nor does it affect the mind or the senses.

In some people, previous treatment with medicines that work by blocking the chemical dopamine in the brain (which can be used to treat a variety of conditions including nausea, vertigo, or anxiety as well as psychiatric conditions such as schizophrenia and depression) can be the cause of oromandibular dystonia.

Such people may also be affected by dystonia elsewhere in the body, and the condition typically comes on after long-term treatment with such drugs.

Another name for dystonia caused in this way is tardive dystonia.

What causes dystonia?

Dystonia is thought to be due to a problem in a part of the brain called the basal ganglia, structures deep in the brain that control movement. Although the precise way in which these structures malfunction

314

is not fully understood, much research is ongoing and is progressing toward a greater understanding of the condition.

How can oromandibular dystonia be treated?

To date, no cure exists for oromandibular dystonia, although a great deal of research is being undertaken around the world. If you decide that you want treatment, then the two main choices are tablets or botulinum toxin injections. Sometimes both can be used together.

A few different drugs can help reduce the severity of symptoms in people with oromandibular dystonia. Although some people get great benefit from such drugs, they are not effective in everyone, and some people experience side effects.

Injections of botulinum toxin can be a very effective treatment for oromandibular dystonia. The botulinum toxin temporarily weakens the muscles it is injected into. Injections will need to be repeated every 3 months or so.

Injections into the muscles that move the mouth can be difficult, as a very precise dose needs to be given to avoid weakening the muscle too much and some muscles can be difficult to inject. Any excessive weakness of the injected muscles is always temporary.

Because of these difficulties, muscles are usually injected using electromyography (EMG)—a tool that helps identify which muscles are affected most by the dystonia.

How do I live with oromandibular dystonia?

Oromandibular dystonia can be a challenging condition to live with. The movements around the mouth can sometimes lead to people feeling self-conscious in social situations. Sensory tricks, such as chewing gum, may help control the spasms for some.

Learning about oromandibular dystonia and talking about it to others who have the condition may help you come to terms with it and find the best way to manage your specific condition. A brief explanation of oromandibular dystonia to others may not only help them to understand your condition, but also, in turn, help you to cope with it.

Chapter 36

Tremor Disorders

Chapter Contents

Section 36.1

Facts about Tremors

From "Tremor Fact Sheet," by the National Institute of
Neurological Disorders and Stroke (NINDS, www.ninds.nih.gov),
part of the National Institutes of Health, December 11, 2007.

What is tremor?

Tremor is an unintentional, somewhat rhythmic, muscle movement involving to-and-fro movements (oscillations) of one or more parts of the body. It is the most common of all involuntary movements and can affect the hands, arms, head, face, vocal cords, trunk, and legs. Most tremors occur in the hands. In some people, tremor is a symptom of another neurological disorder. The most common form of tremor, however, occurs in otherwise healthy people. Although tremor is not life-threatening, it can be embarrassing to some people and make it harder to perform daily tasks.

What causes tremor?

Tremor is generally caused by problems in parts of the brain that control muscles throughout the body or in particular areas, such as the hands. Neurological disorders or conditions that can produce tremor include multiple sclerosis, stroke, traumatic brain injury, and neurodegenerative diseases that damage or destroy parts of the brainstem or the cerebellum. Other causes include the use of some drugs (such as amphetamines, corticosteroids, and drugs used for certain psychiatric disorders), alcohol abuse or withdrawal, mercury poisoning, overactive thyroid, or liver failure. Some forms of tremor are inherited and run in families, while others have no known cause.

What are the characteristics of tremor?

Characteristics may include a rhythmic shaking in the hands, arms, head, legs, or trunk; shaky voice; difficulty writing or drawing; or problems holding and controlling utensils, such as a fork. Some tremors may be triggered by or become exaggerated during times of stress or strong emotion, when the individual is physically exhausted, or during certain postures or movements.

Tremor may occur at any age but is most common in middle-aged and older persons. It may be occasional, temporary, or occur intermittently. Tremor affects men and women equally.

A useful way to understand and describe tremors is to define them according to the following types. **Resting or static tremor** occurs when the muscle is relaxed and the limb is fully supported against gravity, such as when the hands are lying on the lap. It may be seen as a shaking of the limb, even when the person is at rest. This type of tremor is often seen in patients with Parkinson disease. An **action tremor** occurs during any type of movement of an affected body part. There are several subclassifications of action tremor. Postural tremor occurs when the person maintains a position against gravity, such as holding the arms outstretched. Kinetic (or intention) tremor occurs during purposeful voluntary movement, such as touching a finger to one's nose during a medical exam. Task-specific tremor appears when performing highly skilled, goal-oriented tasks such as handwriting or speaking. Isometric tremor occurs during a voluntary muscle contraction that is not accompanied by any movement.

What are the different categories of tremor?

Tremor is most commonly classified by clinical features and cause or origin. Some of the better known forms of tremor, with their symptoms, include the following:

Essential tremor (sometimes called benign essential tremor) is the most common of the more than 20 types of tremor. Although the tremor may be mild and nonprogressive in some people, in others, the tremor is slowly progressive, starting on one side of the body but affecting both sides within 3 years. The hands are most often affected but the head, voice, tongue, legs, and trunk may also be involved. Head tremor may be seen as a "yes-yes" or "no-no" motion. Essential tremor may be accompanied by mild gait disturbance. Tremor frequency may decrease as the person ages, but the severity may increase, affecting the person's ability to perform certain tasks or activities of daily living. Heightened emotion, stress, fever, physical exhaustion, or low blood sugar may trigger tremors and/or increase their severity. Onset is most common after age 40, although symptoms can appear at any age. It may occur in more than one family member. Children of a parent who has essential tremor have a 50 percent chance of inheriting the condition. Essential tremor is not associated with any known pathology.

Parkinsonian tremor is caused by damage to structures within the brain that control movement. This resting tremor, which can occur as an isolated symptom or be seen in other disorders, is often a precursor to Parkinson disease (more than 25 percent of patients with Parkinson disease have an associated action tremor). The tremor, which is classically seen as a "pill-rolling" action of the hands that may also affect the chin, lips, legs, and trunk, can be markedly increased by stress or emotions. Onset of parkinsonian tremor is generally after age 60. Movement starts in one limb or on one side of the body and usually progresses to include the other side.

Dystonic tremor occurs in individuals of all ages who are affected by dystonia, a movement disorder in which sustained involuntary muscle contractions cause twisting and repetitive motions and/or painful and abnormal postures or positions. Dystonic tremor may affect any muscle in the body and is seen most often when the patient is in a certain position or moves a certain way. The pattern of dystonic tremor may differ from essential tremor. Dystonic tremors occur irregularly and often can be relieved by complete rest. Touching the affected body part or muscle may reduce tremor severity. The tremor may be the initial sign of dystonia localized to a particular part of the body.

Cerebellar tremor is a slow, broad tremor of the extremities that occurs at the end of a purposeful movement, such as trying to press a button or touching a finger to the tip of one's nose. Cerebellar tremor is caused by lesions in or damage to the cerebellum resulting from stroke, tumor, or disease such as multiple sclerosis or some inherited degenerative disorder. It can also result from chronic alcoholism or overuse of some medicines. In classic cerebellar tremor, a lesion on one side of the brain produces a tremor in that same side of the body that worsens with directed movement. Cerebellar damage can also produce a "wing-beating" type of tremor called rubral or Holmes' tremor—a combination of rest, action, and postural tremors. The tremor is often most prominent when the affected person is active or is maintaining a particular posture. Cerebellar tremor may be accompanied by dysarthria (speech problems), nystagmus (rapid, involuntary rolling of the eyes), gait problems, and postural tremor of the trunk and neck.

Psychogenic tremor (also called hysterical tremor) can occur at rest or during postural or kinetic movement. The characteristics of this kind of tremor may vary but generally include sudden onset and remission, increased incidence with stress, change in tremor direction and/or body part affected, and greatly decreased or disappearing tremor activity when the patient is distracted. Many patients with psychogenic tremor have a conversion disorder (defined as a psychological disorder that produces physical symptoms) or another psychiatric disease.

Orthostatic tremor is characterized by rhythmic muscle contractions that occur in the legs and trunk immediately after standing. Cramps are felt in the thighs and legs and the patient shakes uncontrollably when asked to stand in one spot. No other clinical signs or symptoms are present and the shaking ceases when the patient sits or is lifted off the ground. Orthostatic tremor may also occur in patients who have essential tremor.

Physiologic tremor occurs in every normal individual and has no clinical significance. It is rarely visible to the eye and may be heightened by strong emotion (such as anxiety or fear), physical exhaustion, hypoglycemia, hyperthyroidism, heavy metal poisoning, stimulants, alcohol withdrawal, or fever. It can be seen in all voluntary muscle groups and can be detected by extending the arms and placing a piece of paper on top of the hands. Enhanced physiologic tremor is a strengthening of physiologic tremor to more visible levels. It is generally not caused by a neurological disease but by reaction to certain drugs, alcohol withdrawal, or medical conditions including an overactive thyroid and hypoglycemia. It is usually reversible once the cause is corrected.

Tremor can result from other conditions as well. Alcoholism, excessive alcohol consumption, or alcohol withdrawal can kill certain nerve cells, resulting in tremor, especially in the hand. (Conversely, small amounts of alcohol may help to decrease familial and essential tremor, but the mechanism behind this is unknown. Doctors may use small amounts of alcohol to aid in the diagnosis of certain forms of tremor but not as a regular treatment for the condition.) Tremor in peripheral neuropathy may occur when the nerves that supply the body's muscles are traumatized by injury, disease, abnormality in the central nervous system, or as the result of systemic illnesses. Peripheral neuropathy can affect the whole body or certain areas, such as the hands, and may be progressive. Resulting sensory loss may be seen as a tremor or ataxia (inability to coordinate voluntary muscle movement) of the affected limbs and problems with gait and balance. Clinical characteristics may be similar to those seen in patients with essential tremor.

How is tremor diagnosed?

During a physical exam a doctor can determine whether the tremor occurs primarily during action or at rest. The doctor will also check for tremor symmetry, any sensory loss, weakness or muscle atrophy, or decreased reflexes. A detailed family history may indicate if the tremor is inherited. Blood or urine tests can detect thyroid malfunction, other metabolic causes, and abnormal levels of certain chemicals that can cause tremor. These tests may also help to identify contributing causes, such as drug interaction, chronic alcoholism, or another condition or disease. Diagnostic imaging using computerized tomography or magnetic resonance imaging may help determine if the tremor is the result of a structural defect or degeneration of the brain.

The doctor will perform a neurological exam to assess nerve function and motor and sensory skills. The tests are designed to determine any functional limitations, such as difficulty with handwriting or the ability to hold a utensil or cup. The patient may be asked to place a finger on the tip of her or his nose, draw a spiral, or perform other tasks or exercises.

The doctor may order an electromyogram to diagnose muscle or nerve problems. This test measures involuntary muscle activity and muscle response to nerve stimulation.

Are there any treatments?

There is no cure for most tremors. The appropriate treatment depends on accurate diagnosis of the cause.

Some tremors respond to treatment of the underlying condition. For example, in some cases of psychogenic tremor, treating the patient's underlying psychological problem may cause the tremor to disappear.

Symptomatic drug therapy is available for several forms of tremor. Drug treatment for parkinsonian tremor involves levodopa and/or dopamine-like drugs such as pergolide mesylate, bromocriptine mesylate, and ropinirole. Other drugs used to lessen parkinsonian tremor include amantadine hydrochloride and anticholinergic drugs.

Essential tremor may be treated with propranolol or other beta blockers (such as nadolol) and primidone, an anticonvulsant drug.

Cerebellar tremor typically does not respond to medical treatment. Patients with rubral tremor may receive some relief using levodopa or anticholinergic drugs.

Dystonic tremor may respond to clonazepam, anticholinergic drugs, and intramuscular injections of botulinum toxin. Botulinum toxin is also prescribed to treat voice and head tremors and several movement disorders.

Clonazepam and primidone may be prescribed for primary orthostatic tremor.

Enhanced physiologic tremor is usually reversible once the cause is corrected. If symptomatic treatment is needed, beta blockers can be used.

Eliminating tremor "triggers" such as caffeine and other stimulants from the diet is often recommended.

Physical therapy may help to reduce tremor and improve coordination and muscle control for some patients. A physical therapist will evaluate the patient for tremor positioning, muscle control, muscle strength, and functional skills. Teaching the patient to brace the affected limb during the tremor or to hold an affected arm close to the body is sometimes useful in gaining motion control. Coordination and balancing exercises may help some patients. Some therapists recommend the use of weights, splints, other adaptive equipment, and special plates and utensils for eating.

Surgical intervention such as thalamotomy and deep brain stimulation may ease certain tremors. These surgeries are usually performed only when the tremor is severe and does not respond to drugs.

Thalamotomy, involving the creation of lesions in the brain region called the thalamus, is quite effective in treating patients with essential, cerebellar, or parkinsonian tremor. This in-hospital procedure is performed under local anesthesia, with the patient awake. After the patient's head is secured in a metal frame, the surgeon maps the patient's brain to locate the thalamus. A small hole is drilled through the skull and a temperature-controlled electrode is inserted into the thalamus. A low-frequency current is passed through the electrode to activate the tremor and to confirm proper placement. Once the site has been confirmed, the electrode is heated to create a temporary lesion. Testing is done to examine speech, language, coordination, and tremor activation, if any. If no problems occur, the probe is again heated to create a 3-mm permanent lesion. The probe, when cooled to body temperature, is withdrawn and the skull hole is covered. The lesion causes the tremor to permanently disappear without disrupting sensory or motor control.

Deep brain stimulation (DBS) uses implantable electrodes to send high-frequency electrical signals to the thalamus. The electrodes are implanted as described above. The patient uses a hand-held magnet to turn on and turn off a pulse generator that is surgically implanted under the skin. The electrical stimulation temporarily disables the tremor and can be "reversed," if necessary, by turning off the implanted electrode. Batteries in the generator last about 5 years and can be replaced surgically. DBS is currently used to treat parkinsonian tremor and essential tremor.

The most common side effects of tremor surgery include dysarthria (problems with motor control of speech), temporary or permanent cognitive impairment (including visual and learning difficulties), and problems with balance.

What research is being done?

The National Institute of Neurological Disorders and Stroke, a unit of the National Institutes of Health (NIH) within the U.S. Department of Health and Human Services, is the nation's leading federal funder of research on disorders of the brain and nervous system. The NINDS sponsors research on tremor both at its facilities at the NIH and through grants to medical centers.

Scientists at the NINDS are evaluating the effectiveness of 1-octanol, a substance similar to alcohol but less intoxicating, for treating essential tremor. Results of two previous NIH studies have shown this agent to be promising as a potential new treatment.

Other NINDS-funded grantees are studying two antidepressant medications, paroxetine and venlafaxine, to see if they can help control depression in Parkinson disease and affect motor symptoms such as tremor, stiffness, slowness, and loss of balance.

An additional NINDS study will examine how dextromethorphan, a drug that alters reflexes of the larynx (voice box), might reduce voice symptoms in people with voice disorders, including vocal tremor. This study will compare the effects of dextromethorphan, lorazepam (a tranquilizer), and a placebo in patients with four types of voice disorders.

Section 36.2

Essential Tremor:
The Most Common Form of Tremor

From "Essential tremor," by the National Library of Medicine,
Genetics Home Reference (ghr.nlm.nih.gov), February 2008.

What is essential tremor?

Essential tremor is a disorder of the nervous system that causes involuntary, rhythmic shaking (tremor), especially in the hands. It involves tremor without any other signs or symptoms, and is distinguished from tremor that results from other disorders or known causes, such as tremors seen with Parkinson disease or head trauma.

Essential tremor usually occurs when the muscles are opposing gravity, such as when the hands are extended, and worsens with movement. This type of tremor is usually not evident at rest.

In addition to the hands and arms, muscles of the trunk, face, head, and neck may also exhibit tremor in this disorder; the legs and feet are not usually involved. Head tremor may appear as a "yes-yes" or "no-no" movement while the affected individual is seated or standing. In some people with essential tremor, voice quality may be affected.

Essential tremor is not considered a dangerous or debilitating condition, and it does not shorten the lifespan. If severe, however, it may interfere somewhat with fine motor skills such as using eating utensils, writing, shaving, or applying makeup. Symptoms of essential tremor may be aggravated by emotional stress, fatigue, hunger, caffeine, cigarette smoking, or extremes of temperature.

Essential tremor may appear at any age, but is most common in the elderly. Some studies have suggested that people with essential tremor may have a higher than average risk of developing Parkinson disease, sensory problems such as hearing loss, or other neurological conditions, while others suggest that essential tremor may be associated with increased longevity.

How common is essential tremor?

Essential tremor is a common disorder, affecting millions of people in the United States. Estimates of its prevalence vary widely because several other disorders, as well as certain medications and other factors, can result in similar tremors. Essential tremor may affect as many as 14 percent of people over the age of 65.

What genes are related to essential tremor?

Essential tremor is a complex disorder. Several genes are believed to help determine an individual's risk of developing this condition. Environmental factors may also be involved.

Some studies have found the DRD3 gene to be associated with essential tremor. The DRD3 gene provides instructions for making a protein called dopamine receptor D3, which is found in the brain. This protein responds to a chemical messenger (neurotransmitter) called dopamine to trigger signals within the nervous system, including signals involved in producing physical movement. A DRD3 variant seen in some families affected by essential tremor may cause the corresponding dopamine receptor D3 protein to respond more strongly to the neurotransmitter, possibly causing the involuntary shaking seen in this condition.

In other studies, the gene HS1BP3 has also been associated with essential tremor. The HS1BP3 gene provides instructions for making a protein called hematopoietic-specific protein 1 binding protein 3. This protein is believed to help regulate chemical signaling in the brain region involved in coordinating movements (the cerebellum) and in specialized nerve cells in the brain and spinal cord that control the muscles (motor neurons). An HS1BP3 variant has been identified in some families affected by essential tremor, but it has also been found in unaffected people. It is unknown what relationship, if any, this genetic change may have to the signs and symptoms of this condition.

How do people inherit essential tremor?

Essential tremor can be passed through generations in families, but the inheritance pattern varies. In most affected families, essential tremor appears to be inherited in an autosomal dominant pattern, which means one copy of the altered gene in each cell is sufficient to cause the disorder. In other families, the inheritance pattern is unclear. Essential tremor may also appear in people with no previous history of the disorder in their family.

Section 36.3

Fragile X Syndrome Causes Tremors

From "Fragile X syndrome," by the National Library of Medicine,
Genetics Home Reference (ghr.nlm.nih.gov), May 2007.

What is fragile X syndrome?

Fragile X syndrome is a genetic condition that causes a range of developmental problems including learning disabilities and mental retardation. Usually, males are more severely affected by this disorder than females.

Males and females with fragile X syndrome may have anxiety and hyperactive behavior such as fidgeting, excessive physical movements, or impulsive actions. They may also have attention deficit disorder, which includes an impaired ability to maintain attention and difficulty focusing on specific tasks. About one third of males with fragile X syndrome also have autism or autistic-like behavior that affects communication and social interaction. Seizures occur in about 15 percent of males and about 5 percent of females with fragile X syndrome.

Many males with fragile X syndrome have characteristic physical features that become more apparent with age. These features include a long and narrow face, large ears, prominent jaw and forehead, unusually flexible fingers, and enlarged testicles (macroorchidism) after puberty.

How common is fragile X syndrome?

Fragile X syndrome occurs in approximately 1 in 4,000 males and 1 in 8,000 females.

What genes are related to fragile X syndrome?

Mutations in the FMR1 gene cause fragile X syndrome. The FMR1 gene provides instructions for making a protein called fragile X mental retardation 1 protein, whose function is not fully understood. This protein likely plays a role in the development of synapses, which are specialized connections between nerve cells. Synapses are critical for relaying nerve impulses.

Nearly all cases of fragile X syndrome are caused by a mutation in which a DNA segment, known as the CGG triplet repeat, is expanded within the FMR1 gene. Normally, this DNA segment is repeated from 5 to about 40 times. In people with fragile X syndrome, however, the CGG segment is repeated more than 200 times. The abnormally expanded CGG segment turns off (silences) the FMR1 gene, which prevents the gene from producing fragile X mental retardation 1 protein. Loss or a shortage (deficiency) of this protein disrupts nervous system functions and leads to the signs and symptoms of fragile X syndrome.

In a small percentage of cases, other types of mutations cause fragile X syndrome. These mutations delete part or all of the FMR1 gene, or change one of the building blocks (amino acids) used to make the fragile X mental retardation 1 protein. As a result, no protein is produced, or the protein's function is impaired because its size or shape is altered.

Males and females with 55 to 200 repeats of the CGG segment are said to have an FMR1 premutation. Most people with a premutation are intellectually normal. In some cases, however, individuals with a premutation have lower than normal amounts of the fragile X mental retardation 1 protein. As a result, they may have mild versions of the physical features seen in fragile X syndrome (such as prominent ears) and may experience emotional problems such as anxiety or depression. Some children with a premutation may have learning disabilities or autistic-like behavior. About 20 percent of women with a premutation have premature ovarian failure, in which menstrual periods stop by age 40. Men, and some women, with a premutation have an increased risk of developing a disorder known as fragile X-associated tremor/ataxia syndrome (FXTAS).

This disorder is characterized by progressive problems with movement (ataxia), tremor, memory loss, loss of sensation in the lower extremities (peripheral neuropathy), and mental and behavioral changes.

How do people inherit fragile X syndrome?

Fragile X syndrome is inherited in an X-linked dominant pattern. A condition is considered X-linked if the mutated gene that causes the disorder is located on the X chromosome, one of the two sex chromosomes. (The Y chromosome is the other sex chromosome.) The inheritance is dominant if one copy of the altered gene in each cell is sufficient to cause the condition.

In women, the FMR1 premutation on the X chromosome can expand to more than 200 CGG repeats in cells that develop into eggs. This means that women with the premutation have an increased risk of having a child with fragile X syndrome. By contrast, the premutation in men does not expand to more than 200 repeats as it is passed to the next generation. (Men pass the premutation only to their daughters. Their sons receive a Y chromosome, which does not include the FMR1 gene.)

What other names do people use for fragile X syndrome?

- FRAXA syndrome
- fra(X) syndrome
- FXS
- Marker X syndrome
- Martin-Bell syndrome
- X-linked mental retardation and macroorchidism

Chapter 37

Choreatic Disorders

Chapter Contents

Section 37.1

What Is Chorea?

Definition

Jerky body movements is a condition in which uncontrolled, purposeless, rapid motions interrupt normal movement or posture.

Considerations

Typical movements of chorea (called tics) include facial grimacing, raising and lowering the shoulders, bending, and extending the fingers and toes. The condition can affect one or both sides of the body.

These involuntary movements are generally not repetitive and can appear purposeful even though they are involuntary and uncontrollable. A person with chorea may be viewed as jittery or restless.

Causes

There are many possible causes of unpredictable, jerky movements, including Sydenham chorea, Huntington disease, and other rare disorders. Some medical illnesses that can cause chorea include anti-cardiolipin antibody syndrome, systemic lupus erythematosus, polycythemia rubra vera, stroke, thyroid disease, and disorders of calcium, glucose, or sodium metabolism.

Some medications such as anti-psychotic drugs, may cause tardive dyskinesia, a movement disorder which may include choreic movements. Rarely, it is inherited in the syndrome called benign hereditary chorea. Some women may develop chorea when pregnant. This is called chorea gravidarum.

Home Care

Therapy is aimed at identifying and treating the underlying cause. If it is due to medication, the drug should be discontinued if possible.

If it is due to medical disease, the disorder should be treated. If the movements are severe and disruptive, medications such as amantadine or tetrabenazine may help control the movements.

Rest helps improve chorea, which can be aggravated by excitement or fatigue. Emotional stress should be minimized.

Safety measures should also be taken to decrease the likelihood of injury from the involuntary movements.

When to Contact a Medical Professional

Call your provider if there is any persistent, unexplained, and uncontrollable bodily motions.

What to Expect at Your Office Visit

The medical history will be obtained and a physical examination performed.

Medical history questions documenting this symptom in detail may include:

- What kind of movement occurs?
- What part of the body is affected?
- What other symptoms are also present?
- Is there irritability?
- Is there weakness or paralysis?
- Is there restlessness?
- Is there emotional instability?
- Are there facial tics?

The physical examination should include an extensive neurological and muscular system examination.

Section 37.2

Tardive Syndromes

"Tardive Dyskinesia," reviewed by Henry A. Nasrallah, M.D., September 2003. © 2003 NAMI: The Nation's Voice on Mental Illness. Reprinted with permission. Reviewed by David A. Cooke, M.D., October 5, 2008.

What is tardive dyskinesia?

Tardive dyskinesia, or TD, is one of the muscular side effects of antipsychotic drugs, especially the older generation like haloperidol. TD does not occur until after many months or years of taking antipsychotic drugs, unlike akathisia (restlessness), dystonia (sudden and painful muscle stiffness), and Parkinsonism (tremors and slowing down of all body muscles), which can occur within hours to days of taking an antipsychotic drug. TD is primarily characterized by random movements in the tongue, lips, or jaw as well as facial grimacing, movements of arms, legs, fingers, and toes, or even swaying movements of the trunk or hips. TD can be quite embarrassing to the affected patient when in public. The movements disappear during sleep. They can be mild, moderate, or severe.

How does an individual get TD?

Essentially, prolonged exposure to antipsychotic treatment (which is necessary for many persons who have chronic schizophrenia) is the major reason that TD occurs in an individual. Some persons get it sooner than others. The risk factors that increase the chances of developing TD are a) duration of exposure to antipsychotics (especially the older generation), b) older age, c) post-menopausal females, d) alcoholism and substance abuse, e) mental retardation, and f) experiencing a lot of EPS [extrapyramidal symptoms] in the acute stage of antipsychotic therapy.

The mechanism of TD is still unknown despite extensive research. However, it is generally believed that long-term blocking of dopamine D_2 receptors (which is what all antipsychotics on the market do) causes an increase in the number of D_2 receptors in the striated region of the brain (which controls muscle coordination). This "up-regulation" of D_2

receptors may cause spontaneous and random muscle contractions or movements throughout the body, but particularly in the peri-oral and facial muscles.

How many individuals currently have TD?

It is not known how many individuals currently have TD. No large scale epidemiological prevalence survey has been done. It would also change because TD can be transient or persistent, and it can be more common in some persons with risk factors than others.

However, there have been several follow-up studies of individuals who start taking antipsychotics in order to measure the annual occurrence (incidence) of TD. Eight studies in young individuals (average age 29 years) receiving the older antipsychotics showed practically the same rate of 5% of those persons develop TD every year, year after year, until eventually almost 50–60% develop TD over their lifetime. The incidence of TD is higher in older individuals (average age 65 years) where our studies have shown that TD occurs in 26% after only one year of exposure to haloperidol, which increases to 52% after two years and up to 60% after three years.

Do the newer generation atypical antipsychotics pose a lower risk of TD?

Yes, the newer atypical antipsychotics are much safer than the older generation when it comes to TD. The first year incidence of TD with risperidone, olanzapine, quetiapine, and ziprasidone in young persons about 0.5%, which is ten-fold lower than with haloperidol. Similarly, the incidence of TD with atypical antipsychotics in the first year in geriatric patients is 2.5%, which is also ten-fold lower than with haloperidol. There is also growing evidence that the incidence is even lower in subsequent years of exposure to atypicals. The problem of TD has been significantly reduced with the advent and widespread use of atypical antipsychotics.

What are the symptoms of TD and is TD reversible?

As described above, the main symptoms of TD are continuous and random muscular movements in the tongue, mouth, and face, but sometimes the limbs and trunks are affected as well. Rarely, the respiration muscles may be affected resulting in grunts and even breathing difficulties. Sometimes, the legs can be so severely affected that walking becomes difficult.

It must be noted that there are many other conditions that resemble TD and must be ruled out before a diagnosis of TD is made. For example, several neurodegenerative brain diseases may cause movement disorders. Very old persons may also develop mouth and facial movements with age that may be mistaken for TD. Blepharospasm is another condition that may be mistaken for TD. It should be emphasized that a history of several months or years of antipsychotic intake must be documented before TD is even considered.

TD is often mild and reversible. The percentage of patients who develop severe or irreversible TD is quite low as a proportion of those receiving long-term antipsychotic therapy.

What should you do if you notice symptoms of TD in yourself or in a family member?

Consult a psychiatrist with an established experience in using antipsychotic drugs or a neurologist who specializes in movement disorders. That physician will take a detailed history and conduct an examination and decide whether you have TD or something else, and will recommend the appropriate management.

The pattern and severity of TD is usually measured on a rating scale called "The Abnormal Involuntary Movement Scale" (AIMS for short). Psychiatrists generally assess patients receiving long-term antipsychotic medication for TD symptoms at least annually using the AIMS.

Are there effective treatments for TD?

There has never been a definitive, validated, and widely accepted treatment for TD. Dozens of drugs have been tested over the past 30 years with mixed results at best. The atypical antipsychotic clozapine has been reported to reverse persistent TD after 6–12 months, possibly through gradual "down-regulation" of supersensitive dopamine D_2 receptors. Some preliminary reports suggest that other atypical antipsychotics may also help reverse TD.

However, given that a large majority of persons who need antipsychotic treatment are now receiving the new atypicals and given the drastically lower incidence of TD with atypical antipsychotics, the issue of developing a treatment for TD may have become a moot one. Preventing the occurrence of TD is much more preferable to treating TD.

Section 37.3

Sydenham Chorea

From "Sydenham Chorea Information Page," by the National Institute
of Neurological Disorders and Stroke (NINDS, www.ninds.nih.gov), part
of the National Institutes of Health, February 14, 2007.

What is Sydenham chorea?

Sydenham chorea (SD) is a neurological disorder of childhood resulting from infection via *Group A beta-hemolytic streptococcus* (GABHS), the bacterium that causes rheumatic fever. SD is characterized by rapid, irregular, and aimless involuntary movements of the arms and legs, trunk, and facial muscles. It affects girls more often than boys and typically occurs between 5 and 15 years of age. Some children will have a sore throat several weeks before the symptoms begin, but the disorder can also strike up to 6 months after the fever or infection has cleared. Symptoms can appear gradually or all at once, and also may include uncoordinated movements, muscular weakness, stumbling and falling, slurred speech, difficulty concentrating and writing, and emotional instability. The symptoms of SD can vary from a halting gait and slight grimacing to involuntary movements that are frequent and severe enough to be incapacitating. The random, writhing movements of chorea are caused by an autoimmune reaction to the bacterium that interferes with the normal function of a part of the brain (the basal ganglia) that controls motor movements. Due to better sanitary conditions and the use of antibiotics to treat streptococcal infections, rheumatic fever, and consequently SD, are rare in North America and Europe. The disease can still be found in developing nations.

Is there any treatment?

There is no specific treatment for SD. For people with the mildest form, bed rest during the period of active movements is sufficient. When the severity of movements interferes with rest, sedative drugs, such as barbiturates or benzodiazepines, may be needed. Antiepileptic medications, such as valproic acid, are often prescribed. Doctors also recommend that children who have had SD take penicillin over the course of the next 10 years to prevent additional manifestations of rheumatic fever.

What is the prognosis?

Most children recover completely from SD, although a small number will continue to have disabling, persistent chorea despite treatment. The duration of symptoms varies, generally from 3 to 6 weeks, but some children will have symptoms for several months. Cardiac complications may occur in a small minority of children, usually in the form of endocarditis. In a third of the children with the disease, SD will recur, typically 1 1/2 to 2 1/2 years after the initial attack. Researchers have noted an association between recurrent SD and the later development of the abrupt onset forms of obsessive-compulsive disorder, attention deficit/hyperactivity disorder, tic disorders, and autism, which they call PANDAS, for Pediatric Autoimmune Neuropsychiatric Disorders Associated with Streptococcus infection. Further studies are needed to determine the nature of the association and the biological pathways that connect streptococcal infection, autoimmune response, and the later development of these specific behavioral disorders.

What research is being done?

The National Institute of Neurological Disorders and Stroke (NINDS) and other institutes of the National Institutes of Health (NIH) conduct research related to SD in laboratories at the NIH, and support additional research through grants to major medical institutions across the country. Currently, researchers are studying how the interplay of genetic, developmental, and environmental factors could determine a child's vulnerability to SD after a GABHS infection. Other researchers are exploring whether children whose symptoms either begin or get worse following a GABHS infection share a common set of abnormal biomolecular pathways responsible for their similar clinical symptoms.

Section 37.4

Paroxysmal Choreoathetosis Disease

From "Paroxysmal Choreoathetosis Information Page," by the National Institutes of Neurological Disorders and Stroke (NINDS, www.ninds.nih .gov), part of the National Institutes of Health, February 14, 2007.

What is paroxysmal choreoathetosis?

Paroxysmal choreoathetosis is a movement disorder characterized by episodes or attacks of involuntary movements of the limbs, trunk, and facial muscles. The disorder may occur in several members of a family, or in only a single family member. Prior to an attack some individuals experience tightening of muscles or other physical symptoms. Involuntary movements precipitate some attacks, and other attacks occur when the individual has consumed alcohol or caffeine, or is tired or stressed. Attacks can last from 10 seconds to over an hour. Some individuals have lingering muscle tightness after an attack. Paroxysmal choreoathetosis frequently begins in early adolescence. A gene associated with the disorder has been discovered. The same gene is also associated with epilepsy.

Is there any treatment?

Drug therapy, particularly carbamazepine, has been very successful in reducing or eliminating attacks of paroxysmal choreoathetosis. While carbamazepine is not effective in every case, other drugs have been substituted with good effect.

What is the prognosis?

Generally, paroxysmal choreoathetosis lessens with age, and many adults have a complete remission. Because drug therapy is so effective, the prognosis for the disorder is good.

Chapter 38

Huntington Disease (HD)

Chapter Contents

Section 38.1

All about Huntington Disease

Excerpted from "Huntington's Disease: Hope Through Research," by the National Institute of Neurological Disorders and Stroke (NINDS, www .ninds.nih.gov), part of the National Institutes of Health, April 15, 2008.

Introduction

In 1872, the American physician George Huntington wrote about an illness that he called "an heirloom from generations away back in the dim past." He was not the first to describe the disorder, which has been traced back to the Middle Ages at least. One of its earliest names was chorea, which, as in "choreography," is the Greek word for dance. The term chorea describes how people affected with the disorder writhe, twist, and turn in a constant, uncontrollable dance-like motion. Later, other descriptive names evolved. "Hereditary chorea" emphasizes how the disease is passed from parent to child. "Chronic progressive chorea" stresses how symptoms of the disease worsen over time. Today, physicians commonly use the simple term Huntington disease (HD) to describe this highly complex disorder that causes untold suffering for thousands of families.

More than 15,000 Americans have HD. At least 150,000 others have a 50 percent risk of developing the disease and thousands more of their relatives live with the possibility that they, too, might develop HD.

Until recently, scientists understood very little about HD and could only watch as the disease continued to pass from generation to generation. Families saw the disease destroy their loved ones' ability to feel, think, and move. In the last several years, scientists working with support from the National Institute of Neurological Disorders and Stroke (NINDS) have made several breakthroughs in the area of HD research. With these advances, our understanding of the disease continues to improve.

This text presents information about HD, and about current research progress, to health professionals, scientists, caregivers, and, most important, to those already too familiar with the disorder: the many families who are affected by HD.

What causes Huntington disease?

HD results from genetically programmed degeneration of nerve cells, called neurons, in certain areas of the brain. This degeneration causes uncontrolled movements, loss of intellectual faculties, and emotional disturbance. Specifically affected are cells of the basal ganglia, structures deep within the brain that have many important functions, including coordinating movement. Within the basal ganglia, HD especially targets neurons of the striatum, particularly those in the caudate nuclei and the pallidum. Also affected is the brain's outer surface, or cortex, which controls thought, perception, and memory.

How is HD inherited?

HD is found in every country of the world. It is a familial disease, passed from parent to child through a mutation or misspelling in the normal gene.

A single abnormal gene, the basic biological unit of heredity, produces HD. Genes are composed of deoxyribonucleic acid (DNA), a molecule shaped like a spiral ladder. Each rung of this ladder is composed of two paired chemicals called bases. There are four types of bases—adenine, thymine, cytosine, and guanine—each abbreviated by the first letter of its name: A, T, C, and G. Certain bases always "pair" together, and different combinations of base pairs join to form coded messages. A gene is a long string of this DNA in various combinations of A, T, C, and G. These unique combinations determine the gene's function, much like letters join together to form words. Each person has about 30,000 genes—a billion base pairs of DNA or bits of information repeated in the nuclei of human cells—which determine individual characteristics or traits.

Genes are arranged in precise locations along 23 rod-like pairs of chromosomes. One chromosome from each pair comes from an individual's mother, the other from the father. Each half of a chromosome pair is similar to the other, except for one pair, which determines the sex of the individual. This pair has two X chromosomes in females and one X and one Y chromosome in males. The gene that produces HD lies on chromosome 4, one of the 22 non-sex-linked, or "autosomal," pairs of chromosomes, placing men and women at equal risk of acquiring the disease.

The impact of a gene depends partly on whether it is dominant or recessive. If a gene is dominant, then only one of the paired chromosomes is required to produce its called-for effect. If the gene is recessive, both parents must provide chromosomal copies for the trait to

343

be present. HD is called an autosomal dominant disorder because only one copy of the defective gene, inherited from one parent, is necessary to produce the disease.

The genetic defect responsible for HD is a small sequence of DNA on chromosome 4 in which several base pairs are repeated many, many times. The normal gene has three DNA bases, composed of the sequence CAG. In people with HD, the sequence abnormally repeats itself dozens of times. Over time—and with each successive generation—the number of CAG repeats may expand further.

Each parent has two copies of every chromosome but gives only one copy to each child. Each child of an HD parent has a 50-50 chance of inheriting the HD gene. If a child does not inherit the HD gene, he or she will not develop the disease and cannot pass it to subsequent generations. A person who inherits the HD gene, and survives long enough, will sooner or later develop the disease. In some families, all the children may inherit the HD gene; in others, none do. Whether one child inherits the gene has no bearing on whether others will or will not share the same fate.

A small number of cases of HD are sporadic, that is, they occur even though there is no family history of the disorder. These cases are thought to be caused by a new genetic mutation—an alteration in the gene that occurs during sperm development and that brings the number of CAG repeats into the range that causes disease.

What are the major effects of the disease?

Early signs of the disease vary greatly from person to person. A common observation is that the earlier the symptoms appear, the faster the disease progresses.

Family members may first notice that the individual experiences mood swings or becomes uncharacteristically irritable, apathetic, passive, depressed, or angry. These symptoms may lessen as the disease progresses or, in some individuals, may continue and include hostile outbursts or deep bouts of depression.

HD may affect the individual's judgment, memory, and other cognitive functions. Early signs might include having trouble driving, learning new things, remembering a fact, answering a question, or making a decision. Some may even display changes in handwriting. As the disease progresses, concentration on intellectual tasks becomes increasingly difficult.

In some individuals, the disease may begin with uncontrolled movements in the fingers, feet, face, or trunk. These movements—which are signs of chorea—often intensify when the person is anxious. HD can also begin with mild clumsiness or problems with balance. Some people develop choreic movements later, after the disease has progressed. They may stumble or appear uncoordinated. Chorea often creates serious problems with walking, increasing the likelihood of falls.

The disease can reach the point where speech is slurred and vital functions, such as swallowing, eating, speaking, and especially walking, continue to decline. Some individuals cannot recognize other family members. Many, however, remain aware of their environment and are able to express emotions.

Some physicians have employed a recently developed Unified HD Rating Scale, or UHDRS, to assess the clinical features, stages, and course of HD. In general, the duration of the illness ranges from 10 to 30 years. The most common causes of death are infection (most often pneumonia), injuries related to a fall, or other complications.

At what age does HD appear?

The rate of disease progression and the age at onset vary from person to person. Adult-onset HD, with its disabling, uncontrolled movements, most often begins in middle age. There are, however, other variations of HD distinguished not just by age at onset but by a distinct array of symptoms. For example, some persons develop the disease as adults, but without chorea. They may appear rigid and move very little, or not at all, a condition called akinesia.

Some individuals develop symptoms of HD when they are very young—before age 20. The terms "early-onset" or "juvenile" HD are often used to describe HD that appears in a young person. A common sign of HD in a younger individual is a rapid decline in school performance. Symptoms can also include subtle changes in handwriting and slight problems with movement, such as slowness, rigidity, tremor, and rapid muscular twitching, called myoclonus. Several of these symptoms are similar to those seen in Parkinson disease, and they differ from the chorea seen in individuals who develop the disease as adults. These young individuals are said to have "akinetic-rigid" HD or the Westphal variant of HD. People with juvenile HD may also have seizures and mental disabilities. The earlier the onset, the faster the disease seems to progress. The disease progresses most rapidly in individuals with juvenile or early-onset HD, and death often follows within 10 years.

Individuals with juvenile HD usually inherit the disease from their fathers. These individuals also tend to have the largest number of CAG repeats. The reason for this may be found in the process of sperm production. Unlike eggs, sperm are produced in the millions. Because DNA is copied millions of times during this process, there is an increased possibility for genetic mistakes to occur. To verify the link between the number of CAG repeats in the HD gene and the age at onset of symptoms, scientists studied a boy who developed HD symptoms at the age of two, one of the youngest and most severe cases ever recorded. They found that he had the largest number of CAG repeats of anyone studied so far—nearly 100. The boy's case was central to the identification of the HD gene and at the same time helped confirm that juveniles with HD have the longest segments of CAG repeats, the only proven correlation between repeat length and age at onset.

A few individuals develop HD after age 55. Diagnosis in these people can be very difficult. The symptoms of HD may be masked by other health problems, or the person may not display the severity of symptoms seen in individuals with HD of earlier onset. These individuals may also show symptoms of depression rather than anger or irritability, or they may retain sharp control over their intellectual functions, such as memory, reasoning, and problem-solving.

There is also a related disorder called senile chorea. Some elderly individuals display the symptoms of HD, especially choreic movements, but do not become demented, have a normal gene, and lack a family history of the disorder. Some scientists believe that a different gene mutation may account for this small number of cases, but this has not been proven.

Is there a treatment for HD?

Physicians may prescribe a number of medications to help control emotional and movement problems associated with HD. It is important to remember however, that while medicines may help keep these clinical symptoms under control, there is no treatment to stop or reverse the course of the disease.

Antipsychotic drugs, such as haloperidol, or other drugs, such as clonazepam, may help to alleviate choreic movements and may also be used to help control hallucinations, delusions, and violent outbursts. Antipsychotic drugs, however, are not prescribed for another form of muscle contraction associated with HD, called dystonia, and may in fact worsen the condition, causing stiffness and rigidity. These medications may also have severe side effects, including sedation, and for that reason should be used in the lowest possible doses.

For depression, physicians may prescribe fluoxetine, sertraline, nortriptyline, or other compounds. Tranquilizers can help control anxiety and lithium may be prescribed to combat pathological excitement and severe mood swings. Medications may also be needed to treat the severe obsessive-compulsive rituals of some individuals with HD.

Most drugs used to treat the symptoms of HD have side effects such as fatigue, restlessness, or hyperexcitability. Sometimes it may be difficult to tell if a particular symptom, such as apathy or incontinence, is a sign of the disease or a reaction to medication.

What kind of care does the individual with HD need?

Although a psychologist or psychiatrist, a genetic counselor, and other specialists may be needed at different stages of the illness, usually the first step in diagnosis and in finding treatment is to see a neurologist. While the family doctor may be able to diagnose HD, and may continue to monitor the individual's status, it is better to consult with a neurologist about management of the varied symptoms.

Problems may arise when individuals try to express complex thoughts in words they can no longer pronounce intelligibly. It can be helpful to repeat words back to the person with HD so that he or she knows that some thoughts are understood. Sometimes people mistakenly assume that if individuals do not talk, they also do not understand. Never isolate individuals by not talking, and try to keep their environment as normal as possible. Speech therapy may improve the individual's ability to communicate.

It is extremely important for the person with HD to maintain physical fitness as much as his or her condition and the course of the disease allows. Individuals who exercise and keep active tend to do better than those who do not. A daily regimen of exercise can help the person feel better physically and mentally. Although their coordination may be poor, individuals should continue walking, with assistance if necessary. Those who want to walk independently should be allowed to do so as long as possible, and careful attention should be given to keeping their environment free of hard, sharp objects. This will help ensure maximal independence while minimizing the risk of injury from a fall. Individuals can also wear special padding during walks to help protect against injury from falls. Some people have found that small weights around the ankles can help stability. Wearing sturdy shoes that fit well can help too, especially shoes without laces that can be slipped on or off easily.

Impaired coordination may make it difficult for people with HD to feed themselves and to swallow. As the disease progresses, persons with HD may even choke. In helping individuals to eat, caregivers should allow plenty of time for meals. Food can be cut into small pieces, softened, or pureed to ease swallowing and prevent choking. While some foods may require the addition of thickeners, other foods may need to be thinned. Dairy products, in particular, tend to increase the secretion of mucus, which in turn increases the risk of choking. Some individuals may benefit from swallowing therapy, which is especially helpful if started before serious problems arise. Suction cups for plates, special tableware designed for people with disabilities, and plastic cups with tops can help prevent spilling. The individual's physician can offer additional advice about diet and about how to handle swallowing difficulties or gastrointestinal problems that might arise, such as incontinence or constipation.

Caregivers should pay attention to proper nutrition so that the individual with HD takes in enough calories to maintain his or her body weight. Sometimes people with HD, who may burn as many as 5,000 calories a day without gaining weight, require five meals a day to take in the necessary number of calories. Physicians may recommend vitamins or other nutritional supplements. In a long-term care institution, staff will need to assist with meals in order to ensure that the individual's special caloric and nutritional requirements are met. Some individuals and their families choose to use a feeding tube; others choose not to.

Individuals with HD are at special risk for dehydration and therefore require large quantities of fluids, especially during hot weather. Bendable straws can make drinking easier for the person. In some cases, water may have to be thickened with commercial additives to give it the consistency of syrup or honey.

Section 38.2

First Drug Treatment Approved for HD Chorea

"FDA Approves First Drug for Treatment of Chorea in
Huntington's Disease," from the U.S. Food and Drug Administration
(FDA, www.fda.gov), August 15, 2008.

The U.S. Food and Drug Administration (FDA) has approved Xenazine (tetrabenazine) for the treatment of chorea in people with Huntington disease. Chorea is the jerky, involuntary movement that occurs in people with this disease.

Xenazine is a new drug and is the first treatment of any kind approved in the United States for any symptom of Huntington disease. Currently there are no other drugs that are FDA-approved to treat chorea.

Serious side effects reported with use of Xenazine include depression and suicidal thoughts and actions. Xenazine should not be used in patients who are actively suicidal or in patients with untreated depression. Concerns about the risk of suicide are heightened in all patients with Huntington disease.

"Xenazine represents hope for patients and families dealing with this difficult disease," said Timothy Coté, M.D., M.P.H., director of FDA's Office of Orphan Products Development. "For the first time, there is a treatment that can help patients with this disease gain some quality of life."

Huntington disease is a rare, inherited neurological disorder affecting about 1 in 10,000 people in the United States. The disease results from genetically programmed degeneration of brain cells. The deterioration causes uncontrolled movements, loss of intellectual faculties, and emotional disturbance. Huntington disease is passed from parent to child through a gene mutation. Each child of a parent with the disease has a 50 percent chance of inheriting the mutation.

About 30,000 people in the United States have Huntington disease and another 200,000 are at risk of developing the condition. Symptoms commonly develop between ages 30 and 50. The disease progresses slowly and a person may live for another 15–20 years after the onset of symptoms.

349

Xenazine decreases the amount of dopamine available to work at relevant synapses in the brain. Dopamine is a chemical that communicates between certain nerve cells in the brain. In patients with Huntington disease, this system is overactive and results in the abnormal movements called chorea. Xenazine decreases the amount of dopamine available to interact with certain nerve cells, thereby decreasing the involuntary movements.

The effectiveness and safety of Xenazine was established primarily in a randomized, double-blind, placebo-controlled multi-center clinical trial. Patients treated with Xenazine had a significant improvement in chorea compared to patients treated with placebo. Other studies provided additional support for this effect.

The most common side effects reported by patients using Xenazine in clinical trials include insomnia, depression, drowsiness, restlessness, and nausea.

While the drug has been shown to decrease chorea in the short-term, it also showed slight worsening in mood, cognition, rigidity, and functional capacity in clinical trials. Health care professionals and family members of patients taking the drug should pay attention to all of the facets of the disease.

Xenazine has been approved with a required Risk Evaluation and Mitigation Strategy (REMS) to ensure that the benefits of the drug outweigh its risks, particularly the risks of depression and suicidal thoughts and actions. REMS is a strategy to manage a known or potential serious risk associated with a drug or biological product.

The REMS includes educational materials for prescribers, pharmacists and patients (and their caregivers) to help minimize adverse effects associated with Xenazine. It also includes a Medication Guide, which informs patients and their caregivers about the risks of depression, suicidal thoughts and actions, and other side effects. The FDA requires that the Medication Guide be handed out with every prescription for the drug dispensed.

Xenazine was granted orphan drug designation by the FDA. A drug is eligible for orphan drug designation if it is intended to treat a disease or condition that affects less than 200,000 people in the United States. A drug is also eligible for orphan drug designation if it is intended to treat a disease or condition that affects more than 200,000 people in the United States, but there is no reasonable expectation that the cost of developing and making available a drug for the disease or condition will be recovered from sales of the drug.

Xenazine is manufactured by Prestwick Pharmaceuticals, Inc., Washington, D.C.

Chapter 39

Movement Disorders during Sleep

Chapter Contents

Section 39.1

Restless Legs Syndrome

Excerpted from "Restless Legs Syndrome Fact Sheet," by the National Institute of Neurological Disorders and Stroke (NINDS, www.ninds.nih .gov), part of the National Institutes of Health, December 11, 2007.

What is restless legs?

Restless legs syndrome (RLS) is a neurological disorder character-ized by unpleasant sensations in the legs and an uncontrollable urge to move when at rest in an effort to relieve these feelings. RLS sen-sations are often described by people as burning, creeping, tugging, or like insects crawling inside the legs. Often called paresthesias (ab-normal sensations) or dysesthesias (unpleasant abnormal sensations), the sensations range in severity from uncomfortable to irritating to painful.

The most distinctive or unusual aspect of the condition is that ly-ing down and trying to relax activates the symptoms. As a result, most people with RLS have difficulty falling asleep and staying asleep. Left untreated, the condition causes exhaustion and daytime fatigue. Many people with RLS report that their job, personal relations, and activi-ties of daily living are strongly affected as a result of their exhaus-tion. They are often unable to concentrate, have impaired memory, or fail to accomplish daily tasks.

Some researchers estimate that RLS affects as many as 12 mil-lion Americans. However, others estimate a much higher occurrence because RLS is thought to be underdiagnosed and, in some cases, misdiagnosed. Some people with RLS will not seek medical attention, believing that they will not be taken seriously, that their symptoms are too mild, or that their condition is not treatable. Some physicians wrongly attribute the symptoms to nervousness, insomnia, stress, arthritis, muscle cramps, or aging.

RLS occurs in both genders, although the incidence may be slightly higher in women. Although the syndrome may begin at any age, even as early as infancy, most patients who are severely affected are middle-aged or older. In addition, the severity of the disorder appears to increase with age. Older patients experience symptoms more frequently and for longer periods of time.

More than 80 percent of people with RLS also experience a more common condition known as periodic limb movement disorder (PLMD). PLMD is characterized by involuntary leg twitching or jerking movements during sleep that typically occur every 10 to 60 seconds, sometimes throughout the night. The symptoms cause repeated awakening and severely disrupted sleep. Unlike RLS, the movements caused by PLMD are involuntary—people have no control over them. Although many patients with RLS also develop PLMD, most people with PLMD do not experience RLS. Like RLS, the cause of PLMD is unknown.

What are common signs and symptoms of restless legs?

As described above, people with RLS feel uncomfortable sensations in their legs, especially when sitting or lying down, accompanied by an irresistible urge to move about. These sensations usually occur deep inside the leg, between the knee and ankle; more rarely, they occur in the feet, thighs, arms, and hands. Although the sensations can occur on just one side of the body, they most often affect both sides.

Because moving the legs (or other affected parts of the body) relieves the discomfort, people with RLS often keep their legs in motion to minimize or prevent the sensations. They may pace the floor, constantly move their legs while sitting, and toss and turn in bed.

Most people find the symptoms to be less noticeable during the day and more pronounced in the evening or at night, especially during the onset of sleep. For many people, the symptoms disappear by early morning, allowing for more refreshing sleep at that time. Other triggering situations are periods of inactivity such as long car trips, sitting in a movie theater, long-distance flights, immobilization in a cast, or relaxation exercises.

The symptoms of RLS vary in severity and duration from person to person. Mild RLS occurs episodically, with only mild disruption of sleep onset, and causes little distress. In moderately severe cases, symptoms occur only once or twice a week but result in significant delay of sleep onset, with some disruption of daytime function. In severe cases of RLS, the symptoms occur more than twice a week and result in burdensome interruption of sleep and impairment of daytime function.

Symptoms may begin at any stage of life, although the disorder is more common with increasing age. Sometimes people will experience spontaneous improvement over a period of weeks or months. Although rare, spontaneous improvement over a period of years also can occur. If these improvements occur, it is usually during the early stages of the disorder. In general, however, symptoms become more severe over time.

People who have both RLS and an associated condition tend to develop more severe symptoms rapidly. In contrast, those whose RLS is not related to any other medical condition and whose onset is at an early age show a very slow progression of the disorder and many years may pass before symptoms occur regularly.

What causes restless legs syndrome?

In most cases, the cause of RLS is unknown (referred to as idiopathic). A family history of the condition is seen in approximately 50 percent of such cases, suggesting a genetic form of the disorder. People with familial RLS tend to be younger when symptoms start and have a slower progression of the condition.

In other cases, RLS appears to be related to the following factors or conditions, although researchers do not yet know if these factors actually cause RLS.

- People with low iron levels or anemia may be prone to developing RLS. Once iron levels or anemia is corrected, patients may see a reduction in symptoms.

- Chronic diseases such as kidney failure, diabetes, Parkinson disease, and peripheral neuropathy are associated with RLS. Treating the underlying condition often provides relief from RLS symptoms.

- Some pregnant women experience RLS, especially in their last trimester. For most of these women, symptoms usually disappear within 4 weeks after delivery.

- Certain medications—such as antinausea drugs (prochlorperazine or metoclopramide), antiseizure drugs (phenytoin or droperidol), antipsychotic drugs (haloperidol or phenothiazine derivatives), and some cold and allergy medications—may aggravate symptoms. Patients can talk with their physicians about the possibility of changing medications.

Researchers also have found that caffeine, alcohol, and tobacco may aggravate or trigger symptoms in patients who are predisposed to develop RLS. Some studies have shown that a reduction or complete elimination of such substances may relieve symptoms, although it remains unclear whether elimination of such substances can prevent RLS symptoms from occurring at all.

How is restless legs syndrome diagnosed?

Currently, there is no single diagnostic test for RLS. The disorder is diagnosed clinically by evaluating the patient's history and symptoms. Despite a clear description of clinical features, the condition is often misdiagnosed or underdiagnosed. In 1995, the International Restless Legs Syndrome Study Group identified four basic criteria for diagnosing RLS: (1) a desire to move the limbs, often associated with paresthesias or dysesthesias, (2) symptoms that are worse or present only during rest and are partially or temporarily relieved by activity, (3) motor restlessness, and (4) nocturnal worsening of symptoms. Although about 80 percent of those with RLS also experience PLMD, it is not necessary for a diagnosis of RLS. In more severe cases, patients may experience dyskinesia (uncontrolled, often continuous movements) while awake, and some experience symptoms in one or both of their arms as well as their legs. Most people with RLS have sleep disturbances, largely because of the limb discomfort and jerking. The result is excessive daytime sleepiness and fatigue.

Despite these efforts to establish standard criteria, the clinical diagnosis of RLS is difficult to make. Physicians must rely largely on patients' descriptions of symptoms and information from their medical history, including past medical problems, family history, and current medications. Patients may be asked about frequency, duration, and intensity of symptoms as well as their tendency toward daytime sleep patterns and sleepiness, disturbance of sleep, or daytime function. If a patient's history is suggestive of RLS, laboratory tests may be performed to rule out other conditions and support the diagnosis of RLS. Blood tests to exclude anemia, decreased iron stores, diabetes, and renal dysfunction should be performed. Electromyography and nerve conduction studies may also be recommended to measure electrical activity in muscles and nerves, and Doppler sonography may be used to evaluate muscle activity in the legs. Such tests can document any accompanying damage or disease in nerves and nerve roots (such as peripheral neuropathy and radiculopathy) or other leg-related movement disorders. Negative results from tests may indicate that the diagnosis is RLS. In some cases, sleep studies such as polysomnography (a test that records the patient's brain waves, heartbeat, and breathing during an entire night) are undertaken to identify the presence of PLMD.

The diagnosis is especially difficult with children because the physician relies heavily on the patient's explanations of symptoms, which, given the nature of the symptoms of RLS, can be difficult for a child to describe. The syndrome can sometimes be misdiagnosed as "growing pains" or attention deficit disorder.

How is restless legs syndrome treated?

Although movement brings relief to those with RLS, it is generally only temporary. However, RLS can be controlled by finding any possible underlying disorder. Often, treating the associated medical condition, such as peripheral neuropathy or diabetes, will alleviate many symptoms. For patients with idiopathic RLS, treatment is directed toward relieving symptoms.

For those with mild to moderate symptoms, prevention is key, and many physicians suggest certain lifestyle changes and activities to reduce or eliminate symptoms. Decreased use of caffeine, alcohol, and tobacco may provide some relief. Physicians may suggest that certain individuals take supplements to correct deficiencies in iron, folate, and magnesium. Studies also have shown that maintaining a regular sleep pattern can reduce symptoms. Some individuals, finding that RLS symptoms are minimized in the early morning, change their sleep patterns. Others have found that a program of regular moderate exercise helps them sleep better; on the other hand, excessive exercise has been reported by some patients to aggravate RLS symptoms. Taking a hot bath, massaging the legs, or using a heating pad or ice pack can help relieve symptoms in some patients. Although many patients find some relief with such measures, rarely do these efforts completely eliminate symptoms.

Physicians also may suggest a variety of medications to treat RLS. Generally, physicians choose from dopaminergics, benzodiazepines (central nervous system depressants), opioids, and anticonvulsants. Dopaminergic agents, largely used to treat Parkinson disease, have been shown to reduce RLS symptoms and PLMD and are considered the initial treatment of choice. Good short-term results of treatment with levodopa plus carbidopa have been reported, although most patients eventually will develop augmentation, meaning that symptoms are reduced at night but begin to develop earlier in the day than usual. Dopamine agonists such as pergolide mesylate, pramipexole, and ropinirole hydrochloride may be effective in some patients and are less likely to cause augmentation.

In 2005, ropinirole became the only drug approved by the U.S. Food and Drug Administration specifically for the treatment of moderate to severe RLS. The drug was first approved in 1997 for patients with Parkinson disease.

Benzodiazepines (such as clonazepam and diazepam) may be prescribed for patients who have mild or intermittent symptoms. These drugs help patients obtain a more restful sleep but they do not fully alleviate RLS symptoms and can cause daytime sleepiness. Because these depressants also may induce or aggravate sleep apnea in some cases, they should not be used in people with this condition.

For more severe symptoms, opioids such as codeine, propoxyphene, or oxycodone may be prescribed for their ability to induce relaxation and diminish pain. Side effects include dizziness, nausea, vomiting, and the risk of addiction.

Anticonvulsants such as carbamazepine and gabapentin are also useful for some patients, as they decrease the sensory disturbances (creeping and crawling sensations). Dizziness, fatigue, and sleepiness are among the possible side effects.

Unfortunately, no one drug is effective for everyone with RLS. What may be helpful to one individual may actually worsen symptoms for another. In addition, medications taken regularly may lose their effect, making it necessary to change medications periodically.

What is the prognosis of people with restless legs?

RLS is generally a lifelong condition for which there is no cure. Symptoms may gradually worsen with age, though more slowly for those with the idiopathic form of RLS than for patients who also suffer from an associated medical condition. Nevertheless, current therapies can control the disorder, minimizing symptoms and increasing periods of restful sleep. In addition, some patients have remissions, periods in which symptoms decrease or disappear for days, weeks, or months, although symptoms usually eventually reappear. A diagnosis of RLS does not indicate the onset of another neurological disease.

Section 39.2

Periodic Limb Movement Disorder

What is periodic limb movement disorder (PLMD)?

Periodic limb movement disorder (PLMD) is a condition that was formerly called sleep myoclonus or nocturnal myoclonus. It is described as repetitive limb movements that occur during sleep and cause sleep disruption. The limb movements usually involve the lower extremities, consisting of extension of the big toe and flexion of the ankle, the knee, and the hip. In some patients, the limb movements can occur in the upper extremities as well.

The limb movements occur most frequently in light non-REM sleep. The repetitive movements are separated by fairly regular intervals of 5 to 90 seconds. There can be significant night-to-night variability to the frequency of limb movements.

What causes PLMD?

The exact cause of PLMD is unknown. However, several medications are known to make PLMD worse. These medications include some antidepressants, antihistamines, and some antipsychotics.

Many individuals have periodic limb movements in sleep (PLMS). This is observed in about 80 percent of patients with restless legs syndrome (RLS). PLMS can occur in over 30 percent of people aged 65 and older and can be asymptomatic. PLMS are very common in patients with narcolepsy, REM behavior disorder, and Parkinson's disease.

True PLMD—the diagnosis of which requires periodic limb movements in sleep that disrupt sleep and are not accounted for by another primary sleep disorder including RLS—is uncommon.

What are some of the symptoms of PLMD?

Most patients are actually not aware of the involuntary limb movements. The limb jerks are more often reported by bed partners. Patients experience frequent awakenings from sleep, non-restorative sleep, daytime fatigue, and/or daytime sleepiness.

How do I know if I have PLMD?

The diagnosis is based on the clinical history as well as an overnight polysomnogram (PSG). This is a test that records sleep and the bioelectrical signals coming from the body during sleep. A thorough neurological examination should be performed. Respiratory monitoring during the PSG allows one to rule out the presence of sleep disordered breathing as a cause for the disrupted sleep and excessive muscle activity. Occasionally, additional sleep laboratory testing is useful. Blood work may be ordered to check on iron status, folic acid, vitamin B12, thyroid function, and magnesium levels.

Who gets PLMD?

PLMD has been less extensively studied than RLS. The exact prevalence is unknown. It can occur at any age; however, the prevalence does increase with increasing age. Unlike RLS, PLMD does not appear to be related to gender.

As with RLS, some medical conditions are associated with PLMD. These include uremia, diabetes, iron deficiency, and spinal cord injury.

How is PLMD treated?

First, certain products and medications should be avoided. Caffeine often intensifies PLMD symptoms. Caffeine-containing products such as chocolate, coffee, tea, and soft drinks should be avoided. Also, many antidepressants can cause a worsening of PLMD in many patients and should be reviewed, discussed, and replaced by your doctor.

Generally, there are several classes of drugs that are used to treat PLMD. These include the Parkinson's disease drugs, anticonvulsant medications, benzodiazepines, and narcotics. Current treatment recommendations consider the anti-Parkinson's medications as a first line of defense. Medical treatment of PLMD often significantly reduces or eliminates the symptoms of these disorders. There is no cure for PLMD and medical treatment must be continued to provide relief.

Chapter 40

Neuroacanthocytosis and Neurodegeneration

Chapter Contents

Section 40.1

Neuroacanthocytosis

"Neuroacanthocytosis Information Page," from the National Institute
of Neurological Disorders and Stroke (NINDS, www.ninds.nih.gov),
part of the National Institutes of Health, February 14, 2007.

What is neuroacanthocytosis?

Neuroacanthocytosis is a rare movement disorder marked by progressive muscle weakness and atrophy, progressive cognitive loss, chorea (involuntary twisting movements of the body), and acanthocytosis (spiked red blood cells associated with several inherited neurological disorders). Other symptoms include facial tics, uncontrolled muscle movement, instability when walking, seizures, biting of the tongue and lips, and changes in personality, comprehension, and judgment. The disorder is due to degeneration of the basal ganglia (a part of the brain that helps control movement) and loss of neurons in the brain and spinal cord. Neuroacanthocytosis has adult and childhood varieties. In adults, onset of classic symptoms usually begins between ages 20 and 50, while in children onset is typically seen in adolescence (but may occur earlier). Adult varieties can involve the heart and immune system. Neuroacanthocytosis is typically an inherited autosomal recessive disorder and is more common in males than in females. Some types of neuroacanthocytosis have been found to be caused by specific gene defects. Parkinsonism has been associated with the disorder in some patients.

Is there any treatment?

Treatment is symptomatic and supportive. Antipsychotic drugs that block dopamine, such as haloperidol, can provide temporary relief from tics and chorea. Drugs used to decrease anxiety, such as diazepam and benzodiazepine, can also decrease movement disorders, which are often made worse by associated stress. Injections of botulinum toxin can relax muscles and reduce unintentional movement. Other drug therapy may include anticonvulsants and antidepressants.

Proper nutrition is required. A feeding tube may be needed for some patients as the disorder progresses. Speech therapy and physical therapy may provide some relief to select patients.

What is the prognosis?

Neuroacanthocytosis is a progressive disease. It is often fatal, generally the result of symptoms that contribute to pneumonia, cardiomyopathy, eating problems, or other complications. Life expectancy following onset of severe symptoms is typically 5–10 years. However, life span may be near normal for patients with no prominent neurologic or cardiac complications.

What research is being done?

The NINDS supports research on disorders such as neuroacanthocytosis, aimed at increasing scientific understanding of the disorders and finding ways to prevent and treat them. The molecular changes responsible for some types of neuroacanthocytosis have recently been identified. Researchers are examining the role of the basal ganglia in neuroacanthocytosis and hope to correlate the specific genetic abnormalities with the clinical features of the disease. Other research is aimed at identifying possible causes of sudden death related to heart muscle abnormality in patients with neuroacanthocytosis.

Section 40.2

Neurodegeneration with Brain Iron Accumulation

"Neurodegeneration with Brain Iron Accumulation Information Page," from the National Institute of Neurological Disorders and Stroke (NINDS, www.ninds.nih.gov), part of the National Institutes of Health, February 14, 2007.

What is neurodegeneration with brain iron accumulation?

Neurodegeneration with brain iron accumulation (NBIA) is a rare, inherited, neurological movement disorder characterized by progressive degeneration of the nervous system. Symptoms, which vary greatly among patients and usually develop during childhood, may include slow writhing, distorting muscle contractions of the limbs, face, or trunk, choreoathetosis (involuntary, purposeless jerky muscle movements), muscle rigidity (uncontrolled tightness of the muscles), spasticity (sudden, involuntary muscle spasms), ataxia (inability to coordinate movements), confusion, disorientation, seizures, stupor, and dementia. Other less common symptoms may include painful muscle spasms, dysphasia (difficulty speaking), mental retardation, facial grimacing, dysarthria (poorly articulated speech), and visual impairment.

Is there any treatment?

There is no cure for NBIA, nor is there a standard course of treatment. Treatment is symptomatic and supportive, and may include physical or occupational therapy, exercise physiology, and/or speech pathology.

What is the prognosis?

Most patients experience periods of rapid deterioration lasting 1–2 months, with relatively stable periods in between. The rate of progression correlates with the age at onset, meaning that children with early symptoms tend to fare more poorly. For those with early onset, dystonia and spasticity can eventually limit the ability to walk, usually leading to use of a wheelchair by the midteens.

Life expectancy is variable, although premature death does occur in NBIA. Premature death usually occurs secondary to dystonia and impaired swallowing, which can lead to poor nutrition or aspiration pneumonia. With improved medical care, however, a greater number of affected individuals reach adulthood. For those with atypical, late-onset NBIA, many are diagnosed as adults and live well into adulthood.

Chapter 41

Spastic Paraplegia

What is hereditary spastic paraplegia (HSP)?

Hereditary spastic paraplegia (HSP) is a group of rare, inherited neurological disorders. Their primary symptoms are progressive spasticity and weakness of the leg and hip muscles. Researchers estimate that some 30 different types of HSP exist; the genetic causes are known for eleven. The HSP incidence rate in the United States is 20,000 people.

The condition is characterized by insidiously progressive lower extremity weakness and spasticity. HSP is classified as uncomplicated or pure if neurological impairment is limited to the lower body. HSP is classified as complicated or complex if other systems are involved or if there are other neurological findings such as seizures, dementia, amyotrophy, extrapyramidal disturbance, or peripheral neuropathy in the absence of other disorders such as diabetes mellitus.

Many different names are used for HSP. The most common are hereditary spastic paraplegia (or paraparesis), familial spastic paraparesis (or paraplegia), and Strümpell-Lorrain disease. Others are spastic paraplegia, hereditary Charcot disease, spastic spinal paralysis, diplegia spinalis progressiva, French Settlement Disease, Troyer syndrome, and Silver syndrome.

The disorder was first identified in the late 1800s by A. Strümpell, a neurologist in Heidelberg, Germany. He observed two brothers and

"Hereditary Spastic Paraplegia: General Information" © 2008 Spastic Paraplegia Foundation. Reprinted with permission. For additional information, visit www.sp-foundation.org.

their father, all of whom had gait disorders and spasticity in their legs. After the death of the brothers, Strümpell showed through autopsy the degeneration of the nerve fibers leading through the spinal cord. HSP was originally named after Strümpell, and later after two Frenchmen, Maurice Lorrain and Jean M. Charcot, who provided more information.

What is (apparently sporadic) spastic paraplegia?

Many individuals with all the signs and symptoms of HSP do not appear to have similarly affected family members. Without proof of a hereditary link, some neurologists call the condition spastic paraplegia or apparently sporadic spastic paraplegia. Other clinicians may diagnose the same condition as primary lateral sclerosis [PLS], which mimics HSP in how it affects the lower body. However, current researcher indicates that PLS eventually affects the arms and speech and swallowing muscles as well as the leg muscles.

There are many reasons why someone with HSP may not have a family history. Recessive and X-linked forms skip generations, which means the disorder may pass silently for generations and then suddenly appear. In addition, the age of onset, progression rate, and severity vary widely so that the disease could have gone undiagnosed in previous generations or an affected individual may have died before symptom onset. Mistaken parentage or new genetic mutations are also possible.

What are the symptoms?

The hallmark of HSP is progressive difficulty walking due to increasingly weak and stiff (spastic) muscles. Symptoms appear in most people between the second and fourth decade of life, but they can start at any age.

Initial symptoms are typically difficulty with balance, stubbing the toe, or stumbling. Changes begin so gradually that other people often notice the change first. As the disease progresses, canes, walkers, and eventually wheelchairs may become needed, although some people never require assistive devices.

Other common symptoms of HSP are urinary urgency and frequency, hyperactive reflexes, difficulty with balance, clonus, Babinski sign, diminished vibration sense in the feet, muscle spasms, and congenital foot problems such as pes cavus (high arched foot). Some people may experience problems with their arms or fine motor control of their fingers but for most people, this is not significant.

Most people with HSP have uncomplicated HSP. There are also rare, complicated forms, which have additional symptoms, such as peripheral neuropathy, ichthyoids (a skin disorder) epilepsy, ataxia, optic neuropathy, retinopathy, dementia, mental retardation, deafness, or problems with speech, swallowing, or breathing. These symptoms may have other causes though, unrelated to HSP. For example, someone with uncomplicated HSP may have peripheral neuropathy caused by diabetes.

Why are my symptoms different from others in my family?

As noted above, the severity of symptoms and age of onset can vary widely, even within the same family. One reason is that HSP is a group of genetically different disorders, not a single disorder. Some differences may be due to genetic mutations. A child may show symptoms before a parent and it's possible for some family members to have very mild symptoms while others have more severe symptoms. This may be due to other genes, environment, nutrition, general health, or factors not yet understood.

In some families, symptoms tend to start at younger ages with each generation. Although rare, HSP sometimes shows incomplete penetrance. This means that occasionally, an individual may have the gene mutation, but for unknown reasons never develop symptoms of HSP. Such individuals can still pass HSP to their children.

How does HSP cause symptoms?

HSP is caused by degeneration of the upper motor neurons in the brain and spinal cord. Upper motor neurons control voluntary movement.

The cell bodies of these neurons are located in the motor cortex area of the brain. They have long, hair-like processes called axons that travel to the brainstem and down the spinal cord. Axons relay the messages to move to lower motor neurons that are located all along the brainstem and spinal cord. Lower motor neurons then carry the messages out to the muscles.

When upper motor neurons degenerate, the correct messages cannot reach the lower motor neurons, and the lower motor neurons cannot transmit the correct messages to the muscles. As the degeneration continues, spasticity and weakness increase. The legs are affected because degeneration occurs primarily at the ends of the longest nerves in the spinal cord, which control the legs. In some cases, the upper body can be minimally affected as well, leading to problems with the arms or speech and swallowing muscles.

How severe will my symptoms get?

There is no way to predict rate of progression or severity of symptoms. Generally, once symptoms begin, progression continues slowly throughout life. For some childhood-onset forms, symptoms become apparent, gradually worsen during childhood, and then stabilize after adolescence. HSP rarely results in complete loss of lower limb mobility.

How is HSP diagnosed?

HSP is diagnosed via a careful clinical examination, by excluding other disorders that cause spasticity and weakness in the legs, and by an observation period to see if other symptoms develop that indicate another condition, such as PLS. Disorders that can be ruled out with testing are ALS [amyotrophic lateral sclerosis], tropical spastic paraparesis (TSP), vitamin deficiencies (B12 or E), thoracic spine herniated disks, and spinal cord tumors or injuries and multiple sclerosis. HSP can resemble cerebral palsy, however, HSP is degenerative and thereby causes increasing spasticity and weakness of the muscles. Two other disorders with spastic paraplegia symptoms termed lathyrism and konzo are caused by toxins in the plants *Lathyrus sativus* and cassava.

HSP is hereditary, and examining family history is important in diagnosing HSP. However, many individuals with all the signs and symptoms of HSP do not have a family history.

What genetic testing is available?

Athena Diagnostics offers testing for five different types of HSP out of the 30 or more different forms of HSP. As more genes are discovered, it is hopeful that such information will lead to greater availability of testing.

Genetic counselors can be found at many major medical centers or by contacting the National Society of Genetic Counselors at 610-872-7608. Gene tests can be used for prenatal testing.

What is the treatment?

No treatments are currently available to prevent, stop, or reverse HSP. Treatment is focused on symptom relief, such as medication to reduce spasticity; physical therapy, and exercise to help maintain flexibility, strength, and range of motion; assistive devices and communications aids; supportive therapy and other modalities.

What is the life expectancy?

Life expectancy is normal. However, complications arising from falls or immobility caused by the symptoms of HSP may inadvertently shorten a person's life.

What is the risk of getting HSP?

There are some thirty different forms of HSP, with three different modes of inheritance: autosomal dominant, autosomal recessive, and X-linked. Each mode has a different risk factor, which ranges from almost none to 50%.

What other conditions cause spasticity and weakness of muscles?

Muscle spasticity and weakness can also be caused by other conditions including (but not limited to) primary lateral sclerosis, spinal cord injury or tumors, cerebral palsy, multiple sclerosis, amyotrophic lateral sclerosis, vitamin absorption, and thoracic spine herniated disks.

There is a virus-caused disease called tropical spastic paraparesis and conditions called lathyrism and konzo caused by toxins in the plants *Lathyrus sativus* and cassava that also cause muscle spasticity and weakness.

Does stress affect symptoms?

Many people find the tightness in their muscles worsens when they are angry, stressed, or upset. This may make it more difficult to walk and speak. It is unknown exactly how emotions affect muscle tone, but it may involve adrenalin levels. Most people also report increased stiffness in cold weather.

Is depression normal?

Periods of feeling down about having HSP are normal and expected. It is not uncommon for people to also experience periods of clinical depression.

Do people with HSP experience memory loss?

Memory disturbance has been reported in some individuals with HSP due to spastin gene mutations. In general, it was mild.

Before attributing memory disturbance to HSP, it is important to consider other causes: stress, anxiety, depression, lack of sleep, medications (including baclofen), and other health conditions including vitamin B12 deficiency.

If memory disturbance is significant, a cause of concern, or worsening, it would be important to discuss this with your primary physician and neurologist.

Are foot problems common?

Yes. Here are a few examples:

- **High arched feet (pes cavus):** High arches occur because there is more weakness in the foot muscles that extend the foot backward and flatten the arch than in the muscles that flex the foot downward.

- **Shortened Achilles tendons:** Achilles tendons are often short, and generally shorten further as HSP progresses.

- **Jumping feet (clonus):** Clonus is an uncontrollable, repetitive jerking of muscles that makes the foot jump rapidly up and down. It occurs when the foot is in a position that causes a disruption of the signals from the brain, leading to an automatic stretch reflex.

- **Hammer toes or bunions:** These may occur due to imbalances in the strength and tone of muscles that maintain proper alignment of joints in the feet.

- **Cold feet and/or foot swelling:** This is most likely caused by poor circulation. Normally, muscle contractions in the legs help pump blood from the legs back to the heart. If the muscles are weakened, or if the person is relatively inactive, the blood flow from the legs may be decreased, and fluids may accumulate.

This can cause swelling, or a sensation of cold feet.

Can my arms be affected?

Some people may experience problems with their arms or fine motor control of their fingers. The degeneration in nerves that supply the arms is mild compared to that which occurs in the nerves that supply the legs. For most people, this is not significant.

Can HSP affect sexual function?

The short answer appears to be yes, although it is important to remember that sexual desire and/or function can be affected by many other factors such as age, stress, depression, fatigue, medical disorders, or medications.

Some people report that stiffness, spasms, and cramps that are part of HSP may either inhibit (or intensify) orgasm, or that orgasm may bring on leg stiffness, spasms, or clonus. Stiffness of the legs or arms may cause difficulty using certain positions for intercourse.

Is HSP an ataxia?

No. The group of disorders known as ataxias (such as Friedreich ataxia) are spino-cerebellar disorders in which there is a disturbance either in the part of the brain known as the cerebellum or in the connections to it. HSP does not involve the cerebellum. Ataxias can be hereditary or sporadic.

The term "ataxia" means without coordination, and can also refer to a symptom in which there is a lack of muscle control resulting in a jerky or unsteady movement. People with HSP may have incoordination as a symptom. This does not mean they have ataxia.

Can I donate blood?

HSP cannot be passed to others through donation of blood. There is no medical reason why a person with HSP cannot donate blood.

When was HSP identified?

In the late 1800s, A. Strümpell, a neurologist in Heidelberg, Germany, described this disorder. He observed two brothers and their father, who had gait disorders and spasticity in their legs. After the death of the brothers, Strümpell was able to show through autopsy the degeneration of the nerve fibers leading through the spinal cord. The disorder was originally named after Strümpell, and after two Frenchmen who later provided more information about the disorder, Lorrain and Charcot.

Is HSP more prevalent in certain ethnic groups?

There is no evidence that HSP is more prevalent in one ethnic group than another.

373

Chapter 42

Tourette Syndrome

What is Tourette syndrome?

Tourette syndrome (TS) is a neurological disorder characterized by repetitive, stereotyped, involuntary movements and vocalizations called tics. The disorder is named for Dr. Georges Gilles de la Tourette, the pioneering French neurologist who in 1885 first described the condition in an 86-year-old French noblewoman.

The early symptoms of TS are almost always noticed first in childhood, with the average onset between the ages of 7 and 10 years. TS occurs in people from all ethnic groups; males are affected about three to four times more often than females. It is estimated that 200,000 Americans have the most severe form of TS, and as many as one in 100 exhibit milder and less complex symptoms such as chronic motor or vocal tics or transient tics of childhood. Although TS can be a chronic condition with symptoms lasting a lifetime, most people with the condition experience their worst symptoms in their early teens, with improvement occurring in the late teens and continuing into adulthood.

What are the symptoms?

Tics are classified as either simple or complex. Simple motor tics are sudden, brief, repetitive movements that involve a limited number of

From "Tourette Syndrome Fact Sheet," by the National Institute of Neurological Disorders and Stroke (NINDS, www.ninds.nih.gov), part of the National Institutes of Health, June 2008.

375

muscle groups. Some of the more common simple tics include eye blinking and other vision irregularities, facial grimacing, shoulder shrugging, and head or shoulder jerking. Simple vocalizations might include repetitive throat-clearing, sniffing, or grunting sounds. Complex tics are distinct, coordinated patterns of movements involving several muscle groups. Complex motor tics might include facial grimacing combined with a head twist and a shoulder shrug. Other complex motor tics may actually appear purposeful, including sniffing or touching objects, hopping, jumping, bending, or twisting. Simple vocal tics may include throat-clearing, sniffing/snorting, grunting, or barking. More complex vocal tics include words or phrases. Perhaps the most dramatic and disabling tics include motor movements that result in self-harm such as punching oneself in the face or vocal tics including coprolalia (uttering swear words) or echolalia (repeating the words or phrases of others). Some tics are preceded by an urge or sensation in the affected muscle group, commonly called a premonitory urge. Some with TS will describe a need to complete a tic in a certain way or a certain number of times in order to relieve the urge or decrease the sensation.

Tics are often worse with excitement or anxiety and better during calm, focused activities. Certain physical experiences can trigger or worsen tics, for example tight collars may trigger neck tics, or hearing another person sniff or throat-clear may trigger similar sounds. Tics do not go away during sleep but are often significantly diminished.

What is the course of TS?

Tics come and go over time, varying in type, frequency, location, and severity. The first symptoms usually occur in the head and neck area and may progress to include muscles of the trunk and extremities. Motor tics generally precede the development of vocal tics and simple tics often precede complex tics. Most patients experience peak tic severity before the mid-teen years with improvement for the majority of patients in the late teen years and early adulthood. Approximately 10 percent of those affected have a progressive or disabling course that lasts into adulthood.

Can people with TS control their tics?

Although the symptoms of TS are involuntary, some people can sometimes suppress, camouflage, or otherwise manage their tics in an effort to minimize their impact on functioning. However, people

with TS often report a substantial buildup in tension when suppressing their tics to the point where they feel that the tic must be expressed. Tics in response to an environmental trigger can appear to
be voluntary or purposeful but are not.

What causes TS?

Although the cause of TS is unknown, current research points to
abnormalities in certain brain regions (including the basal ganglia,
frontal lobes, and cortex), the circuits that interconnect these regions,
and the neurotransmitters (dopamine, serotonin, and norepinephrine)
responsible for communication among nerve cells. Given the often complex presentation of TS, the cause of the disorder is likely to be equally
complex.

What disorders are associated with TS?

Many with TS experience additional neurobehavioral problems
including inattention; hyperactivity and impulsivity (attention deficit hyperactivity disorder—ADHD); and related problems with reading, writing, and arithmetic; and obsessive-compulsive symptoms such
as intrusive thoughts/worries and repetitive behaviors. For example,
worries about dirt and germs may be associated with repetitive hand-
washing, and concerns about bad things happening may be associated
with ritualistic behaviors such as counting, repeating, or ordering and
arranging. People with TS have also reported problems with depression or anxiety disorders, as well as other difficulties with living, that
may or may not be directly related to TS. Given the range of potential complications, people with TS are best served by receiving medical care that provides a comprehensive treatment plan.

How is TS diagnosed?

TS is a diagnosis that doctors make after verifying that the patient has had both motor and vocal tics for at least 1 year. The exist-
ence of other neurological or psychiatric conditions can also help
doctors arrive at a diagnosis. Common tics are not often misdiagnosed
by knowledgeable clinicians. But atypical symptoms or atypical presentation (for example, onset of symptoms in adulthood) may require
specific specialty expertise for diagnosis. There are no blood or laboratory tests needed for diagnosis, but neuroimaging studies, such as
magnetic resonance imaging (MRI), computerized tomography (CT),

and electroencephalogram (EEG) scans, or certain blood tests may be used to rule out other conditions that might be confused with TS.

It is not uncommon for patients to obtain a formal diagnosis of TS only after symptoms have been present for some time. The reasons for this are many. For families and physicians unfamiliar with TS, mild and even moderate tic symptoms may be considered inconsequential, part of a developmental phase, or the result of another condition. For example, parents may think that eye blinking is related to vision problems or that sniffing is related to seasonal allergies. Many patients are self-diagnosed after they, their parents, other relatives, or friends read or hear about TS from others.

How is TS treated?

Because tic symptoms do not often cause impairment, the majority of people with TS require no medication for tic suppression. However, effective medications are available for those whose symptoms interfere with functioning. Neuroleptics are the most consistently useful medications for tic suppression; a number are available but some are more effective than others (for example, haloperidol and pimozide). Unfortunately, there is no one medication that is helpful to all people with TS, nor does any medication completely eliminate symptoms. In addition, all medications have side effects. Most neuroleptic side effects can be managed by initiating treatment slowly and reducing the dose when side effects occur. The most common side effects of neuroleptics include sedation, weight gain, and cognitive dulling. Neurological side effects such as tremor, dystonic reactions (twisting movements or postures), parkinsonian-like symptoms, and other dyskinetic (involuntary) movements are less common and are readily managed with dose reduction. Discontinuing neuroleptics after long-term use must be done slowly to avoid rebound increases in tics and withdrawal dyskinesias. One form of withdrawal dyskinesia called tardive dyskinesia is a movement disorder distinct from TS that may result from the chronic use of neuroleptics. The risk of this side effect can be reduced by using lower doses of neuroleptics for shorter periods of time.

Other medications may also be useful for reducing tic severity, but most have not been as extensively studied or shown to be as consistently useful as neuroleptics. Additional medications with demonstrated efficacy include alpha-adrenergic agonists such as clonidine and guanfacine. These medications are used primarily for hypertension but are also used in the treatment of tics. The most common side effect from these medications that precludes their use is sedation.

Effective medications are also available to treat some of the associated neurobehavioral disorders that can occur in patients with TS. Recent research shows that stimulant medications such as methylphenidate and dextroamphetamine can lessen ADHD symptoms in people with TS without causing tics to become more severe. However, the product labeling for stimulants currently contraindicates the use of these drugs in children with tics/TS and those with a family history of tics. Scientists hope that future studies will include a thorough discussion of the risks and benefits of stimulants in those with TS or a family history of TS and will clarify this issue. For obsessive-compulsive symptoms that significantly disrupt daily functioning, the serotonin reuptake inhibitors (clomipramine, fluoxetine, fluvoxamine, paroxetine, and sertraline) have been proven effective in some patients.

Psychotherapy may also be helpful. Although psychological problems do not cause TS, such problems may result from TS. Psychotherapy can help the person with TS better cope with the disorder and deal with the secondary social and emotional problems that sometimes occur. More recently, specific behavioral treatments that include awareness training and competing response training, such as voluntarily moving in response to a premonitory urge, have shown effectiveness in small controlled trials. Larger and more definitive NIH-funded studies are underway.

Is TS inherited?

Evidence from twin and family studies suggests that TS is an inherited disorder. Although early family studies suggested an autosomal dominant mode of inheritance (an autosomal dominant disorder is one in which only one copy of the defective gene, inherited from one parent, is necessary to produce the disorder), more recent studies suggest that the pattern of inheritance is much more complex. Although there may be a few genes with substantial effects, it is also possible that many genes with smaller effects and environmental factors may play a role in the development of TS. Genetic studies also suggest that some forms of ADHD and OCD are genetically related to TS, but there is less evidence for a genetic relationship between TS and other neurobehavioral problems that commonly co-occur with TS. It is important for families to understand that genetic predisposition may not necessarily result in full-blown TS; instead, it may express itself as a milder tic disorder or as obsessive-compulsive behaviors. It is also possible that the gene-carrying offspring will not develop any TS symptoms.

379

The sex of the person also plays an important role in TS gene expression. At-risk males are more likely to have tics and at-risk females are more likely to have obsessive-compulsive symptoms.

People with TS may have genetic risks for other neurobehavioral disorders such as depression or substance abuse. Genetic counseling of individuals with TS should include a full review of all potentially hereditary conditions in the family.

What is the prognosis?

Although there is no cure for TS, the condition in many individuals improves in the late teens and early 20s. As a result, some may actually become symptom-free or no longer need medication for tic suppression. Although the disorder is generally lifelong and chronic, it is not a degenerative condition. Individuals with TS have a normal life expectancy. TS does not impair intelligence. Although tic symptoms tend to decrease with age, it is possible that neurobehavioral disorders such as depression, panic attacks, mood swings, and antisocial behaviors can persist and cause impairment in adult life.

What is the best educational setting for children with TS?

Although students with TS often function well in the regular classroom, ADHD, learning disabilities, obsessive-compulsive symptoms, and frequent tics can greatly interfere with academic performance or social adjustment. After a comprehensive assessment, students should be placed in an educational setting that meets their individual needs. Students may require tutoring, smaller or special classes, and in some cases special schools.

All students with TS need a tolerant and compassionate setting that both encourages them to work to their full potential and is flexible enough to accommodate their special needs. This setting may include a private study area, exams outside the regular classroom, or even oral exams when the child's symptoms interfere with his or her ability to write. Untimed testing reduces stress for students with TS.

What research is being done?

Within the federal government, the leading supporter of research on TS and other neurological disorders is the National Institute of Neurological Disorders and Stroke (NINDS). The NINDS, a part of the National Institutes of Health (NIH), is responsible for supporting and conducting research on the brain and central nervous system.

NINDS sponsors research on TS both in its laboratories at the NIH and through grants to major medical institutions across the country. The National Institute of Mental Health, the National Center for Research Resources, the National Institute of Child Health and Human Development, the National Institute on Drug Abuse, and the National Institute on Deafness and Other Communication Disorders also support research of relevance to TS. And another component of the Department of Health and Human Services, the Centers for Disease Control and Prevention, funds professional education programs as well as TS research.

Knowledge about TS comes from studies across a number of medical and scientific disciplines, including genetics, neuroimaging, neuropathology, clinical trials (medication and non-medication), epidemiology, neurophysiology, neuroimmunology, and descriptive/diagnostic clinical science.

Genetic studies: Currently, NIH-funded investigators are conducting a variety of large-scale genetic studies. Rapid advances in the technology of gene finding will allow for genome-wide screening approaches in TS, and finding a gene or genes for TS would be a major step toward understanding genetic risk factors. In addition, understanding the genetics of TS genes will strengthen clinical diagnosis, improve genetic counseling, lead to the clarification of pathophysiology, and provide clues for more effective therapics.

Neuroimaging studies: Within the past 5 years, advances in imaging technology and an increase in trained investigators have led to an increasing use of novel and powerful techniques to identify brain regions, circuitry, and neurochemical factors important in TS and related conditions.

Neuropathology: Within the past 5 years, there has been an increase in the number and quality of donated postmortem brains from TS patients available for research purposes. This increase, coupled with advances in neuropathological techniques, has led to initial findings with implications for neuroimaging studies and animal models of TS.

Clinical trials: A number of clinical trials in TS have recently been completed or are currently underway. These include studies of stimulant treatment of ADHD in TS and behavioral treatments for reducing tic severity in children and adults. Smaller trials of novel approaches to treatment such as dopamine agonist and GABAergic medications also show promise.

Epidemiology and clinical science: Careful epidemiological studies now estimate the prevalence of TS to be substantially higher than previously thought with a wider range of clinical severity. Furthermore, clinical studies are providing new findings regarding TS and co-existing conditions. These include subtyping studies of TS and OCD, an examination of the link between ADHD and learning problems in children with TS, a new appreciation of sensory tics, and the role of coexisting disorders in rage attacks. One of the most important and controversial areas of TS science involves the relationship between TS and autoimmune brain injury associated with group A beta-hemolytic streptococcal infections or other infectious processes. There are a number of epidemiological and clinical investigations currently underway in this intriguing area.

Chapter 43

Other Hyperkinetic Movement Disorders

Chapter Contents

Section 43.1

Angelman Syndrome

"Angelman Syndrome" is from the National Library of Medicine,
Genetics Home Reference (ghr.nlm.nih.gov), November 2006.

What is Angelman syndrome?

Angelman syndrome is a complex genetic disorder that affects the
nervous system. Characteristic features of this condition include developmental delay or mental retardation, severe speech impairment,
seizures, small head size (microcephaly), and problems with movement
and balance (ataxia). Delayed development can be noted by 6 months
to 12 months of age, and other common signs and symptoms usually
become apparent in early childhood. People with Angelman syndrome
typically have a happy, excitable demeanor with frequent smiling and
laughter, a short attention span, and hand-flapping movements. Some
affected individuals also have unusually fair skin and light-colored
hair.

How common is Angelman syndrome?

Angelman syndrome affects an estimated 1 in 12,000 to 20,000
people.

What are the genetic changes related to Angelman syndrome?

Angelman syndrome is related to chromosome 15. Mutations in the
UBE3A gene cause Angelman syndrome. The OCA2 gene is associated with Angelman syndrome.

People normally inherit one copy of the UBE3A gene from each
parent. Both copies of this gene are active in many of the body's tissues. In the brain, however, only the copy inherited from a person's
mother (the maternal copy) is active. This parent-specific gene activation is called genomic imprinting. If the maternal copy of the
UBE3A gene is lost because of a chromosomal change or a gene mutation, a person will have no active copies of the gene in the brain.

This loss of gene function likely causes many of the characteristic features of Angelman syndrome.

Several different genetic mechanisms can result in the inactivation or absence of the maternal copy of the UBE3A gene. Most cases of Angelman syndrome (about 70 percent) occur when a segment of the maternal chromosome 15 containing this gene is deleted. In other cases (about 11 percent), Angelman syndrome is caused by a mutation in the maternal copy of the UBE3A gene.

In a small percentage of cases, a person with Angelman syndrome inherits two copies of chromosome 15 from his or her father (paternal copies) instead of one copy from each parent. This phenomenon is called paternal uniparental disomy. Rarely, Angelman syndrome can also be caused by a chromosomal rearrangement called a translocation, or by a mutation or other defect in the DNA region that controls activation of the UBE3A gene. Both of these genetic changes can abnormally inactivate UBE3A or other genes on the maternal copy of chromosome 15.

The OCA2 gene is located on the segment of chromosome 15 that is often deleted in Angelman syndrome. The protein produced from this gene helps determine the coloring (pigmentation) of the skin, hair, and eyes. A deletion of the OCA2 gene is associated with light-colored hair and fair skin in some people with this condition.

The causes of Angelman syndrome are unknown in 10 to 15 percent of cases. Changes involving other genes or chromosomes may be responsible for the features of Angelman syndrome in these cases.

Can Angelman syndrome be inherited?

Most cases of Angelman syndrome are not inherited, particularly those caused by a deletion in the maternal chromosome 15 or by paternal uniparental disomy. These genetic changes occur as random events during the formation of reproductive cells or in early fetal development. Affected people typically have no history of the disorder in their family.

Rarely, a genetic change responsible for Angelman syndrome can be inherited. For example, it is possible for a mutation in the UBE3A gene or in the nearby DNA region that controls gene activation to be passed from one generation to the next.

Section 43.2

Wilson Disease

"Wilson disease" is from the National Library of Medicine, *Genetics Home Reference* (ghr.nlm.nih.gov), February 2007.

What is Wilson disease?

Wilson disease is an inherited disorder in which excessive amounts of copper accumulate in the body, particularly in the liver, brain, and eyes. Typically, signs and symptoms of Wilson disease first appear between the ages of 6 and 40, but most often begin during the teenage years.

Liver disease is usually the initial feature of Wilson disease in people between the ages of 6 and 45. Signs and symptoms of liver disease include yellowing of the skin or the whites of the eye (jaundice), fatigue, loss of appetite, and abdominal swelling. Psychiatric or nervous system problems commonly occur in young adults with Wilson disease. Signs and symptoms of these problems can include clumsiness, trembling, difficulty walking, speech problems, deteriorating school work, depression, anxiety, and mood swings. In many individuals with Wilson disease, copper deposits form a green-to-brownish ring, called the Kayser-Fleischer ring, around the cornea (the front surface of the eye). Abnormalities in eye movements, such as the restricted ability to gaze upwards, may also occur.

How common is Wilson disease?

Wilson disease is a rare disorder that affects approximately 1 in 30,000 individuals.

What genes are related to Wilson disease?

Mutations in the ATP7B gene cause Wilson disease.

Normal variations in the PRNP gene modify the course of Wilson disease.

The ATP7B gene provides instructions for making a protein that plays a role in the transport of copper from the liver to other parts of the body. This protein is particularly important for the elimination of excess copper from the body. Mutations in the ATP7B gene prevent the transport protein from functioning properly. With a shortage of functional protein, excess copper is not removed from the body. As a result, copper accumulates to toxic levels that can damage tissues and organs, particularly the liver and brain.

A normal variation in the PRNP gene may delay the age of onset of Wilson disease and affect the type of symptoms that develop. The PRNP gene provides instructions for making prion protein, which is active in the brain and other tissues. This protein also appears to be involved in transporting copper. Studies have focused on the effects of a PRNP gene variation that affects position 129 of the prion protein. At this position, the protein building block (amino acid) methionine or valine is used. Among people who have mutations in the ATP7B gene, it appears that the onset of symptoms of Wilson disease is delayed by several years if they have methionine (instead of valine) at position 129 in the prion protein. Research findings also suggest that methionine, instead of valine, at position 129 may be associated with an increased occurrence of symptoms that affect the nervous system, particularly tremors. Larger studies are needed, however, before the effects of this PRNP variation on Wilson disease can be established.

How do people inherit Wilson disease?

This condition is inherited in an autosomal recessive pattern, which means both copies of the gene in each cell have mutations. The parents of an individual with an autosomal recessive condition each carry one copy of the mutated gene, but they typically do not show signs and symptoms of the condition.

What other names do people use for Wilson disease?

- Copper storage disease
- Hepatolenticular degeneration syndrome
- WD
- Wilson's disease

Part Five

Diagnosis and Treatment of Movement Disorders

Chapter 44

Neurological Tests and Procedures Used to Diagnose Movement Disorders

Diagnostic tests and procedures are vital tools that help physicians confirm or rule out the presence of a neurological disorder or other medical condition. A century ago, the only way to make a positive diagnosis for many neurological disorders was by performing an autopsy after a patient had died. But decades of basic research into the characteristics of disease, and the development of techniques that allow scientists to see inside the living brain and monitor nervous system activity as it occurs, have given doctors powerful and accurate tools to diagnose disease and to test how well a particular therapy may be working.

Perhaps the most significant changes in diagnostic imaging over the past 20 years are improvements in spatial resolution (size, intensity, and clarity) of anatomical images and reductions in the time needed to send signals to and receive data from the area being imaged. These advances allow physicians to simultaneously see the structure of the brain and the changes in brain activity as they occur. Scientists continue to improve methods that will provide sharper anatomical images and more detailed functional information.

Researchers and physicians use a variety of diagnostic imaging techniques and chemical and metabolic analyses to detect, manage, and treat neurological disease. Some procedures are performed in

"Neurological Diagnostic Tests and Procedures" is from the National Institute of Neurological Disorders and Stroke (NINDS, www.ninds.nih.gov), part of the National Institutes of Health, April 8, 2008.

specialized settings, conducted to determine the presence of a particular disorder or abnormality. Many tests that were previously conducted in a hospital are now performed in a physician's office or at an outpatient testing facility, with little if any risk to the patient. Depending on the type of procedure, results are either immediate or may take several hours to process.

What are some of the more common screening tests?

Laboratory screening tests of blood, urine, or other substances are used to help diagnose disease, better understand the disease process, and monitor levels of therapeutic drugs. Certain tests, ordered by the physician as part of a regular check-up, provide general information, while others are used to identify specific health concerns. For example, blood and blood product tests can detect brain and/or spinal cord infection, bone marrow disease, hemorrhage, blood vessel damage, toxins that affect the nervous system, and the presence of antibodies that signal the presence of an autoimmune disease. Blood tests are also used to monitor levels of therapeutic drugs used to treat epilepsy and other neurological disorders. Genetic testing of DNA extracted from white cells in the blood can help diagnose Huntington disease and other congenital diseases. Analysis of the fluid that surrounds the brain and spinal cord can detect meningitis, acute and chronic inflammation, rare infections, and some cases of multiple sclerosis. Chemical and metabolic testing of the blood can indicate protein disorders, some forms of muscular dystrophy and other muscle disorders, and diabetes. Urinalysis can reveal abnormal substances in the urine or the presence or absence of certain proteins that cause diseases including the mucopolysaccharidoses.

Genetic testing or counseling can help parents who have a family history of a neurological disease determine if they are carrying one of the known genes that cause the disorder or find out if their child is affected. Genetic testing can identify many neurological disorders, including spina bifida, in utero (while the child is inside the mother's womb). Genetic tests include the following:

- **Amniocentesis**, usually done at 14–16 weeks of pregnancy, tests a sample of the amniotic fluid in the womb for genetic defects (the fluid and the fetus have the same DNA). Under local anesthesia, a thin needle is inserted through the woman's abdomen and into the womb. About 20 milliliters of fluid (roughly 4 teaspoons) is withdrawn and sent to a lab for evaluation. Test results often take 1–2 weeks.

- **Chorionic villus sampling**, or CVS, is performed by removing and testing a very small sample of the placenta during early pregnancy. The sample, which contains the same DNA as the fetus, is removed by catheter or fine needle inserted through the cervix or by a fine needle inserted through the abdomen. It is tested for genetic abnormalities and results are usually available within 2 weeks. CVS should not be performed after the 10th week of pregnancy.

- **Uterine ultrasound** is performed using a surface probe with gel. This noninvasive test can suggest the diagnosis of conditions such as chromosomal disorders.

What is a neurological examination?

A **neurological examination** assesses motor and sensory skills, the functioning of one or more cranial nerves, hearing and speech, vision, coordination and balance, mental status, and changes in mood or behavior, among other abilities. Items including a tuning fork, flashlight, reflex hammer, ophthalmoscope, and needles are used to help diagnose brain tumors, infections such as encephalitis and meningitis, and diseases such as Parkinson disease, Huntington disease, amyotrophic lateral sclerosis (ALS), and epilepsy. Some tests require the services of a specialist to perform and analyze results.

X-rays of the patient's chest and skull are often taken as part of a neurological work-up. X-rays can be used to view any part of the body, such as a joint or major organ system. In a conventional x-ray, also called a radiograph, a technician passes a concentrated burst of low-dose ionized radiation through the body and onto a photographic plate. Since calcium in bones absorbs x-rays more easily than soft tissue or muscle, the bony structure appears white on the film. Any vertebral misalignment or fractures can be seen within minutes. Tissue masses such as injured ligaments or a bulging disk are not visible on conventional x-rays. This fast, noninvasive, painless procedure is usually performed in a doctor's office or at a clinic.

Fluoroscopy is a type of x-ray that uses a continuous or pulsed beam of low-dose radiation to produce continuous images of a body part in motion. The fluoroscope (x-ray tube) is focused on the area of interest and pictures are either videotaped or sent to a monitor for viewing. A contrast medium may be used to highlight the images. Fluoroscopy can be used to evaluate the flow of blood through arteries.

What are some diagnostic tests used to diagnose neurological disorders?

Based on the result of a neurological exam, physical exam, patient history, x-rays of the patient's chest and skull, and any previous screening or testing, physicians may order one or more of the following diagnostic tests to determine the specific nature of a suspected neurological disorder or injury. These diagnostics generally involve either nuclear medicine imaging, in which very small amounts of radioactive materials are used to study organ function and structure, or diagnostic imaging, which uses magnets and electrical charges to study human anatomy.

The following list of available procedures—in alphabetical rather than sequential order—includes some of the more common tests used to help diagnose a neurological condition.

Angiography is a test used to detect blockages of the arteries or veins. A cerebral angiogram can detect the degree of narrowing or obstruction of an artery or blood vessel in the brain, head, or neck. It is used to diagnose stroke and to determine the location and size of a brain tumor, aneurysm, or vascular malformation. This test is usually performed in a hospital outpatient setting and takes up to 3 hours, followed by a 6- to 8-hour resting period. The patient, wearing a hospital or imaging gown, lies on a table that is wheeled into the imaging area. While the patient is awake, a physician anesthetizes a small area of the leg near the groin and then inserts a catheter into a major artery located there. The catheter is threaded through the body and into an artery in the neck. Once the catheter is in place, the needle is removed and a guide wire is inserted. A small capsule containing a radiopaque dye (one that is highlighted on x-rays) is passed over the guide wire to the site of release. The dye is released and travels through the bloodstream into the head and neck. A series of x-rays is taken and any obstruction is noted. Patients may feel a warm to hot sensation or slight discomfort as the dye is released.

Biopsy involves the removal and examination of a small piece of tissue from the body. Muscle or nerve biopsies are used to diagnose neuromuscular disorders and may also reveal if a person is a carrier of a defective gene that could be passed on to children. A small sample of muscle or nerve is removed under local anesthetic and studied under a microscope. The sample may be removed either surgically, through a slit made in the skin, or by needle biopsy, in which a thin hollow needle is inserted through the skin and into the muscle. A small piece of muscle or nerve remains in the hollow needle when it is removed from the body. The biopsy is usually performed at an outpatient testing facility. A brain biopsy, used to determine tumor type, requires surgery to remove a small piece of the brain or tumor. Performed in a hospital, this operation is riskier than a muscle biopsy and involves a longer recovery period.

Brain scans are imaging techniques used to diagnose tumors, blood vessel malformations, or hemorrhage in the brain. These scans are used to study organ function or injury or disease to tissue or muscle. Types of brain scans include computed tomography, magnetic resonance imaging, and positron emission tomography.

Cerebrospinal fluid analysis involves the removal of a small amount of the fluid that protects the brain and spinal cord. The fluid is tested to detect any bleeding or brain hemorrhage, diagnose infection to the brain and/or spinal cord, identify some cases of multiple sclerosis and other neurological conditions, and measure intracranial pressure.

The procedure is usually done in a hospital. The sample of fluid is commonly removed by a procedure known as a lumbar puncture, or spinal tap. The patient is asked to either lie on one side, in a ball position with knees close to the chest, or lean forward while sitting on a table or bed. The doctor will locate a puncture site in the lower back, between two vertebrate, then clean the area and inject a local anesthetic. The patient may feel a slight stinging sensation from this injection. Once the anesthetic has taken effect, the doctor will insert a special needle into the spinal sac and remove a small amount of fluid (usually about 3 teaspoons) for testing. Most patients will feel a sensation of pressure only as the needle is inserted.

A common after-effect of a lumbar puncture is headache, which can be lessened by having the patient lie flat. Risk of nerve root injury or infection from the puncture can occur but it is rare. The entire procedure takes about 45 minutes.

Computed tomography, also known as a CT scan, is a noninvasive, painless process used to produce rapid, clear two-dimensional images of organs, bones, and tissues. Neurological CT scans are used to view

395

the brain and spine. They can detect bone and vascular irregularities, certain brain tumors and cysts, herniated disks, epilepsy, encephalitis, spinal stenosis (narrowing of the spinal canal), a blood clot or intracranial bleeding in patients with stroke, brain damage from head injury, and other disorders. Many neurological disorders share certain characteristics and a CT scan can aid in proper diagnosis by differentiating the area of the brain affected by the disorder.

Scanning takes about 20 minutes (a CT of the brain or head may take slightly longer) and is usually done at an imaging center or hospital on an outpatient basis. The patient lies on a special table that slides into a narrow chamber. A sound system built into the chamber allows the patient to communicate with the physician or technician. As the patient lies still, x-rays are passed through the body at various angles and are detected by a computerized scanner. The data is processed and displayed as cross-sectional images, or "slices," of the internal structure of the body or organ. A light sedative may be given to patients who are unable to lie still and pillows may be used to support and stabilize the head and body. Persons who are claustrophobic may have difficulty taking this imaging test.

Occasionally a contrast dye is injected into the bloodstream to highlight the different tissues in the brain. Patients may feel a warm or cool sensation as the dye circulates through the bloodstream or they may experience a slight metallic taste.

Although very little radiation is used in CT, pregnant women should avoid the test because of potential harm to the fetus from ionizing radiation.

Discography is often suggested for patients who are considering lumbar surgery or whose lower back pain has not responded to conventional treatments. This outpatient procedure is usually performed at a testing facility or a hospital. The patient is asked to put on a metal-free hospital gown and lie on an imaging table. The physician numbs the skin with anesthetic and inserts a thin needle, using x-ray guidance, into the spinal disk. Once the needle is in place, a small amount of contrast dye is injected and CT scans are taken. The contrast dye outlines any damaged areas. More than one disk may be imaged at the same time. Patient recovery usually takes about an hour. Pain medicine may be prescribed for any resulting discomfort.

An **intrathecal contrast-enhanced CT scan** (also called cisternography) is used to detect problems with the spine and spinal nerve roots. This test is most often performed at an imaging center. The patient is asked to put on a hospital or imaging gown. Following application of a topical anesthetic, the physician removes a small sample of the spinal fluid via lumbar puncture. The sample is mixed with a contrast dye and injected into the spinal sac located at the base of the lower back. The patient is then asked to move to a position that will allow the contrast fluid to travel to the area to be studied. The dye allows the spinal canal and nerve roots to be seen more clearly on a CT scan. The scan may take up to an hour to complete. Following the test, patients may experience some discomfort and/or headache that may be caused by the removal of spinal fluid.

Electroencephalography, or EEG, monitors brain activity through the skull. EEG is used to help diagnose certain seizure disorders, brain tumors, brain damage from head injuries, inflammation of the brain and/or spinal cord, alcoholism, certain psychiatric disorders, and metabolic and degenerative disorders that affect the brain. EEGs are also used to evaluate sleep disorders, monitor brain activity when a patient has been fully anesthetized or loses consciousness, and confirm brain death.

This painless, risk-free test can be performed in a doctor's office or at a hospital or testing facility. Prior to taking an EEG, the person must avoid caffeine intake and prescription drugs that affect the nervous system. A series of cup-like electrodes are attached to the patient's scalp, either with a special conducting paste or with extremely fine needles. The electrodes (also called leads) are small devices that are attached to wires and carry the electrical energy of the brain to a machine for reading. A very low electrical current is sent through the electrodes and the baseline brain energy is recorded. Patients are then exposed to a variety of external stimuli—including bright or flashing light, noise, or certain drugs—or are asked to open and close the eyes, or to change breathing patterns. The electrodes transmit the resulting changes in brain wave patterns. Since movement and nervousness can change brain wave patterns, patients usually recline in a chair or on a bed during the test, which takes up to an hour. Testing for certain disorders requires performing an EEG during sleep, which takes at least 3 hours.

In order to learn more about brain wave activity, electrodes may be inserted through a surgical opening in the skull and into the brain to reduce signal interference from the skull.

Electromyography, or EMG, is used to diagnose nerve and muscle dysfunction and spinal cord disease. It records the electrical activity from the brain and/or spinal cord to a peripheral nerve root (found in the arms and legs) that controls muscles during contraction and at rest.

During an EMG, very fine wire electrodes are inserted into a muscle to assess changes in electrical voltage that occur during movement and when the muscle is at rest. The electrodes are attached through a series of wires to a recording instrument. Testing usually takes place at a testing facility and lasts about an hour but may take longer, depending on the number of muscles and nerves to be tested. Most patients find this test to be somewhat uncomfortable.

An EMG is usually done in conjunction with a **nerve conduction velocity (NCV) test**, which measures electrical energy by assessing the nerve's ability to send a signal. This two-part test is conducted most often in a hospital. A technician tapes two sets of flat electrodes on the skin over the muscles. The first set of electrodes is used to send small pulses of electricity (similar to the sensation of static electricity) to stimulate the nerve that directs a particular muscle. The second set of electrodes transmits the responding electrical signal to a recording machine. The physician then reviews the response to verify any nerve damage or muscle disease. Patients who are preparing to take an EMG or NCV test may be asked to avoid caffeine and not smoke for 2 to 3 hours prior to the test, as well as to avoid aspirin and non-steroidal anti-inflammatory drugs for 24 hours before the EMG. There is no discomfort or risk associated with this test.

Electronystagmography (ENG) describes a group of tests used to diagnose involuntary eye movement, dizziness, and balance disorders, and to evaluate some brain functions. The test is performed at an imaging center. Small electrodes are taped around the eyes to record eye movements. If infrared photography is used in place of electrodes, the patient wears special goggles that help record the information. Both versions of the test are painless and risk-free.

Evoked potentials (also called evoked response) measure the electrical signals to the brain generated by hearing, touch, or sight. These tests are used to assess sensory nerve problems and confirm neurological conditions including multiple sclerosis, brain tumor, acoustic neuroma (small tumors of the inner ear), and spinal cord injury. Evoked potentials are also used to test sight and hearing (especially in infants and young children), monitor brain activity among coma patients, and confirm brain death.

Testing may take place in a doctor's office or hospital setting. It is painless and risk-free. Two sets of needle electrodes are used to test for nerve damage. One set of electrodes, which will be used to measure the electrophysiological response to stimuli, is attached to the patient's scalp using conducting paste. The second set of electrodes is attached to the part of the body to be tested. The physician then records the amount of time it takes for the impulse generated by stimuli to reach the brain. Under normal circumstances, the process of signal transmission is instantaneous.

Auditory evoked potentials (also called brain stem auditory evoked response) are used to assess high-frequency hearing loss, diagnose any damage to the acoustic nerve and auditory pathways in the brainstem, and detect acoustic neuromas. The patient sits in a soundproof room and wears headphones. Clicking sounds are delivered one at a time to one ear while a masking sound is sent to the other ear. Each ear is usually tested twice, and the entire procedure takes about 45 minutes.

Visual evoked potentials detect loss of vision from optic nerve damage (in particular, damage caused by multiple sclerosis). The patient sits close to a screen and is asked to focus on the center of a shifting checkerboard pattern. Only one eye is tested at a time; the other eye is either kept closed or covered with a patch. Each eye is usually tested twice. Testing takes 30–45 minutes.

Somatosensory evoked potentials measure response from stimuli to the peripheral nerves and can detect nerve or spinal cord damage or nerve degeneration from multiple sclerosis and other degenerating diseases. Tiny electrical shocks are delivered by electrode to a nerve in an arm or leg. Responses to the shocks, which may be delivered for more than a minute at a time, are recorded. This test usually lasts less than an hour.

Magnetic resonance imaging (MRI) uses computer-generated radio waves and a powerful magnetic field to produce detailed images of body structures including tissues, organs, bones, and nerves. Neurological uses include the diagnosis of brain and spinal cord tumors, eye disease, inflammation, infection, and vascular irregularities that may lead to stroke. MRI can also detect and monitor degenerative disorders such as multiple sclerosis and can document brain injury from trauma.

The equipment houses a hollow tube that is surrounded by a very large cylindrical magnet. The patient, who must remain still during the test, lies on a special table that is slid into the tube. The patient will be asked to remove jewelry, eyeglasses, removable dental work, or other items that might interfere with the magnetic imaging. The patient should wear a sweat shirt and sweat pants or other clothing free of metal eyelets or buckles. MRI scanning equipment creates a magnetic field around the body strong enough to temporarily realign water molecules in the tissues. Radio waves are then passed through the body to detect the "relaxation" of the molecules back to a random alignment and trigger a resonance signal at different angles within the body. A computer processes this resonance into either a three-dimensional picture or a two-dimensional "slice" of the tissue being scanned, and differentiates between bone, soft tissues, and fluid-filled spaces by their water content and structural properties. A contrast dye may be used to enhance visibility of certain areas or tissues. The patient may hear grating or knocking noises when the magnetic field is turned on and off. (Patients may wear special earphones to block out the sounds.) Unlike CT scanning, MRI does not use ionizing radiation to produce images. Depending on the part(s) of the body to be scanned, MRI can take up to an hour to complete. The test is painless and risk-free, although persons who are obese or claustrophobic may find it somewhat uncomfortable. (Some centers also use open MRI machines that do not completely surround the person being tested and are less confining. However, open MRI does not currently provide the same picture quality as standard MRI and some tests may not be available using this equipment). Due to the incredibly strong magnetic field generated by an MRI, patients with implanted medical devices such as a pacemaker should avoid the test.

Functional MRI (fMRI) uses the blood's magnetic properties to produce real-time images of blood flow to particular areas of the brain. An fMRI can pinpoint areas of the brain that become active and note how long they stay active. It can also tell if brain activity within a region occurs simultaneously or sequentially. This imaging process is used to assess brain damage from head injury or degenerative disorders such as Alzheimer disease and to identify and monitor other neurological disorders, including multiple sclerosis, stroke, and brain tumors.

Myelography involves the injection of a water- or oil-based contrast dye into the spinal canal to enhance x-ray imaging of the spine. Myelograms are used to diagnose spinal nerve injury, herniated disks, fractures, back or leg pain, and spinal tumors.

The procedure takes about 30 minutes and is usually performed in a hospital. Following an injection of anesthesia to a site between two vertebrae in the lower back, a small amount of the cerebrospinal fluid is removed by spinal tap and the contrast dye is injected into the spinal canal. After a series of x-rays is taken, most or all of the contrast dye is removed by aspiration. Patients may experience some pain during the spinal tap and when the dye is injected and removed. Patients may also experience headache following the spinal tap. The risk of fluid leakage or allergic reaction to the dye is slight.

Positron emission tomography (PET) scans provide two- and three-dimensional pictures of brain activity by measuring radioactive isotopes that are injected into the bloodstream. PET scans of the brain are used to detect or highlight tumors and diseased tissue, measure cellular and/or tissue metabolism, show blood flow, evaluate patients who have seizure disorders that do not respond to medical therapy and patients with certain memory disorders, and determine brain changes following injury or drug abuse, among other uses. PET may be ordered as a follow-up to a CT or MRI scan to give the physician a greater understanding of specific areas of the brain that may be involved with certain problems. Scans are conducted in a hospital or at a testing facility, on an outpatient basis. A low-level radioactive isotope, which binds to chemicals that flow to the brain, is injected into the bloodstream and can be traced as the brain performs different functions. The patient lies still while overhead sensors detect gamma rays in the body's tissues. A computer processes the information and displays it on a video monitor or on film. Using different compounds, more than one brain function can be traced simultaneously. PET is painless and relatively risk-free. Length of test time depends on the part of the body to be scanned. PET scans are performed by skilled technicians at highly sophisticated medical facilities.

A **polysomnogram** measures brain and body activity during sleep. It is performed over one or more nights at a sleep center. Electrodes are pasted or taped to the patient's scalp, eyelids, and/or chin. Throughout the night and during the various wake/sleep cycles, the electrodes record brain waves, eye movement, breathing, leg and skeletal muscle activity, blood pressure, and heart rate. The patient may be videotaped to note any movement during sleep. Results are then used to identify any characteristic patterns of sleep disorders, including restless legs syndrome, periodic limb movement disorder, insomnia, and breathing disorders such as obstructive sleep apnea. Polysomnograms are non-invasive, painless, and risk-free.

Single photon emission computed tomography (SPECT), a nuclear imaging test involving blood flow to tissue, is used to evaluate

401

certain brain functions. The test may be ordered as a follow-up to an MRI to diagnose tumors, infections, degenerative spinal disease, and stress fractures. As with a PET scan, a radioactive isotope, which binds to chemicals that flow to the brain, is injected intravenously into the body. Areas of increased blood flow will collect more of the isotope. As the patient lies on a table, a gamma camera rotates around the head and records where the radioisotope has traveled. That information is converted by computer into cross-sectional slices that are stacked to produce a detailed three-dimensional image of blood flow and activity within the brain. The test is performed at either an imaging center or a hospital.

Thermography uses infrared sensing devices to measure small temperature changes between the two sides of the body or within a specific organ. Also known as digital infrared thermal imaging, thermography may be used to detect vascular disease of the head and neck, soft tissue injury, various neuromusculoskeletal disorders, and the presence or absence of nerve root compression. It is performed at an imaging center, using infrared light recorders to take thousands of pictures of the body from a distance of 5 to 8 feet. The information is converted into electrical signals which results in a computer-generated two-dimensional picture of abnormally cold or hot areas indicated by color or shades of black and white. Thermography does not use radiation and is safe, risk-free, and noninvasive.

Ultrasound imaging, also called ultrasound scanning or sonography, uses high-frequency sound waves to obtain images inside the body. Neurosonography (ultrasound of the brain and spinal column) analyzes blood flow in the brain and can diagnose stroke, brain tumors, hydrocephalus (build-up of cerebrospinal fluid in the brain), and vascular problems. It can also identify or rule out inflammatory processes causing pain. It is more effective than an x-ray in displaying soft tissue masses and can show tears in ligaments, muscles, tendons, and other soft tissue masses in the back. Transcranial Doppler ultrasound is used to view arteries and blood vessels in the neck and determine blood flow and risk of stroke.

During ultrasound, the patient lies on an imaging table and removes clothing around the area of the body to be scanned. A jelly-like lubricant is applied and a transducer, which both sends and receives high-frequency sound waves, is passed over the body. The sound wave echoes are recorded and displayed as a computer-generated real-time visual image of the structure or tissue being examined. Ultrasound is painless, noninvasive, and risk-free. The test is performed on an outpatient basis and takes between 15 and 30 minutes to complete.

What lies ahead?

Scientists funded by the NINDS seek to develop additional and improved screening methods to more accurately and quickly confirm a specific diagnosis and allow scientists to investigate other factors that might contribute to disease. Technological advances in imaging will allow researchers to better see inside the body, at less risk to the patient. These diagnostics and procedures will continue to be important clinical research tools for confirming a neurological disorder, charting disease progression, and monitoring therapeutic effect.

Chapter 45

Working with Your Doctor

Chapter Contents

Section 45.1

The Role of the Neurologist

What Is a Neurologist?

A neurologist is a medical doctor with specialized training in diagnosing, treating, and managing disorders of the brain and nervous system. Neurologists do not perform surgery.

A neurologist's training includes an undergraduate degree, 4 years of medical school, a 1-year internship, and 3 years of specialized training. Many neurologists also have additional training in one area of neurology such as stroke, epilepsy, or movement disorders. This is called a subspecialty.

What Does a Neurologist Treat?

Common neurological disorders include:

- Stroke
- Pain
- Headache
- Epilepsy
- Tremor
- Sleep disorders
- Alzheimer's disease
- Parkinson disease
- Multiple sclerosis
- Brain and spinal cord injuries
- Brain tumors
- Amyotrophic lateral sclerosis (ALS), also called Lou Gehrig's Disease

What Is the Role of a Neurologist?

Neurologists are principal care providers or consultants to other doctors. When a person has a neurological disorder that requires frequent care, a neurologist is often the principal care provider. People with disorders, such as Parkinson disease, Alzheimer's disease, seizure disorders, or multiple sclerosis may use a neurologist as their principal care doctor.

In a consulting role, a neurologist will diagnose and treat a neurological disorder and then advise the primary care doctor managing the person's overall health. For example, a neurologist may act in a consulting role for conditions such as stroke, concussion, or headache.

Neurologists can recommend surgical treatment, but they do not perform surgery. When treatment includes surgery, neurologists may monitor the patients and supervise their continuing treatment. Neurosurgeons are medical doctors who specialize in performing surgical treatments of the brain or nervous system.

Diagnosis and Treatment of Neurological Disorders

An accurate diagnosis is the first step toward effective treatment. Diagnosis involves getting a detailed health history of the patient, and neurological tests for vision, strength, coordination, reflexes, and sensation. Sometimes, further tests are needed to reach a diagnosis.

Some common neurological tests are:

- Computerized tomography or computer-assisted tomography (CT or CAT scan)
- Magnetic resonance imaging (MRI)
- Transcranial Doppler (TCD)
- Neurosonography
- Electroencephalogram (EEG)
- Electromyogram (EMG)
- Evoked potentials
- Sleep studies
- Cerebral spinal fluid analysis (spinal tap or lumbar puncture)

Computerized tomography or computer assisted tomography (CT of CAT scan): This test uses x-rays and computers to create multidimensional images of selected body parts. Dye may be injected into a patient's vein to obtain a clearer view. Other than needle insertion for the dye, this test is painless.

Magnetic resonance imaging (MRI): An MRI is an advanced way of taking pictures of the inner brain. It is harmless and involves magnetic fields and radio waves. It is performed when a patient is lying in a small chamber for about 30 minutes. It is painless, but may be stressful for individuals with claustrophobia (fear of closed areas). A physician can offer options to help you relax.

Transcranial Doppler (TCD): This test uses sound waves to measure blood flow in the vessels of the brain. A microphone is placed on different parts of the head to view the blood vessels. This test is painless.

Neurosonography: This test uses ultra high frequency sound wave to analyze blood flow and blockage in the blood vessels in or leading to the brain. This test is painless.

Electroencephalogram (EEG): The EEG records the brain's continuous electrical activity through electrodes attached to the scalp. It is used to help diagnose structural diseases of the brain and episodes such as seizures, fainting, or blacking out. This test is painless.

Electromyogram (EMG): An EMG measures and records electrical activity in the muscles and nerves. This may be helpful in determining the cause of pain, numbness, tingling, or weakness in the muscles or nerves. Small needles are inserted into the muscle and mild electrical shocks are given to stimulate the nerve. Discomfort may be associated with this test.

Evoked potentials: This test records the brain's electrical response to visual, auditory, and sensory stimulation. This test is useful in evaluating and diagnosing symptoms of dizziness, numbness, and tingling, as well as visual disorders. Discomfort may be associated with this test.

Sleep studies: These tests are used to diagnose specific causes of sleep problems. To perform the tests, it is often necessary for a patient to spend the night in a sleep laboratory. Brain wave activity, heart rate, electrical activity of the heart, breathing, and oxygen in the blood are all measured during the sleep test. The test is painless.

Cerebrospinal fluid analysis (spinal tap or lumbar puncture): This test is used to check for bleeding, hemorrhage, infection, or other disorder of the brain, spinal cord, and nerves. In this test, the lower back is numbed with local anesthesia and a thin needle is placed into the space that contains the spinal fluid. The amount of spinal fluid that is needed for the tests is removed and the needle is withdrawn. Discomfort may be associated with this test.

Section 45.2

Making the Most of Your Doctor Visit

Stone, K. "Making the Most of Your Doctor Visit," *Neurology Now* Summer 2005; 1(2): 39-40. ©2 2005 American Academy of Neurology. Reprinted with permission of Lippincott Williams and Wilkins.

If you want the best health care possible, be prepared and informed. Doing both can also save you money. Just ask Mary Elizabeth McNary.

She was diagnosed with multiple sclerosis (MS) in the late 1980s and now works as a rehabilitation counselor in the National Multiple Sclerosis Society's Washington, D C. office.

You are a consumer of health care, she advises people who are newly diagnosed with MS. You owe it to yourself to take 15 to 20 minutes to list your questions for your doctor visit, she tells them. And don't you dare leave that office until all questions are asked, she adds. She also suggests keeping a calendar of tests and procedures performed for cross-referencing when the billing statement arrives.

Of course, in an emergency situation, there isn't time to sit down and note questions or to write down a personal health history. That's why it's important to maintain a health record that can be shared with a doctor at each visit, she says.

Take a Team Approach

What you do during a doctor's visit can mean the difference between a productive meeting or a frustrating experience, says University of

Alabama at Birmingham psychologist Joshua Klapow, Ph.D. Bring a list of your symptoms and medications and prioritize your concerns. Leave with a plan. Write it down and repeat it back to the doctor. If you don't understand the plan, ask for clarification, he advises.

Sometimes the responsibility for asking falls to a parent or caregiver. Sue Mielenhausen's 12-year-old son was diagnosed with epilepsy at age five. The Mielenhausens, of St. Paul, Minnesota, consider themselves part of a collaborative decision-making team with their son's pediatric neurologists.

"No one knows your child like you do," says Mielenhausen. Part of having a good working relationship with health care providers extends beyond the doctor to the clinic staff, she says. "It's important to be able to get through on the phone. We've had a good experience with the triage nurse. She returns calls immediately."

She makes sure her son is involved as well.

"It's really important that the child be engaged during conversations with the doctor. A child is going to feel more comfortable asking questions if they've been involved in conversations," she adds.

Mielenhausen keeps records of her son's care. "I've tried to keep a good record, noting dates and times of reoccurrences."

The American Academy of Neurology (AAN) also offers tips on working with your neurologist on The Brain Matters, a website for patients. The tips include asking a relative or friend to come with you, because sometimes a second pair of ears may be helpful. Your companion can also jot down notes during the visit, which can be extremely helpful afterwards, the site notes.

Good Personal Health Records Ensure Safety

Maureen Callaghan, M.D., a general neurologist in Olympia, Washington, estimates that only about one-third of her patients come in prepared. Sharing pertinent health records is a matter of patient safety, Dr. Callaghan says. This helps prevent the prescription of medications that may counteract with existing prescriptions. Good records can also avoid ordering redundant and expensive diagnostic tests.

Neurologists also need to be aware of all existing conditions, such as high blood pressure or diabetes. Bringing along a health record of other conditions and names of other health care providers makes providing care easier.

Stacey Rudnicki, M.D., an associate professor of Neurology at the University of Arkansas for Medical Sciences Medical Center in Little Rock, Ark., routinely sends new patients a questionnaire that covers symptoms, family medical history, previous tests, prior surgeries, alcohol use, and cigarette smoking history and medications.

Many patients assume they will have only 15 to 20 minutes with their doctor at each visit. But Dr. Rudnicki advises new patients that a neurological exam is usually more involved and requires more time than other office visits. Neurologists tend to spend more time with patients than the average doctor. "We might meet for 30 minutes to 90 minutes. They should come in with the mindset that they may be in a little longer," says Dr. Rudnicki.

Kathy Stone is a freelance science and health writer whose articles appear in the *Applied Neurology* magazine, and in several newspapers, including the *St. Paul Pioneer Press* in St. Paul, Minnesota.

Chapter 46

Managing Spasticity

Introduction

Spasticity is one of the most mysterious of all MS [multiple sclerosis] symptoms. It comes and goes. It feels different to different people—and even to the same person at different times. There are even occasions when a physician finds spasticity, but the person affected has no symptoms. There's also an inherent paradox. Spasticity is not all negative. The stiffness it may give the legs can be a real help in moving about or transferring from bed to chairs, to car seats, on and off a toilet, and more.

What is spasticity?

The word spasticity refers to involuntary muscle stiffness or spasms (sudden muscle contractions).

In any coordinated movement, some muscles relax while others contract. Spasticity occurs when this coordination is impaired and too many muscles contract at the same time. MS-related spasticity can cause a leg to lock up and refuse to bend.

Spasticity is not completely understood. Doctors believe the problem is caused by increased sensitivity in the parts of muscles responsible for tightening, relaxing, and stretching. This likely occurs as a result of demyelination of the nerves connected to these muscles. This may lead to excessive firing of the nerves that control muscles.

"Controlling Spasticity in MS," © 2007 National Multiple Sclerosis Society (www.nationalmssociety.org). Reprinted with permission.

In mild cases, the condition is noticeable only as a feeling of tight or stiff muscles. When the condition is severe, the person can experience painful spasms or twisted limbs, which can impede mobility and other physical functions.

There are two types of MS-related spasms: flexor and extensor. Flexor spasticity is defined as an involuntary bending of the hips or knees (mostly involving the hamstring muscles on the back of the upper leg). The hips and knees bend up toward the chest. Extensor spasticity is an involuntary straightening of the legs. Extensor spasticity involves the quadriceps (muscles on the front of the upper leg) and the adductors (inner thigh muscles). The hips and knees remain straight with the legs very close together or crossed over at the ankles.

How common is spasticity?

Spasticity is one of the more common symptoms of MS. If all degrees of spasticity are taken together, it occurs in an estimated 80 percent of people with the disease. The question of degree is important. For one person, spasticity may cause a stiff leg, while in another, it makes walking impossible. For many people, the extra effort needed to move around when muscles are spastic contributes significantly to fatigue. On the other hand, spasticity can also compensate for muscle weakness, making it easier to stand, walk, and move. Spasticity may also occur in the arms. Although this is less common in MS, it can significantly interfere with use of the hands in important activities such as bathing and eating.

Treatment

The Treatment Partnership

Because the condition is so individual, successful treatment of spasticity demands a true partnership between you and your doctor, nurse, physical therapist, and/or occupational therapist. Your family also plays an important role. The first step in building a good treatment partnership is knowing that treatment strategies are possible.

"Treating spasticity is not a matter of the doctor writing out a prescription for pills and saying come back in 3 months," said Charles R. Smith, M.D., former director of the Multiple Sclerosis Comprehensive Care Centers at White Plains Hospital in White Plains, New York, and at Bronx Lebanon Hospital in the Bronx, New York.

A doctor can identify the presence and degree of spasticity by stretching your legs to check for involuntary resistance. For example, if your leg is spastic, your muscles will automatically resist when the doctor quickly bends your knee. If spasticity is mild, the doctor will feel barely any resistance; if the spasticity is severe, your leg may be so stiff that the doctor cannot bend it at all.

Treatment begins with the doctor recommending ways to relieve the symptoms. Strategies may include medication, exercise, or changes in daily activities. To individualize the plan, and to adjust the dosage of any medication to its most effective level, your doctor will need to follow your progress. She or he may also make referrals to other health-care professionals, such as a physical therapist (PT) or occupational therapist (OT).

Nurses normally have responsibility for health education and for learning in detail how patients' daily lives are affected by their symptoms and are an important part of this process. Take the time to ask your nurse questions and provide personal information. Both your doctor and nurse will guide you through the sometimes tricky process of medication adjustment. In addition, the PT and OT can provide individualized training with specific exercises and ways to make daily activities easier.

Self-Help

Spasticity, like other aspects of your MS, is in many ways unique to you. As with other MS symptoms, it tends to come and go and to be worse under certain conditions. Typical triggers include cold temperatures, high humidity, tight clothing, tight shoes, constipation, poor posture, and having a viral infection such as a cold or the flu, or a bacterial infection including skin sores or bladder infections.

In time you will become aware of the triggers that affect you most. Some, like tight shoes, can be avoided. Others triggers merit an intervention.

Effective self-help means:

- Don't assume that nothing can be done. Spasticity does not have to be tolerated. Improvement is usually possible.

- Make sure an appropriate exercise program is a regular part of your routine. The National MS Society's illustrated booklets *Stretching for People with MS* and *Stretching with a Helper for People with MS* include exercises specifically for spasticity. Ask your physical therapist, nurse, or doctor for suggestions.

- Explore complementary relaxation techniques such as progressive muscle relaxation, yoga, meditation, or deep-breathing exercises.

None of these is a cure, but they can make it easier to sleep at night and face the next day's problems with a clearer head and reduced spasticity.

- If your doctor agrees, explore massage. You may even receive some insurance reimbursement depending on your plan. Massage can help relax muscles and enhance range of motion and may be helpful in preventing pressure sores. Massage should not be used if pressure sores or reddened areas of skin are present. The American Massage Therapy Association has a national locator service and can supply names of qualified therapists. Call 877-905-2700 or visit their website at http://www.amtamassage .org/findamassage/locator.aspx.

- Be patient but persistent through adjustments in daily activities, the types and doses of medication, the type and timing of exercise, and the use of devices, gadgets, and adaptations.

Treatment Goals

Spasticity interferes with daily activities, so the primary goal of treatment is to reduce the negative effects as much as possible. Sections of this text detail what can be accomplished by medication, physical therapy, orthotic devices (splints or braces), and occupational therapy. Some strategies seek to relieve the affected muscles; others involve learning to work around spasticity by adopting new ways to do things.

Treatment also aims at preventing the serious complications of spasticity. These include contractures (frozen or immobilized joints) and pressure sores. Since these complications also act as spasticity triggers, they can set off a dangerous escalation of symptoms. In fact, surgical measures are considered for those rare cases of spasticity that defy all other treatments.

Contractures are not only painful and disabling, but if left untreated, they become permanent, leaving legs that can never be straightened and limiting joint mobility in such places as the shoulder. Treatment (and prevention) of contractures usually combines treatment of spasticity with medication and physical therapy, prescribed and tailored to the individual by the physician.

Pressure Sores

Pressure sores, sometimes called bed sores, or pressure ulcers, occur in people who spend much of their day sitting or lying down. The

416

term, "bed sore," is misleading. One does not need to be in bed all the time to be at risk for a pressure sore. MS reduces the thousands of small movements people ordinarily make both in sleep and while sitting down. MS can dull sensation in the buttocks or legs, eliminating the usual sensory cues for shifting position.

Spasticity contributes to pressure sores by making normal movement more difficult and by causing posture changes that create pressure points. Another cause of pressure sores is "shearing," which occurs when the person is receiving positioning assistance from someone, and the movement is more sliding or dragging than lifting.

Pressure sores begin innocently enough, as small reddened areas. The spot may not even feel painful or tender. However, there may already be significant damage to the soft tissues underneath reddened areas of skin. If pressure on the area is not relieved, the skin will break down, forming a sore. These sores can deepen quickly. They are prone to infection, and they can eventually destroy large areas of underlying tissue and even bone. Your nurse or doctor can provide instruction in prevention and early detection. Controlling spasticity is part of good pressure sore prevention. Complicated infected pressure sores are contributing factors in some MS-related deaths.

Rehabilitation

Physical Therapy

A physical therapist (PT) recommends and teaches specific exercises and movements that can increase flexibility and relieve spasticity. First, you will have several tests that measure muscle tone, resistance, strength, and coordination. You'll also be asked about your general functioning in routine daily activities.

In addition to stretching exercises you do yourself, PTs also relieve spasticity with specific exercises (done with the help of another person) to stretch and relax shortened muscle fibers, increase joint movement, extend contracted muscles, and improve circulation. Some of these techniques may be taught to a family member or helper so that they can be performed on a routine basis at home.

Strengthening exercises prescribed by the PTs are also important because a muscle that is spastic is not necessarily strong.

Physical therapy can help maintain range of motion to prevent contractures. Strengthening the spastic muscles, and those that oppose the spastic ones, may be particularly beneficial. This is like making sure that both the "push" and the "pull" are in good condition.

417

PTs may also recommend hydrotherapy (therapy using water) and local application of cold packs. Hydrotherapy is a very effective way to temporarily relax spastic limbs, especially when used in combination with gentle stretching.

For those who are unable to stand independently, a standing frame allows for stretching of leg muscles, as well as pressure on the leg bones, which helps limit bone mineral loss (osteoporosis).

Orthotic Devices

Orthotic devices (such as braces and splints) maintain the extremity in a better position, which makes it easier to move around or get into a more comfortable position. They should be fitted by a professional. A common example is the ankle-foot orthosis (AFO—which places the ankle in a better alignment). Although many drugstores and catalogs offer them over-the-counter, ill-fitting devices can aggravate spasticity and cause pressure sores or pain. Trained PTs can direct you to the best options and teach you how to use them.

Occupational Therapy

Occupational therapists (OTs) are experts in modifications that make daily life with spasticity more comfortable and enhance independence. That might include replacing small drawer pulls with large knobs, spraying drawer tracks with silicone to make the drawers glide, or lowering the clothes bar in your closets. OTs will recommend assistive devices and let you try out samples. You may be amazed at the ingenuity of the available devices.

Here is a small sample:

- **Dressing aids:** These include sock pullers, long shoehorns, and shoe and boot removers, all of which help you dress with a minimum of bending. There are elastic shoelaces that let you slip in and out of shoes without having to retie them, zipper pulls with long handles, and more.

- **Toiletry and grooming aids:** In addition to electric shavers and electric toothbrushes, there are easy-grip handles for shaving-cream cans, combs, or brushes, and palm or wrist cuffs to hold either regular bath brushes or bent-handled brushes, to extend your reach.

For people who use wheelchairs, OTs may also recommend positioning changes that minimize spasticity. Sometimes simple adjustments in the height of a footrest or the width of a seat can make a world of difference. OTs can also develop exercise programs for your hands and arms, and may recommend splints that position the hands for best functional use.

Medications

Drug Therapy

There are two medications approved for the treatment of spasticity and other medications that can serve well in certain situations. The most effective dosage will depend on striking a balance between the drug's good and bad effects. An effective dosage tends to vary from time to time. An infection, cold weather, an ingrown toenail—whatever triggers your spasticity—will also influence the amount of medication needed to control it.

Typically, the doctor will increase the dose of medication gradually until the full benefit is evident, and reduce the dose if side effects occur. In addition, people on your health-care team can suggest timing your medication in specific situations. For example, taking an antispasticity medication an hour before sexual activity can prevent painful spasms during orgasm.

Baclofen: Baclofen (Lioresal®) is a muscle relaxant that works in the spinal cord. It is most often taken three or four times a day, and common side effects are drowsiness and muscle weakness. Baclofen relaxes normal as well as spastic muscles. Nausea, a less common side effect, can usually be avoided by taking baclofen with food. The drug has a good safety record with long-term use. The side effects don't build up or become worse over time. At high doses, this medication reduces concentration and contributes to fatigue.

Because it usually restores flexibility within a short period, baclofen may allow other treatment, such as physical therapy, to be more effective. Baclofen does not cure spasticity or improve coordination or strength. A gradual increase in dosing often allows for higher and more effective doses to be taken. It should not be greatly reduced or stopped suddenly without consulting with your physician.

Intrathecal baclofen: Some people require a higher dose of baclofen but cannot tolerate the increased side effects. A surgically implanted pump can administer very small amounts of the drug directly and continuously to the spinal cord (specifically, to the fluid which surrounds the cord).

The baclofen pump has been extremely successful. The pump can improve (or at least maintain) a person's level of functioning. It may even help some people remain ambulatory. And it permits people with very limited mobility to be positioned to minimize pain and the risk of skin breakdown.

The computer-controlled, battery-operated pump, which weighs about 6 ounces, is surgically implanted under the skin of the abdomen. A tube runs from the pump to the spinal canal. The pump is programmed to release a pre-set dose specific for the individual. People who use the pump are seen by their physician or nurse for a new drug supply and a check of the computer program every 1 to 3 months. New drug is injected into the pump through the skin. The little computer can be reprogrammed painlessly by radio signals. When the battery wears out (in 3 to 7 years) the pump itself is surgically removed and replaced. The tube remains in place.

Tizanidine: Tizanidine (Zanaflex®) works quickly to calm spasms and relax tightened muscles, but may cause greater sedation than other medications. Tizanidine is typically taken three times a day. In addition to drowsiness, dry mouth is a common and usually temporary side effect. Hypotension (low blood pressure) is another potential side effect although less frequent.

This drug also has a good safety record with long-term use. It does not cure spasticity or improve muscle coordination or strength. A combination of baclofen and tizanidine may give the best results. Tizanidine should be used with caution with ciprofloxacin HCI [hydrochloride-containing] (Cipro®), which is used to prevent or treat urinary tract infections, since increased drowsiness or sleepiness can occur.

Diazepam: Spasticity can also be treated with diazepam (Valium®), generally in small doses. This drug is not as effective as those mentioned above, but it has the benefit of relieving anxiety, making it easier for someone who is restless or has disturbing night-time spasms to relax and get a good night's sleep.

Drowsiness and potential dependency with long-term use make diazepam a less desirable choice. However, in some circumstances, diazepam and another antispasticity drug may be prescribed together. People for whom this works say that they would rather be a bit sluggish and fully flexible than wide awake and spastic. Clonazepam (Klonopin®), can also help control spasms, particularly at night.

Gabapentin: Gabapentin (Neurontin®) is used to control some types of seizures in epilepsy. In MS it controls certain types of pain and can reduce spasticity. The most common side effects include blurred or double vision, dizziness, and drowsiness. Once you've started on it, gabapentin should not be stopped without consulting your physician.

Dantrolene: Dantrolene sodium (Dantrium®) is generally used only if other drugs (alone or in combination) have been ineffective. It works by partially paralyzing muscles, making it a poor choice for people who walk. Dantrolene can produce serious side effects, including liver damage and blood abnormalities. The longer a person takes this drug, the more these problems are likely to develop. People taking dantrolene must have periodic blood tests.

Levetiracetam: Levetiracetam (Keppra®) is another drug used for seizure control in some forms of epilepsy. In MS, it can sometimes be helpful in improving spasticity and spasms. Side effects and treatment considerations are similar to those seen with gabapentin.

Botulinum toxin: Injection of botulinum toxin (Botox®) has been shown to help spasticity. However, the benefit is limited to the injected muscles, and the treatment must be repeated every 3 to 6 months. Only small amounts of the drug can be injected into the body at any one time. Otherwise, the immune system might create antibodies against it. For these reasons, Botox is not a good choice when many muscles are spastic or the spastic muscles are large. It is a very good choice when muscles of the arm are spastic, as these muscles are small and do not require a lot of medication. Side effects include weakness of the injected muscle and some nearby muscles, and a brief "flulike" syndrome. Despite the drug's effectiveness, the FDA [U.S. Food and Drug Administration] has not yet approved Botox for MS-related spasticity, and the drug is very expensive.

Phenol: Another treatment is the injection of a nerve block called phenol. This treatment also needs to be repeated every 3 to 6 months, and is often effective when oral agents have had unsatisfactory results.

A Final Option: Severe Spasticity

Enormous progress has been made in controlling spasticity in the past 2 decades. If none of the treatments discussed above have helped, surgery might be recommended for relief. The relief is permanent, but so is the resulting disability. The techniques include severing tendons (tenotomy) or nerve roots (rhizotomy) in order to relax cramped-up muscles. These measures are only undertaken after serious consideration and for the most difficult cases of spasticity.

Chapter 47

Botulinum Toxin (Botox) Injections for Treatment of Muscle Spasticity

Chapter Contents

Section 47.1

Understanding Botox

From "Understanding Botox," a fact sheet from the Office
of Women's Health and the U.S. Food and Drug Administration
(FDA, www.fda.gov), August 2005.

Botox™ is used to make lines or wrinkles between the eyebrows look better. It only lasts for a short time.

What is Botox?

Botox comes from a kind of bacteria. The bacteria can make you very sick. But doctors have found that a chemical in Botox can also help treat some health problems. They have been using it safely for many years.

How was this found?

FDA (Food and Drug Administration) approved Botox over 10 years ago to treat certain problems with the eye muscle. Doctors noticed that some wrinkles around the eyes looked better, too. The company that makes Botox tested it. They showed the FDA that Botox worked and was safe for treating some kinds of wrinkles.

How does Botox work?

Wrinkles may be caused when a muscle tightens. Botox is injected through the skin into the muscle. The Botox keeps the muscle from tightening. When the muscle can't tighten, the wrinkle doesn't show as much.

You mean you can't move your muscles?

A doctor trained in the use of Botox will inject small amounts of Botox into the muscle. Only the treated muscle can't move.

What happens over time?

Botox works for about four months. As the muscle returns to normal, you will see the wrinkle again.

Are there any side effects?

Yes. Side effects may include:

- droopy eyelids, which can last for a few weeks;
- feeling like you have the flu; and
- headache and upset stomach.

Risk of botulism (a life or death illness that makes it hard for a person to move the arms and legs or to breathe) is low with Botox, if used the right way.

Remember—Botox is a drug, not a cosmetic.

What should I do if I want to try Botox?

- Ask about how Botox could help or hurt you.
- Make sure your doctor is trained in the use of Botox.
- Make sure you get treatment in a doctor's office or clinic.
- Emergency equipment should be on hand in case of a problem.
- Do not use if you are pregnant or think you might be pregnant.
- Do not use if you are breastfeeding.
- Tell your doctor if you are taking antibiotics.
- Tell your doctor if you have any problems with nerves or muscles.

Are "Botox parties" safe?

No. You should only get Botox in a clinic or doctor's office. You should never share a tube of Botox.

Can I use Botox on other wrinkles?

Botox is only approved to treat wrinkles between the eyebrows.

Can I get Botox at any age?

Botox is only approved for people 18–65 years old. It has not been tested on people under 18 or over 65.

Section 47.2

Is Botox Safe?

From "Early Communication about an Ongoing Safety Review: Botox and Botox Cosmetic (Botulinum toxin Type A) and Myobloc (Botulinum toxin Type B)," from the U.S. Food and Drug Administration's (FDA) Center for Drug Evaluation and Research (CDER, www.fda.gov/cder), February 8, 2008.

This information reflects FDA's current analysis of available data concerning these drugs. This information does not mean that FDA has concluded there is a causal relationship between the drug products and the emerging safety issue. Nor does it mean that FDA is advising healthcare professionals to discontinue prescribing these products. FDA is considering, but has not reached a conclusion about whether this information warrants any regulatory action. FDA intends to update this text when additional information or analyses become available.

FDA has received reports of systemic adverse reactions including respiratory compromise and death following the use of botulinum toxins types A and B for both FDA-approved and unapproved uses. The reactions reported are suggestive of botulism, which occurs when botulinum toxin spreads in the body beyond the site where it was injected. The most serious cases had outcomes that included hospitalization and death, and occurred mostly in children treated for cerebral palsy-associated limb spasticity. Use of botulinum toxins for treatment of limb spasticity (severe arm and leg muscle spasms) in children or adults is not an approved use in the United States.

These serious systemic adverse reactions occurred following treatment of a variety of conditions using a wide range of botulinum toxin doses. FDA is currently reviewing safety data from clinical studies submitted by the manufacturers of Botox, Botox Cosmetic, and Myobloc, as well as post-marketing adverse event reports and the medical literature.

Botox (botulinum toxin type A) is approved for treatment of conditions such as blepharospasm (spasm of the eyelids), cervical dystonia (severe neck muscle spasms), and severe primary axillary hyperhydrosis (excess sweating). Botox Cosmetic, also botulinum toxin Type A, is approved for temporary improvement in the appearance of moderate to severe facial frown lines.

Myobloc (botulinum toxin Type B) is approved for the treatment of adults with cervical dystonia; the safety and effectiveness of Myobloc for cervical dystonia in children have not been established.

FDA is aware of the body of literature describing the use of botulinum toxins to treat limb spasticity in children and adults. The safety, efficacy, and dosage of botulinum toxins have not been established for the treatment of limb spasticity of cerebral palsy or for use in any condition in children less than 12 years of age.

The current prescribing information (labeling) for Botox, Botox Cosmetic, and Myobloc describes adverse reactions occurring in regions near the site of injection for each product's approved uses, such as dysphagia (difficulty swallowing) after injections to treat cervical dystonia, or ptosis (drooping eye lids) after injections for glabellar frown lines or for strabismus and blepharospasm.

The Warnings sections of the labeling for both botulinum toxin products note that important systemic adverse effects, including severe difficulty swallowing and difficulty breathing have occurred in patients with neuromuscular disorders after local injection of typical doses of botulinum toxin. FDA now has evidence that similar, potentially life-threatening systemic toxicity from the use of botulinum toxin products can also result after local injection in patients with other underlying conditions such as those with cerebral palsy associated limb spasticity. Systemic toxicity has been reported in children, several of whom required feeding tubes and/or ventilation (breathing) support.

Until such time that FDA has completed its review, healthcare professionals who use medicinal botulinum toxins should:

- Understand that potency determinations expressed in "Units" or "U" are different among the botulinum toxin products; clinical doses expressed in units are not comparable from one botulinum product to the next.

- Be alert to the potential for systemic effects following administration of botulinum toxins such as: dysphagia, dysphonia, weakness, dyspnea, or respiratory distress.

- Understand that these effects have been reported as early as one day and as late as several weeks after treatment.

- Provide patients and caregivers with the information they need to be able to identify the signs and symptoms of systemic effects after receiving an injection of a botulinum toxin.

- Tell patients they should receive immediate medical attention if they have worsening or unexpected difficulty swallowing or talking, trouble breathing, or muscle weakness.

What does FDA know now about these data?

The FDA has reviewed post-marketing cases from its Adverse Event Reporting System (AERS) database and from the medical literature of pediatric and adult patients diagnosed with botulism following a local injection with a marketed botulinum toxin product.

The pediatric botulism cases occurred in patients less than 16 years old, with reported symptoms ranging from dysphagia to respiratory insufficiency requiring gastric feeding tubes and ventilatory support. Serious outcomes included hospitalization and death. The most commonly reported use of botulinum toxin among these cases was treatment of limb muscle spasticity associated with cerebral palsy.

For Botox, doses ranged from 6.25 to 32 Units/kilogram (U/kg) in these cases. For Myobloc, reported doses were from 388 to 625 U/kg. The reports of adult botulism cases described symptoms including patients experiencing difficulty holding up their heads, dysphagia, and ptosis. Some reports described systemic effects that occurred distant from the site of injection and included weakness and numbness of the lower extremities. Among the adult cases that were serious, including hospitalization, none required intubation or ventilatory support. No deaths were reported. The doses for Botox ranged from 100 to 700 Units and for Myobloc from 10,000 to 20,000 U.

This early communication is in keeping with FDA's commitment to inform the public about its ongoing safety reviews of drugs. FDA will communicate to the public its conclusions, resulting recommendations, and any regulatory actions after the review of the data are completed.

Report serious adverse events to FDA's MedWatch reporting system by completing a form on line at www.fda.gov/medwatch/report/hcp.htm, by faxing (800-FDA-0178), by mail using the postage-paid address form provided online (5600 Fishers Lane, Rockville, MD 20853-9787), or by telephone (800-FDA-1088).

Chapter 48

Treating Spasticity in Children and Adolescents

Chapter Contents

Section 48.1

Nonsurgical Treatment Options for Children and Adolescents with Spasticity

Occupational Therapy

Occupational therapy [OT] recommendations are often, but not always, in conjunction with other intervention such as a spasticity reduction and/ or orthopedic surgery. The occupational therapy services in the community are often recommended to address upper extremity impairment, difficulty with self-care skills (such as dressing and self-feeding) and/or visual motor delay. The OT can also address any oral motor/feeding issues at the evaluation. Specific OT recommendations that can be made are as follows:

- **Splinting:** Patients with range of motion (ROM) limitations may benefit from splinting such as a resting hand split or an elbow split to preserve the ROM available. Splints can be fabricated from a low temperature plastic or can be a soft splint made from neoprene.

- **Serial casting:** This is more commonly used in patients who need to gain ROM in the lower extremities but can also be used in the upper extremities, most often to gain elbow extension. Typically, a cast is placed on the arm at the maximum or near maximum position that can be achieved. The cast is changed weekly with the hope of increasing range of motion each week for approximately 3–4 weeks.

- **Constraint induced therapy:** This involved restraining the strong arm for brief periods to encourage more voluntary and refined movement in the weaker arm for patients with hemiparesis.

A cast or splint is often used to restrain the strong arm and the patient is provided with established activities to do with the weaker arm.

- **Therapeutic horseback riding:** This is an excellent activity to improve balance and overall strength. Therapists will ride with a patient (to provide head and/or trunk control) or walk along side the patient who can sit independently on the horse.

- **Assistive technology evaluation:** A referral for this type can assist in determining if wheelchair modifications, communication devices, or other adaptive equipment can be utilized to optimize function.

Oral Medications

All oral medications act systemically, that is, they affect the whole body and reduce spasticity or other abnormal movements throughout the body. They are usually mildly effective and usually more effective in young children than in older ones. No medication is effective for every individual.

- **Baclofen (Lioresal):** Baclofen is a medication quite similar to a chemical, GABA, that is deficient in people who have spasticity and is probably the most helpful and is used most often. Baclofen is usually given three times a day. When taken by mouth, a relatively small amount of baclofen gets into the spinal cord (where it needs to be to be effective. Baclofen is usually given in increasing doses up to a dose that depends on body size and weight. The medication is given in three divided doses and is increased until there is benefit, unacceptable side effects, or until a target dose is reached without benefit. The main side effect of oral baclofen is drowsiness. That side effect can be lessened if baclofen doses are started at low levels and increased slowly (e.g., every 5–14 days). Confusion and unsteadiness are less common side effects. Baclofen is not addicting and may be taken for years with minimal risk of it affecting other body organs. Baclofen is also effective in the treatment of dystonia.

- **Dantrolene (Dantrium):** Dantrolene is a medication used to treat spasticity. It is the only medication that acts on the muscles themselves rather than on the brain and for this reason, it causes less sedation than baclofen or diazepam although it may cause diarrhea, weakness, or a rash. Dantrolene may cause muscle

431

weakness in high doses. Usual doses for spasticity range from 50–100 mg/day. Because Dantrolene occasionally causes liver damage, blood work is done approximately every 6 months to test liver function.

- **Tizanidine (Zanaflex):** Tizanidine is a relatively new medication that appears to be mildly effective but its use in children is often complicated by unacceptable drowsiness. Doses range from 4–24 mg/ day. Side effects include drowsiness, dizziness, and low blood pressure.

- **Diazepam (Valium):** Diazepam is mildly effective in reducing spasticity and athetosis. It also acts in the brain and also affects the release of GABA. Its effects last for far longer than the other medications. Unfortunately, diazepam is habituating, i.e., children who take it for several months get used to it and may require several months of slowly decreasing doses to get off of it.

- **Clonazepam (Klonopin):** Clonazepam is a medication similar to diazepam but has a shorted time of activity and is more easily discontinued. It may be given to treat dystonia or chorea. Doses range from 0.5 mg/twice daily to 2 mg three times a day.

- **Trihexyphenidyl (Artane):** This medication is frequently given to treat dystonia. It is given three times a day, beginning at perhaps 2 mg three times a day and increasing every 3–5 days up to 6–7 mg three times a day, and sometimes higher. Artane may cause dry mouth or urinary hesitancy but causes drowsiness infrequently.

- **L-dopa/Carbidopa (Sinemet):** This medication is often given briefly to children with dystonia for two reasons. First, there is a rare condition called dopa-responsive dystonia that may mimic CP [cerebral palsy] and is dramatically improved by low doses of Sinemet. Secondly, some people with other forms of dystonia—including dystonic CP—are improved by Sinemet.

Intramuscular Injections

Intramuscular injections are given to patients who have spasticity or dystonia that is more severe in one or more areas and that is not satisfactorily treated by oral medications. The most common intramuscular medication is botulinum toxin; the most commonly used form of botulinum toxin is Botox. Recently, another form of botulinum toxin has become available, Myobloc; it is used mainly for children who do not respond to Botox injections. The medication can be injected directly into a spastic or dystonic muscle to decrease the tightness in those muscles. These medications weaken only the injected muscle and rarely cause any kind of central nervous system side effects.

Whenever intramuscular medications are used, they are usually injected in several different areas of the affected muscles. It is not unusual to inject 4–6 muscles at one time. Because of the multiple injections that are required, some type of anesthetic is usually used, either a topical anesthetic to numb the skin over the muscles to be injected, or children can be given an anesthetic gas to sedate them for the 5 minutes or so needed for the injections.

- **Botox:** Botox is a purified protein from the botulinum toxin. It comes frozen and is dissolved in saline then injected into the muscle through small needles. The amount to be given is determined by how tight the individual muscles are and by the weight of the child. Doses of 10–15 units/kilogram of body weight are commonly used and some experts use higher doses than that. The effects begin about 2–3 days after the Botox is injected, hit a peak about 3 weeks later, and usually wear off in about 3 months. Injections are often repeated for 2–4 years. Botox has minimal side effects. Rarely, children may become unusually floppy for a few days or weeks after high doses of Botox.

- **Myobloc:** Myobloc is a purified protein from a different form of botulinum toxin. It has been available for the past two years and there is less information on its use than for Botox. Myobloc comes already is a liquid form and is refrigerated until it is used. Doses of Myobloc are approximately 50 units of Myobloc to 1 unit of Botox. It can be given into any affected muscles and appears to have similar effectiveness and safety to Botox. The costs of the two medications are similar.

- **Alcohol and phenol:** These two medications were used fairly often before Botox and Myobloc were available but are used infrequently now. They are injected into spastic muscles near nerves and temporarily injure the muscle or nerve. Their effects last somewhat longer: 6–12 months. They may cause unpleasant sensations (feeling) in areas around the injected nerves.

Follow-up: After injections, physical therapists often perform serial casting and initiate therapy to increase range of motion. It is important for your therapist to follow up with the team with regard to the effectiveness of the injections. Injections may be repeated several times, although effectiveness sometimes decreases after multiple injections.

Section 48.2

Surgical Treatment Options for Children and Adolescents with Spasticity

"Surgical Treatment Options for Spasticity and Other Movement Disorders," © 2008 Children's Hospital of Pittsburgh Spasticity and Movement Disorder Clinic. Reprinted with permission.

Intrathecal Baclofen

Baclofen is a drug that helps reduce spasticity and dystonia. Taken orally, little baclofen enters the spinal fluid, spinal cord, or brain. If baclofen is given directly into the spinal fluid, it soaks into the spinal cord and is far more effective, with far fewer side effects.

Selective Rhizotomy

A rhizotomy is an operation in which a nerve or part of a nerve is intentionally cut. Lumbar rhizotomies are operations on the lower back to partially divide nerves from the legs. Selective lumbar rhizotomies are operations in which the neurosurgeon divides the various nerves coming into the spine from the legs into several branches, tests each branch with an electrical stimulus, then cuts the branches which give abnormal responses. There is debate as to whether selective lumbar rhizotomies give better results than non-selective rhizotomies. The problem in deciding is that both operations are effective and no one knows if one is better.

Screening/Selection Criteria

Candidates for a rhizotomy are usually young (4 to 8 years old), have relatively good leg strength, and do not have severe leg contractures.

The primary goal of surgery is often to improve walking. Rhizotomy can be done at any age to facilitate care. Rhizotomies will relieve the spasticity but will not improve contractures (shortening of muscles and tendons) that are already present, nor will they improve dystonia.

Surgery

Rhizotomy surgery generally lasts about 2 to 3 hours. The procedure involves a midline incision about 3–4 inches long in the lumbar region. Muscles are separated away from the spine and the nerve roots coming and going to the legs are exposed. Each nerve root divided into 3–5 branches and is tested with special monitoring equipment to identify nerves that give abnormal responses when they are electrically stimulated. The nerve roots that give abnormal responses are cut; usually 50–60% of the top half of each nerve is divided.

Expectations

Children are at bed rest for 2–3 days postoperatively. They are hospitalized for 3–5 days and then go home. We ask them to wait for 1 month after operation to start intensive physical therapy [PT]. The frequency of PT varies with the goals, from 1–2 times a week if the goal is to improve range of motion to 4–5 times a week if the goals are to improve strength and walking.

Myths/Facts

Myth: Selective rhizotomy is usually permanent but the effects sometimes wear off.

Fact: Whenever children get significantly tighter a few months or years after rhizotomy, it is almost always because they have dystonia (which is not improved by rhizotomy) rather than because their spasticity has returned.

Myth: Rhizotomies have a high complication rate.

Fact: The complication rate is surprisingly low: 5–10%, lover than the rate of complications for insertion of baclofen pumps.

Deep Brain Stimulation

Deep brain stimulation (DBS) is a method of treating dystonia and tremor that involves an operation in which thin blunt wires (electrodes) are surgically implanted precisely into a small area deep in the brain. If the abnormal movement affects one side of the body, one electrode is inserted (on the opposite side of the brain than the body is affected). If both sides of the body are affected, bilateral (both sides) electrodes are inserted. The electrodes are tunneled under the skin down the neck and are connected to an electrical stimulator unit than can be programmed with a computer to stimulate the area of the brain at the tip of the electrode. The idea behind DBS is that fast electrical stimulation (130 times a second) interrupts the abnormal electrical circuit within the brain that is causing the abnormal movements.

At the present time, we have an FDA [U.S. Food and Drug Administration]-approved protocol to study the use of DBS in children 12–21 with severe dystonia. We have also used DBS to treat tremor in a few teenagers. DBS is not presently approved for the general (non-research) treatment of movement disorders in children.

Screening/Selection Criteria

Candidates for DBS usually have severe dystonia that has not responded adequately to oral medications or to ITB [intrathecal baclofen]. They are 12–21 years old (at present) and do not have any other medical condition that might increase the risks of DBS.

Implantation

The operation in children is done under a general anesthetic. Patients are anesthetized then a stereotactic frame (a metal frame marked like a ruler) is attached to their head and an MR [magnetic resonance] scan is done. The target for the electrodes is determined by selecting its location on the MR scan, then calculations are made based on markings on the frame to determine the trajectory and depth the electrodes need to be inserted. A small hole is drilled in the skull and the electrode is guided to the desired spot, which is usually within 1 mm of the desired location. The wires are then tunneled under the skin and connected to the stimulator. The stimulator is turned on the next day and is adjusted frequently during the first few weeks after operations to improve the movements as much as possible.

Follow-Up

Patients are seen approximately every 2 weeks for adjustments postoperatively, then at 1, 2, and 3 years.

Expectations

DBS is too new to know how well it will work. Based on studies done in Europe, it appears to be very beneficial for children with primary (genetic) dystonia and somewhat less effective for dystonia due to CP [cerebral palsy] or head injuries, but the numbers of patients treated so far are too small to come to any firm conclusions.

Orthopedic Surgery

Surgery is performed to increase the ease of care, improve function, and on occasion, particularly in the upper extremity, to improve the appearance. Both bony and soft tissue surgery are involved. All four extremities can have surgery at the same setting. Although quite time consuming and initially a bit more uncomfortable, it allows the patient to recover more appropriately because most of the deformities have been corrected at once.

Procedures

The major soft tissue procedure involves lengthening the muscle-tendon unit. This usually involves cutting the tendon where it overlaps the muscle belly. This stretches the entire unit which improves the length of the extremity. On occasion, particularly at the Achilles tendon, the tendon is partially cut in three areas through tiny stab wounds during the skin. This allows the tendon to lengthen appropriately without a large incision. Postoperatively, casting is needed for both methods for 4–6 weeks.

Bony surgery (osteotomy) is performed at the upper femur (thigh bone) to reposition the femoral head (ball) into the acetabulum (cup) and to realign inappropriate rotational deformities. Osteotomies are also performed at the lower tibia (shin bone) to correct malrotation deformities. Internal fixation of some sort is needed to hold the bones together until they heal. Sometimes, and particularly in the tibia, additional external support is needed with a cast.

Spine surgery is sometimes needed to correct deformities as well. If needed, the patients are referred to our spine surgery colleagues.

Expectations

Because the cerebral palsy still exists, the patient cannot ever be returned to a normal status. However, at a minimum, care is usually significantly improved. In ambulatory patients, their gait is usually improved. In the upper extremities, the appearance and care are improved. By testing, assuming independent activity is present, the function is usually improved. However, unless this is the dominant extremity, the overall function may not be improved. Postoperatively, physical and occupational therapy are necessary to regain the strength and agility needed to gain the appropriate level of function. This may take 3–12 months depending on how much surgery is done. At the hip, when repositioned and especially when done early, the risk of degenerative arthritis is significantly diminished. If the hip remains out of position, arthritis will occur and lead to pain and leg deformity.

Follow-Up

Postoperative follow up is needed for cast removal and x-ray evaluation to determine the healing of the osteotomies. Additional follow-up is needed to access the progression of the therapy. For patients who live far away from Pittsburgh, we do try to arrange follow-up visits with a local orthopedic surgeon if they are willing to do so.

Myths/Facts

Myth: Surgery corrects everything and makes the patient normal.

Fact: Surgery will improve the alignment of the extremities. If decent function is present, function should improve but it depends on how well the muscles can be controlled and how well the patient works with therapy.

Myth: Surgery only needs to be done one time.

Fact: With soft tissue surgery, the younger the patient, the more likely that it may have to be repeated in several years, especially at the Achilles tendon. However with spasticity reduction (baclofen pump/ rhizotomy), the incidence of recurrent surgery has significantly diminished.

Myth: It is okay to leave a partially dislocated hip alone for a long time.

Fact: The longer the hip is partially dislocated, the more serious the deformity becomes and the more degeneration will occur. The earlier the deformity is corrected, the more remodeling may occur and the more likely the hip will become nearly, if not completely normal. Sometimes, when done early enough, only soft tissue surgery is needed.

If done late, sometimes bony surgery will need to be done on both the femur and pelvic sides of the hip.

Section 48.3

Selective Dorsal Rhizotomy for Cerebral Palsy

Introduction

Of all the surgical procedures currently performed on patients with cerebral palsy, selective dorsal rhizotomy (SDR) has undergone more thorough scientific scrutiny than any other (including orthopaedic). Accumulated evidence and our own experience indicate that SDR is an excellent option for selected patients with spastic CP [cerebral palsy]. We think parents and patients need to inquire about SDR as a part of the management of CP before the patient undergoes orthopedic surgery.

The first report of dorsal rhizotomy in 1913 clearly illustrated reduction of spasticity and marked improvement in walking, standing, and sitting in children with spastic CP. However, the operation received no attention from neurosurgeons until the 1970s, when the procedure was refined and named functional dorsal rhizotomy. In the late 1980s, pediatric neurosurgeons in the United States began to employ SDR for treatment for CP spasticity, and our Center has been performing SDR on patients with CP since 1987.

Outline of the SDR Procedure

SDR involves sectioning (cutting) of some of the sensory nerve fibers that come from the muscles and enter the spinal cord.

Two groups of nerve roots leave the spinal cord and lie in the spinal canal. The ventral spinal roots send information to the muscle; the dorsal spinal roots transmit sensation from the muscle to the spinal cord.

At the time of the operation, the neurosurgeon divides each of the dorsal roots into 3–5 rootlets and stimulates each rootlet electrically.

By examining electromyographic (EMG) responses from muscles in the lower extremities, the surgical team identifies the rootlets that cause spasticity. The abnormal rootlets are selectively cut, leaving the normal rootlets intact. This reduces messages from the muscle, resulting in a better balance of activities of nerve cells in the spinal cord, and thus reduces spasticity.

Details of Our SDR Procedure

Different surgical techniques are utilized to perform SDR. Neurosurgeons typically perform SDR after removing the lamina (laminectomy) from 5–7 vertebrae. That technique was also used at our Center to perform SDR on over 140 children with CP. However, we were concerned about possible problems that can arise from removal of such a large amount of bone from the spine. Additionally, because of the extensive removal of the bone, we could not offer SDR to children with weak trunk muscles or to adults. Thus, in 1991, we developed a less invasive surgical technique, which requires removal of the lamina from only 1–2 vertebrae. We refined the technique further and currently remove the lamina from a single lumbar vertebra.

SDR begins with a 1- to 2-inch incision along the center of the lower back just above the waist. The spinous processes and a portion of the lamina are removed to expose the spinal cord and spinal nerves. Ultrasound and an x-ray locate the tip of the spinal cord, where there is a natural separation between sensory and motor nerves. A rubber pad is placed to separate the motor from the sensory nerves. The sensory nerve roots that will be tested and cut are placed on top of the pad and the motor nerves beneath the pad, away from the operative field.

After the sensory nerves are exposed, each sensory nerve root is divided into 3–5 rootlets. Each rootlet is tested with EMG [electromyography], which records electrical patterns in muscles. Rootlets are ranked from 1 (mild) to 4 (severe) for spasticity. The severely abnormal rootlets are cut. This technique is repeated for rootlets between spinal nerves L2 and S2. Half of the L1 dorsal root fibers are cut without EMG testing.

When testing and cutting are complete, the dura mater is closed, and fentanyl is given to bathe the sensory nerves directly. The other layers of tissue, muscle, fascia, and subcutaneous tissue are sewn. The skin is closed with glue. There are no stitches to be removed from the back. Surgery takes approximately 4 hours. The patient goes to the recovery room for 1–2 hours before being transferred to the intensive care unit overnight.

Advantages of Our Technique over Other Techniques for SDR

We believe that our SDR procedure has these significant advantages over others:

1. Reduced risk of spinal deformities in later years

2. Decreased postrhizotomy motor weakness

3. Reduced hip flexor spasticity by sectioning the first lumbar dorsal root

4. Shorter-term, less intense back pain

5. Earlier resumption of vigorous physical therapy

Possible Complications

The dorsal rhizotomy is a long and complex neurosurgical procedure. As in other major neurosurgical procedures, it presents some risks. Paralysis of the legs and bladder, impotence, and sensory loss are the most serious complications. Wound infection and meningitis are also possible, but they are usually controlled with antibiotics. Leakage of the spinal fluid through the wound is another risk.

Abnormal sensitivity of the skin on the feet and legs is relatively common after SDR, but usually resolves within 6 weeks. There is no way to prevent the abnormal sensitivity in the feet. Transient change in bladder control may occur, but this also resolves within a few weeks. A few of our patients have experienced urinary tract infections and pneumonia.

Complications in Our Patients

In our more than 1,700 patients, only one adult patient had a spinal fluid leak that required surgical repair. A few children had spinal fluid collection under the skin but no surgery was needed. One patient developed angulation of the spine (kyphosis) that required spine fusion. There were no long-term complications in any of patients who underwent surgery as early as 1987. Our results indicate the long term safety of SDR.

Outcome of SDR

As mentioned in our overview, SDR has been tested more thoroughly than any other surgical procedure for treatment of CP. On the basis of reported studies and our own experience, we believe that SDR can greatly benefit selected patients with spastic CP. All parents and patients should be informed of this option when surgical treatment is considered.

Spasticity: At present, SDR is the only surgical procedure that can provide permanent reduction of spasticity in CP. In our patients with spastic diplegia, SDR always reduced spasticity, and recurrences have been rare. Return of spasticity in later years is highly unlikely after its reduction over many years.

In patients with spastic quadriplegia, however, SDR can fail to reduce spasticity. Recurrence of spasticity is relatively common in severely involved nonambulatory patients with spastic quadriplegia. In patients who can walk with an assistive device, the risk for recurrent spasticity is less than in nonambulatory patients, and even if it does recur, it is less severe than before the operation.

It is our opinion that patients with CP do not depend on spasticity for any activities. Their case is different from that of patients with spasticity associated with spinal cord injury, in whom the spasticity sometimes does help with standing and taking steps.

Strength: SDR does not cause permanent weakness. However, patients will experience transient motor weakness that may last a few weeks to months after SDR. It should be remembered that a varying degree of motor weakness is always present in CP. When spasticity is reduced or eliminated, the motor weakness underlying spasticity becomes more noticeable, but the impression that SDR produces motor weakness is incorrect.

Patients who walk independently always resume independent walking within a few weeks after SDR. Patients who walk with crutches will also resume crutch walking within several weeks after SDR. Patients who walk well with a walker prior to SDR resume assisted walking within several weeks. Patients who use a walker and assistance require much longer to resume the level of walking they were capable of before SDR.

After spasticity is reduced, it becomes easier for patients to increase strength with therapy and exercise. Adolescents and adults can start treadmill and other types of exercise that were impossible before SDR.

It is important to note that SDR does not result in floppy extremities, even immediately after the operation.

Motor function: SDR results in improvements in sitting, standing, walking, and balance control in walking. In three randomized studies of changes in gross motor functions after SDR, two of the studies showed improvements and one did not find significant benefits from SDR. All three studies are, however, far short of conclusive. They assessed outcomes using measures of gross motor function, which do not allow assessment of changes in quality of motor functions or of children whose impairment is relatively mild. Also, the follow-up studies of these patients were too short to address the long-term benefits of SDR, the effects of reduced spasticity on deformities, and the need for orthopaedic surgery. In our view, the study by McLaughlin et al., which failed to find any beneficial effect from SDR, is flawed by various limitations, so no conclusion can be drawn from it.

Typically, improvements in motor function are most noticeable during the first 6 months after SDR. After that, improvements are slow but steady. In children, these improvements can continue up to 10 years of age. In adults and adolescents, improvements continue for approximately 2 years after SDR.

Deformities: Patients with CP almost invariably have some deformities in the lower extremities. Common deformities are hip subluxation, hamstring and heel cord contractures, foot deformities, and in-toeing. These deformities can be improved by SDR.

Hip subluxation can progress if left untreated. In most patients, SDR can halt the progression; certainly it does not exacerbate or increase the risk of hip subluxation. However, some children under 5 years of age who have poorly developed hip joints do show progression of hip subluxation regardless of treatment.

SDR reduces the severity of hamstring and heel cord contractures. It is common to see improvements in in-toeing gait and in other abnormal gait patterns after SDR. Also, the lack of spasticity makes it easy to stretch the tight muscles. When contractures have been present for years, however, the affected muscles and tendons are shortened. It takes many months to improve such contractures, and in older children and adults, it is often impossible to do so except through surgical release.

Early SDR, at 2–4 years of age, can prevent the development of deformities. For this reason, we favor early surgery. Also, SDR will reduce deformities and makes it easier to treat deformities later with orthopaedic surgery.

Orthopaedic surgery: Many patients with spastic CP require multiple orthopaedic operations. Our study showed that early SDR may reduce the rate of subsequent orthopaedic procedures. It is important to remember that deformities are due not only to spasticity but also to motor impairment and consequent limited muscle stretching in daily activities. That is, muscles without spasticity can still develop contractures if they are not used and stretched fully. Therefore, many patients will still require follow-up with orthopaedic surgeons after SDR.

We favor SDR prior to orthopaedic surgery. Muscle and tendon release procedures increase a range of joint movements but weaken the muscles permanently. Since SDR can increase the range of joint movement without causing muscle weakness, we recommend SDR prior to muscle releases. Persistent muscle and tendon contractures after SDR are treated with vigorous stretching, night splints, and serial casting. If all the nonsurgical treatments fail to resolve the contractures, we recommend orthopaedic surgery as a last resort.

Upper extremity functions: SDR is performed to improve the lower extremity functions, but it can also improve the gross range of motion of the upper extremities. It does not improve fine motor skills. The upper extremity improvements are seen in children with relatively severe quadriplegic CP. If the upper extremity involvement is mild, SDR will not result in noticeable improvements.

Potty training: Spastic CP can be associated with small bladder capacity and also with difficulties in sitting, which can delay potty training in young children. From time to time, we have seen children complete potty training soon after SDR.

Cognitive improvements: We have seen children who showed marked changes in cognitive functions after SDR, and in our earlier study we found significant increase in the speed of visual recognition.

Speech improvement: SDR can be followed by significant improvements of speech. We attribute this to improved sitting posture, reduced distraction by spasticity, and improved cognitive functions. However, it is difficult to predict which patients will show speech improvements.

Emotional improvements: Parents often note that their children become much less irritable and more loving after SDR. We attribute this to decreased mental distraction by tight muscles.

Chapter 49

Treating Tremor

Chapter Contents

Section 49.1

Overview of Tremor Treatments

Two conditions make up the largest numbers of patients with movement disorders who might be suitable for radiosurgical treatment. These diseases are Parkinson's disease and essential tremor (familial tremor). In unusual circumstances, movement disorders may also be due to head injuries, brain infections such as encephalitis, or following strokes. Movement disorders take a wide variety of forms. One of the most common movement disorders is tremor.

Parkinson's Disease and Essential Tremor

In Parkinson's disease, the tremor or shaking usually involves the arms and hands and is most prominent when the patient is at rest. In essential or familial tremor, the hands and arms are usually quiet at rest, but if the patient attempts to perform a task, such as picking up a glass of water or writing, then the tremor becomes very noticeable. Tremor can sometimes involve the head and neck and also sometimes involves the legs. Tremor interferes with many normal activities. Patients may be unable to write their name and, for instance, sign checks. They may be unable to drink from a cup or glass without spilling, and they may be unable to cut food with a knife and fork. In addition, patients may be unable to feed themselves, button clothing, comb their hair, or perform almost any movement that involves coordinated control of the hands, fingers, and arms.

In essential or familial tremor, the movement disorder is the only aspect of the disease. The only difference between essential tremor and familial tremor is that in the latter, there is a family history with tremor being present in other generations, whereas in essential tremor, there is not. The actual tremor itself is identical in both conditions.

In Parkinson's disease, there are often other movement abnormalities in addition to tremor. These may include bradykinesia (slowness of movement) and rigidity or stiffness in the muscles, which make movements difficult. Also, in Parkinson's disease, there is frequently difficulty with walking because of the slowness and stiffness of movement and because of poor balance and a tendency to fall.

Nonsurgical Treatment

Medications are available for initial treatment of movement disorders. In Parkinson's disease, medications containing L-dopa (levodopa) are the most commonly used. A variety of newer medications may also be effective in the control of Parkinson's disease symptoms. In essential tremor, the beta-blocker family of drugs, which includes Inderal (propranolol) and Mysoline (primidone), may be effective. In general, surgical treatment of any kind, including radiosurgery, is usually reserved for patients whose symptoms cannot be effectively controlled with medications.

Surgical Treatment

Various forms of surgical treatment are available to control movement disorders when medications are ineffective. The surgical procedures available generally fall into two categories: 1) ablative or destructive procedures such as thalamotomy or pallidotomy, and 2) stimulation procedures performed by the implantation of stimulating electrodes within the brain.

Although the exact mechanism of movement disorders is not completely understood, it is clear that in most cases, overactivity in one of two structures within the brain causes movement disorders. This overactivity is located either in the thalamus or in the globus pallidus. Recently, suppression of movement disorders by electrical stimulation in another area, the subthalamic nucleus, has been suggested, but stimulation in this area remains under clinical investigation.

Radiosurgical versus Radiofrequency Methods

Excessive activity of brain cells in a small part of the thalamus called the ventral intermediate nucleus (VIM) is thought to be responsible for both the tremor of Parkinson's disease and the tremor seen in essential or familial tremor. Its involvement in other forms of tremor varies. The classical surgical method of dealing with tremor has been to destroy this small group of cells (thalamotomy) by passing an especially designed needle into the area and then heating the needle tip with radiofrequency electrical current. The correct area of the brain can be identified by a combination of imaging studies (usually MRI [magnetic resonance imaging] scanning) and electrical recordings made with a tiny wire electrode (microelectrode).

In the 1960s, Lars Leksell, a Swedish neurosurgeon, began to experiment with destroying this area using radiosurgery. Since that time, there has been considerable experience in using radiosurgical methods to treat movement disorders, rather than radiofrequency methods. The advantage of the radiofrequency method is the presumed ability to more carefully locate the exact target using the electrical recording and stimulation methods mentioned previously.

The disadvantage is that it requires passage of a needle electrode through the brain tissue resulting in the possibility of complications such as bleeding and infection, either within or upon the surface of the brain. Unintended injury to other normal structures can lead to complications such as paralysis, loss of feeling, or interference with speech, among others.

Radiosurgical treatment does not require placing any invasive device within the body and must rely therefore on imaging studies such as MRI scanning to correctly localize the target. Some people have felt that the inability to use microelectrode recording and stimulation when radiosurgical procedures are performed is a drawback of those procedures. As we will see, however, the outcome of Gamma Knife radiosurgical procedures is equally effective as that of radiofrequency procedures performed in the thalamus and is considerably safer. Those complications that directly surround an operation such as anesthetic complications, hemorrhage, and infection, do not occur with radiosurgical treatment.

It should be strongly noted that radiosurgery with the LINAC [linear accelerator] technology is not recommended for any type of movement disorder as the machines can not reach the precision of the Gamma Knife and potential harm will be done to the patient.

Thalamotomy

Both radiofrequency and radiosurgical thalamotomy can be expected to relieve tremor in about 85% of patients. In some patients, the tremor is markedly suppressed but not totally relieved and in other patients, the tremor is completely relieved. Examples of a patient's handwriting before and after a thalamotomy was performed with the Gamma Knife machine. Virtually all of the treatment of movement disorders using radiosurgery has been with the Gamma Knife. There is little or no experience in using the other forms of radiosurgery, that is, the linear accelerator or heavy particle beam radiosurgery, to make such lesions for treatment of movement disorders.

Therefore, results achieved with Gamma Knife may not be indicative of results achieved with other types of radiosurgical equipment. The Gamma Knife is designed to perform this type of treatment. We have performed more than 200 thalamotomies for the relief of tremor over a period of more than 8 years. Only two relatively mild side effects have been seen in these 200 patients. Both involve mild weakness or coordination difficulty in the side of the body opposite to the thalamotomy. No other complications of any kind have been seen in any of the other patients.

For radiofrequency thalamotomy, the complication rate has been variously estimated from as low as five percent to as high as 20% or 25%. These complications can include paralysis, loss of feeling, difficulties with speech and, in a rare case, severe hemorrhage requiring a major operation (craniotomy) to remove a large blood clot within the brain or on the surface of the brain. It is our belief that radiosurgical thalamotomy with the Gamma Knife offers the safest method for treatment of tremor.

Deep Brain Stimulation

Recently, there has been considerable attention to the use of deep brain stimulation to treat tremor. The success rate with this method is about equal to that of thalamotomy performed either by the radiofrequency or radiosurgical method. Deep brain stimulation requires, however, a permanent implantation of stimulating hardware (wires and battery) within the brain and the body. The potential for hardware-related complications such as wire breakage, dislocation of the wires, the need for frequent reprogramming of the batteries, and the eventual failure and need for replacement of the batteries, in addition to the relatively high cost of the hardware, in our opinion, limit the practical usage of deep brain stimulation.

Deep brain stimulation may be particularly useful if a thalamotomy has been performed previously on one side and one is interested in controlling tremor on the other side. Performing a bilateral or two-sided thalamotomy increases the risk considerably. This risk may be lowered by performing a thalamotomy on one side and then placing a deep brain stimulator on the other side.

Pallidotomy

The other area of the brain involved in movement disorders is the globus pallidus. Overactivity in this structure generally produces the slowness of movement and stiffness seen in Parkinson's disease patients. The globus pallidus generally is not thought to play any role in familial or essential tremor. The pallidotomy procedure, which destroys a portion of the globus pallidus, can be performed by either radiofrequency or Gamma Knife approaches. Once again, we are unaware of any significant experience with either linear accelerator or particle beam radiosurgery for the performance of pallidotomy.

We have performed nearly 100 pallidotomies in the past eight years using the Gamma Knife. The success rate closely approximates that which can be obtained with the radiofrequency method. As the radiosurgical pallidotomy technique was being developed, some complications occurred more frequently than one would have expected with the radiofrequency method. However, during the past 60 patients, only a single complication, a partial visual loss, has occurred. No other complications of any kind have been seen. We believe that radiosurgical pallidotomy is as effective as radiofrequency pallidotomy and considerably safer.

Recently, information has been published on the use of deep brain stimulation in the globus pallidus, as well. This method has been employed primarily in Europe and is currently not approved by the Food & Drug Administration of the United States for use here. As mentioned previously, there has been recent interest in deep brain stimulation in an area called the subthalamic nucleus. Most of this work has also been done in Europe and currently deep brain stimulation also is not approved for use in the United States, although some experimental applications are currently being carried out.

Summary

By the end of 1998, it had been reported that 814 patients had received Gamma Knife treatment for Parkinson's disease at all Gamma Knife centers throughout the world, and a significant number of additional patients had received treatment for essential tremor and other forms of tremor. The interest in using radiosurgery to treat movement disorders is increasing. It is attractive to patients and their families because of its effectiveness and safety. Many radiosurgical centers perform the procedures on an outpatient basis and, at maximum, an overnight stay is required. Patients are able to return to normal activities immediately without the recovery period generally required after an open skull procedure, such as a radiofrequency thalamotomy or deep brain stimulator implantation.

Section 49.2

Gamma Knife Surgery for Tremor

The Gamma Knife is a remarkable tool that allows neurosurgeons to operate on abnormal areas of the brain without making an incision. Using a technique called stereotactic radiosurgery, the Gamma Knife is designed to precisely target and destroy abnormalities within the skull using highly focused gamma radiation. Patients experience minimal pain and, in most cases, can resume regular activities the day after treatment.

Gamma Knife treatment is not experimental. The Gamma Knife has been in use for over 30 years, and has been used successfully to treat more than 100,000 patients worldwide. It is one of the most advanced techniques in the treatment of disorders affecting the brain and its adjacent structures. It's not surprising that the Gamma Knife is regarded as the "gold standard" for stereotactic radiosurgery.

How Does the Gamma Knife Work?

The Gamma Knife uses ionizing radiation (gamma rays) produced by 201 cobalt-60 sources to target and destroy a tumor, a blood vessel abnormality such as an arteriovenous malformation (AVM) within or adjacent to brain tissue, or to treat the symptoms of Parkinson's disease and trigeminal neuralgia (an excruciatingly painful facial condition) with extreme accuracy. Since each individual gamma ray is of relatively weak intensity, the normal brain tissue surrounding the abnormality is protected as the full dose of radiation is focused only at the point where all 201 beams converge. This explains why side effects are rare and usually temporary. Since the procedure is noninvasive, or "bloodless," the risks of postoperative complications, such as infection and hemorrhage, are eliminated.

Treatment with the Gamma Knife is accomplished by a multidisciplinary team consisting of a neurosurgeon, a radiation oncologist, and a radiation physicist. The referring physician is an active partner in the treatment process, and patients accepted for Gamma Knife treatment remain in their primary physician's care.

Providing regular reports on patient status, the Gamma Knife team maintains ongoing communication with referring physicians through evaluation, treatment, follow-up, and outcome studies.

Risks and Advantages

The advantages associated with Gamma Knife treatment are numerous. Unlike traditional neurosurgery, prolonged hospitalization is avoided and the effects of a general anesthetic are eliminated. Patients unable to undergo brain surgery because of their underlying medical condition can undergo Gamma Knife surgery with minimal risk. Costs are usually a fraction of the cost of traditional open surgery, and are even more favorable when the cost of dealing with immediate postoperative complications is considered. Since the Gamma Knife does not result in immediate destruction of an arteriovenous malformation (AVM) or brain tumor, follow-up evaluations and imaging studies at regular intervals are essential in order to determine whether the condition treated is responding as expected.

Chapter 50

Dystonia Treatments

Section 50.1

Oral Medications for Dystonia

There are many medications that have been shown to improve dystonia. No single drug works for every individual, and several trials of medications may be necessary to determine which is most appropriate for you. Working with your physician to determine the drugs best suited for your case may be challenging, but finding the right drug(s) can result in a dramatic improvement in symptoms.

There are several categories of medications used in the treatment of dystonia. These categories include:

- anticholinergics;
- benzodiazepines;
- baclofen;
- dopaminergic agents/Dopamine-depleting agents;
- tetrabenazine.

Anticholinergics: Anticholinergics include such drugs as Artane® (trihexyphenidyl), Cogentin® (benztropine), or Parsitan® (ethopropazine) which block a neurotransmitter called acetylcholine. Use of these drugs is sometimes limited by central side effects such as confusion, drowsiness, hallucination, personality change, and memory difficulties, and peripheral side effects such as dry mouth, blurred vision, urinary retention, and constipation.

Benzodiazepines: Benzodiazepines, such as Valium® (diazepam), Klonopin® (clonazepam), and Ativan® (lorazepam) affect the nervous system's ability to process a neurotransmitter called GABA-A [gamma-aminobutyric acid A]. A primary side effect is sedation, but others include depression, personality change, and drug addiction. Rapid discontinuation can result in a withdrawal syndrome. Some dystonia patients tolerate very high doses without apparent adverse effects.

Baclofen: Baclofen (Lioresal®) stimulates the body's ability to process a neurotransmitter called GABA-B. Intrathecal forms of baclofen, in which a steady dose of medication is fed into the nervous system by a surgically implanted device, are also available. Side effects may include confusion, dizziness or lightheadedness, drowsiness, nausea, and muscle weakness.

Dopaminergic agents/dopamine-depleting agents. Some patients with primary dystonia respond to drugs which increase the neurotransmitter dopamine. These drugs are called dopaminergic agents and include Sinemet® (levodopa) or Parlodel® (bromocriptine). Side effects may include parkinsonism, hypotension, and depression. Ironically, however, many patients respond to agents which block or deplete dopamine. Many of these drugs are antipsychotic agents like Clozaril® (clozapine), Nitoman® (tetrabenazine), or Reserpine®.

Tetrabenazine: Tetrabenazine is a drug that decreases dopamine and may help some patients. It is not generally available in the United States, but some physicians at major research centers are occasionally granted exemptions for use in the patients, particularly for research purposes.

Most of the medications used to treat dystonia work by affecting the neurotransmitter chemicals in the nervous system that execute the brain's instructions for muscle movement and the control of movement. Patients are typically started on a very low dose of medication, and the dose is gradually increased until the benefit is fully realized and/or side effects warrant a lower dose.

It is very important that you follow your physician's instructions about how and when to take these medications and to not abruptly stop taking them unless under the guidance of the prescribing physician.

If you do not understand the prescription directions or are unsure of the dosing, call your physician's office for clarification. Report all side effects to your physician.

Section 50.2

Surgical Interventions for Dystonia

Surgical treatments for dystonia may be an option for individuals whose symptoms do not respond to oral medications or botulinum toxin injections. Researchers are actively refining current techniques and collecting information about which patients may benefit the most from surgical treatments.

Peripheral Surgeries

The symptoms of dystonia occur when muscles of the body receive faulty information from the brain causing them to contract involuntarily. These faulty messages originate most commonly in a part of the brain called the basal ganglia. These messages are conveyed over brain pathways to the spinal cord and, from the spinal cord, reach the muscles via nerves.

Peripheral surgeries occur outside the brain and generally target the specific nerves and muscles affected by the incorrect messages from the brain. Peripheral surgeries are generally used to treat focal dystonia. An exception is intrathecal baclofen, which targets the spinal cord and is used to treat generalized or hemidystonia. However, for the purpose of this discussion, intrathecal baclofen is included under the category of peripheral surgeries.

Cervical Dystonia: The Bertrand Procedure (Selective Peripheral Denervation)

Selective peripheral denervation surgery for cervical dystonia is commonly referred to as the Bertrand procedure. In the 1970s, Dr. Claude Bertrand, with the collaboration of Dr. Pedro Molina-Negro, developed this procedure as a peripheral approach to treat cervical dystonia. The term selective refers to the care taken to identify the muscles of the neck affected by dystonia, and the term denervation refers to cutting the nerves that supply those muscles. The purpose of the Bertrand procedure is to reduce abnormal contractions in the affected muscles by severing the nerves to these muscles. The goal of the procedure is to leave intact the supply of nerves to unaffected or less-affected muscles.

This procedure is tailored to address the unique needs and symptoms of each patient. The initial approach is often to denervate the muscles causing the most prominent dystonic movement, knowing that some residual movements may remain from lesser-affected muscles. If the results do not sufficiently alleviate symptoms, a second procedure may be performed. In many cases, the initial surgery is enough to significantly improve the abnormal posture. More aggressive surgeries, in which all cervical muscles involved in the dystonia are denervated in a single operation, may result in excessive weakness in the neck.

An essential part of the procedure is the preoperative evaluation to properly identify the muscles involved and to assess if the procedure will benefit the individual. Patients who may be eligible for the surgery are observed clinically by the physician and with EMG [electromyography] equipment to monitor muscle activity and pinpoint the muscles affected by the dystonia.

One basic element of the Bertrand procedure is to cut rootlets of the spinal accessory nerve, which supply sternocleidomastoid muscles in the neck, and to spare the nerves to the trapezius muscle. The spinal accessory nerve is one of 12 cranial nerves that originate in the brainstem, which is the junction of the brain and the spinal cord. A second element of the Bertrand procedure is cutting the posterior rami (branch) of one or more spinal nerves along the cervical vertebrae. (This element of the procedure is called posterior ramisectomy.) Spinal nerves are arranged in pairs along the length of the spinal cord and supply muscles and organs. Some research suggests that the ramisectomy increases the improvement in persons who have become resistant to botulinum toxin therapy.

To date over 2,000 cervical dystonia patients have undergone this procedure. Some centers report significant improvement in as many as 88% of cases. Although the procedure may benefit individuals with a range of symptoms, the categories of patients who may have the best results from the Bertrand procedure are individuals in which:

- symptoms mainly affect the neck;
- symptoms have stabilized for 3 years;

- the head turns to one side (rotational torticollis);
- the head is tilted (laterocollis);
- the head turns and is pulled backward (rotational torticollis with superior retrocollis);
- the head turns and tilts forward (rotational torticollis with superior antecollis);
- the head is pulled back (superior retrocollis).

Dystonia in which the head turns both to the side and either back or forward may have the best outcome. Individuals who respond to botulinum toxin therapy as well as nonresponders may be eligible. The procedure may also be an option for a small number of patients with generalized dystonia who have very defined symptoms in the neck.

Side effects may include numbness in the back of the head, tightness at the surgery site, some remaining movements, difficulty swallowing, and lack of benefit. Patients are often able to go home after two or three nights in the hospital.

Studies have demonstrated that the Bertrand procedure can significantly improve the posture of the neck with a better range of motion. Physical therapy following the procedure is very important to preserve range of motion.

Laryngeal Dystonia: Selective Laryngeal Denervation and Reinnervation

Selective laryngeal adduction denervation and reinnervation (SLAD/R) is a surgical procedure to treat adductor spasmodic dysphonia/laryngeal dystonia by cutting (denervating) selected end branches of the recurrent laryngeal nerve, which is a branch of the vagus cranial nerve.

The first attempts to reduce the spasms of spasmodic dysphonia by severing the laryngeal nerve took place in the 1970s. Cutting the laryngeal nerve paralyzed the muscles controlling one side of the larynx so that the larynx could not contract excessively. Early results were good, but symptoms reappeared in many patients. Subsequent pioneers in the field sought to improve the procedure by varying the method by which the nerve was separated from the muscle. Recurrence of symptoms as well as breathy voice continued to be a problem in many patients.

The element that distinguishes SLAD/R from previous incarnations of the surgery is that, after the recurrent laryngeal nerve is cut

458

away from the thyroarytenoid and lateral cricoarytenoid muscles, the muscle's nerves are hooked up to another nerve (reinnervated), one that is not associated with the dystonia. Supplying the muscle with another nerve prevents the problematic branch of laryngeal nerve from growing back and reconnecting to the muscle. Preventing the laryngeal nerve from communicating to the muscle prevents the spasms from returning and helps to change the closing forces of the larynx. It is important to note that the procedure is performed on both sides of the vocal cords, unlike previous nerve operations performed for adductor SD.

The procedure is accomplished through an incision in the neck and by creating a small window into the laryngeal cartilage to expose the underlying nerves and muscles. An operating microscope is often used to aid in identification and suturing of the tiny nerve branches. The procedure takes 3 or 4 hours to complete. Great care is taken to preserve the back part of the cartilage that protects the nerve branches to the breathing muscles.

SLAD/R is best suited for individuals with spasmodic dysphonia without a tremor. It may be an option for persons who are not satisfied with botulinum toxin treatments. Hundreds of people with spasmodic dysphonia have undergone SLAD/R. During the initial recovery period, all patients experience temporary voice breathiness and some experience swallowing difficulty. These issues resolve over a few months and the patient is left with an improved voice. Studies have indicated that as many as 85–90% of patients are very satisfied with the results of surgery, and the results, so far, have been life long.

Laryngeal Dystonia: Thyroplasty

Thyroplasty surgeries include a group of surgical techniques to modify the cartilage surrounding the larynx. These adjustable and reversible procedures involve manipulating the cartilage by implanting wedges or shims to hold the tissue in place. A number of variations of this procedure are currently used and are effective for restoration of the voice after paralysis or in changing the pitch of the voice.

Type I thyroplasty has been used for the abductor variety of laryngeal dystonia/spasmodic dysphonia. In this procedure, the vocal cords are brought closer together in hopes of decreasing the effect of the abductor spasms. Results are mixed, with some patients getting good relief, and others having minimal effect.

Type II thyroplasty is a procedure for adductor spasmodic dysphonia that involves spreading the vocal cords apart by inserting a shim that prevents them from contacting each other during the spasms that occur with this disorder. Although some have reported good relief of vocal strain, others feel the trade off to a breathy and weak voice is too excessive.

Researchers in the United States and abroad continue to investigate thyroplasty procedures. The advantage of these procedures is that they are largely nondestructive and do not alter the muscles or nerve supply of the larynx. They work through adjustment of biomechanics alone and are theoretically reversible, although in practice the reversibility may be limited by scarring.

Blepharospasm: Myectomy Surgery

Surgical removal of the eyelid and brow-squeezing muscles is referred to as a myectomy procedure and is used to treat blepharospasm. Myectomy prevents the muscles surrounding the eyes from being stimulated by removing the muscle.

Before the availability of botulinum toxin, myectomy was essentially the only treatment option for blepharospasm. The introduction of botulinum toxin injections in 1989 benefited many persons with blepharospasm thereby changing the population of individuals eligible for myectomy. Candidates for myectomy became those for whom botulinum toxin is not sufficient.

Just as the patient selection changed, the procedure itself evolved. Initially, the procedure involved removing all eyelid-squeezing muscles in both upper and lower lids as well as the brow area at one time. At the present time, the procedure is tailored to the needs of the patients. It is most common for the surgeon to remove the muscle in the upper eyelids and brow (full upper myectomy) and then reevaluate the need for a lower myectomy at a later date. Patients heal faster when the procedure is done in stages, and some individuals do not require the lower myectomy.

The full upper myectomy may be done entirely through an eyebrow incision. The incision lies immediately adjacent to the brow hair and allows access to the upper lid orbicularis muscle, and part of the lower lid orbicularis muscle as well as the procerus and corrugator muscles in the brow area. Most of the orbicularis muscle is removed during the eyelid surgery. A strip of dense muscle is left at the margin of the upper eyelid to help maintain some voluntary closure and to protect the eyelash roots.

A limited upper myectomy is a partial upper myectomy. It is available for those individuals who are benefiting from botulinum toxin

460

but need something extra to restore function of the eyes. It may be helpful for those patients who have apraxia (difficulty opening the eyes) or for those who in addition to blepharospasm have ptosis (drooping lids). Partial removal of the orbicularis may subsequently decrease the need for botulinum toxin in these patients. A limited myectomy is done through an upper eyelid crease incision and involves removal of the orbicularis muscle within the upper lid area only. Because there is less tissue removal than the full upper myectomy, patients recover in less time. A limited myectomy also gives more predictable cosmetic improvement because less tissue is removed. It is not designed to replace a full upper myectomy. Most patients will still require botulinum toxin injections following the limited myectomy procedure.

Persons who have stopped responding to botulinum toxin as well as those rare individuals who fail to respond at all may be eligible for myectomy. Individual surgical centers have treated hundreds of blepharospasm patients with myectomy. Techniques used for cosmetic surgery, such as sculpting the fat beneath the brow and manipulating the placement of the brow, may be implemented to provide a beneficial aesthetic as well as functional result.

Myectomy surgery can be done under local or general anesthesia. The healing process following a myectomy may take up to a year. In most cases, the patients are able to keep their eyes open immediately following the operation. However, considerable swelling, hematomas (blood accumulation in lid), lymphedema (tissue fluid), and bruising may be present early in the postoperative period and prevent complete eyelid opening. Cool compresses in the first 4 to 5 days followed by warm compresses are very helpful at settling the lid swelling and bruising.

There are numerous potential side effects associated with myectomy surgery that are predictable and, to some degree, occur in most patients. Numbness of the forehead region often occurs and is usually temporary but may last a year or more. Loss of tissue volume in the eyelid area may occur with the muscle removal, but the improved brow, lid position, and decreased eyelid wrinkling generally gives an improved cosmetic appearance. Decreased eyelid closure occurs as a result of eyelid muscle removal and may require the need for additional artificial tears and lubricating ointment. As the eyelid swelling resolves, the eyelid closure improves and the dry eye symptoms generally improve. Chronic lid swelling which may last 6 months or longer in some patients can be a chronic and troublesome complication. Chronic lid swelling is much less severe and persistent in the modern myectomy practices in which upper and lower lid myectomies are performed separately. Infection, hematoma, brow hair loss, and abnormal positioning of the lower lid can occasionally occur but are uncommon.

Patients continue to improve in function as well as in appearance for about 6 months to a year after myectomy surgery. Reports have shown that visual disability is improved in approximately 90% of patients. Some patients have more improvement than others. Touch-up procedures are required in some cases, and some individuals continue to require botulinum toxin injections.

Generalized Dystonia and Hemidystonia: Intrathecal Baclofen (The Baclofen Pump)

Baclofen (Lioresal®) is a medication introduced in the late 1960s as a treatment for spasticity. The medication is also commonly used to treat select cases of dystonia. Baclofen in the spinal fluid around the brain and spinal cord supplements the body's supply of a chemical neurotransmitter called GABA [gamma-aminobutyric acid], which relaxes muscle movement. The drug may be given orally, but very high doses must often be used to ensure that the drug saturates the blood stream and reaches the spinal fluid. High doses of oral baclofen may cause intolerable side effects such as muscle weakness and fatigue. A surgically implanted baclofen pump delivers baclofen directly to the spinal fluid, and only very small doses are needed. (The term intrathecal means in the spinal fluid.)

Intrathecal baclofen therapy is a nondestructive, adjustable, and reversible treatment. Several hundred dystonia patients have been treated with intrathecal baclofen. It has been used for children and adults with generalized dystonia (both primary and secondary) and hemidystonia who respond to oral baclofen. Many persons treated with intrathecal baclofen have a combination of dystonia and cerebral palsy. Intrathecal baclofen may be used to treat dystonia affecting the upper and lower limbs.

In order to determine if an individual is eligible for intrathecal baclofen, he/she will undergo a screening test to observe the body's response to baclofen. A response to the oral drug may necessitate a screening test to observe the body's response to a small dose injected directly into the spinal fluid. The medication is injected using a standard lumbar puncture. The screening test procedure involves injection of the medication followed by several hours of observation. Relaxation of the muscles indicates that an implanted baclofen pump will likely be effective. The effects of the screening test are temporary and may last several hours after the injection. If a patient does not respond at all to the screening test, a second test using the same procedure may be tried the next day or at a later date.

Some physicians use a continuous intrathecal infusion of baclofen as a screening method, since more patients respond to continuous infusion than to single injection screening doses. In the infusion technique, a small catheter is inserted into the spinal fluid and is connected to an external pump that infuses baclofen in increasing doses over 2 to 3 days.

Starting intrathecal baclofen therapy involves surgically implanting a pacemaker-like device into the abdomen. The device is usually placed either to the right or left of the belly button, beneath the skin and fat of the abdomen. The pump is connected to a thin tube that is tunneled around the side of the body to the back. A small needle introduces the tube to the spinal canal. Once the surgical incisions are closed, the pump is adjusted by a remote computerized device to deliver the amount of medication appropriate for the individual. The procedure takes 1 to 2 hours, and hospital stay may range from 4 to 7 days. Modest improvement of symptoms may be noticeable before the individual is discharged from the hospital, and it may take 6 months or more to achieve the full extent of benefit.

Regular maintenance is a key component of intrathecal baclofen therapy. Regular exams and physical therapy may be a component of postoperative care. Pumps must be refilled every 1 to 4 months in the physician's office as a straightforward outpatient procedure. The pump is refilled by inserting a thin needle through the skin, into the pump. The frequency of refilling the pump depends on the dose required. If necessary, the doctor may adjust the delivery rate of the pump at the time of the refill by remote control. The pump battery needs to be replaced about every 7 years.

Baclofen in the spinal fluid relaxes muscles throughout the body, and appears especially effective for targeting dystonia in both the upper and lower half of the body. Intrathecal baclofen may be more effective for treating secondary dystonia than for primary dystonia.

Studies have shown that intrathecal baclofen can dramatically improve symptoms and quality of life. Some centers have reported significant improvement in as much as 85% of patients. However, like any surgery, the procedure is not without risks. Hardware complications may also arise including infection and catheter breakage and disconnection. In a small percentage of cases, patients may lose effect within the first year of therapy or experience a worsening of symptoms. The most common side effects are constipation, decreased muscle control, and drowsiness.

Brain Surgeries

The goals of brain surgery for persons with dystonia are to decrease muscle spasms, increase mobility and function, and improve pain.

There are currently two categories of brain surgery for dystonia: lesioning procedures, which involve selective destruction of targeted, abnormal brain tissue, and deep brain stimulation (DBS), which mimics the effects of lesioning by manipulating selective brain areas with nondestructive electrical pulses.

Although risks exist, case studies have shown that both lesioning procedures and DBS can result in marked improvement of dystonia with minimal complications. Some patients are able to decrease or altogether stop drug therapy following surgery.

Dystonia most often originates in a part of the brain called the basal ganglia, which are involved in the coordination and control of muscle movements. The basal ganglia are a group of structures that include the globus pallidus (also called the pallidum), the thalamus, and the subthalamic nucleus. Lesioning procedures for dystonia usually target the globus pallidus or the thalamus; deep brain stimulation usually targets the globus pallidus or subthalamic nucleus. The globus pallidus is responsible for the output of messages from the basal ganglia. The recipient of this output is the thalamus. The subthalamic nucleus is a tiny structure located directly beneath the thalamus and is connected to the globus pallidus.

Different parts of the brain work together to help the body accomplish a specific task, such as tapping the foot. The parts of the brain communicate via circuits or pathways of individual brain cells that transmit chemical messages from one to the other. In an individual with dystonia, the circuits that facilitate the movement of the foot are disrupted by abnormal activity. The goal of brain surgery is to free up the circuits so that the brain and body may accomplish the intended function—in this case, moving the foot.

Brain surgery may be performed unilaterally (on one side of the brain) or bilaterally (on both sides). The effects of surgery occur on the side of the body opposite to the surgical site.

To date, most persons who have undergone brain surgery for dystonia were treated for generalized dystonia. However, individuals who may be eligible for brain surgery include persons with focal, segmental, or generalized dystonia with significant, disabling symptoms that do not respond satisfactorily to other therapies. Adults as well as children with primary and secondary dystonia may be eligible.

Based on the limited available data, different categories of patients may respond differently to brain surgery. Although cases of both secondary dystonias (including tardive dystonia) and focal dystonias may be eligible, it appears as though persons with DYT-1 [DYT stands for dystonia] generalized dystonia are the best candidates for brain surgery—either lesioning or DBS. Studies have shown as much as 60–90% improvement in DYT-1 patients treated with lesioning or DBS. Patients with secondary hemidystonia may be eligible for brain surgery, though they may not benefit as much as those with DYT-1 dystonia. Researchers are examining the possibility that persons with secondary dystonia may get greater benefit from lesioning or DBS to the thalamus rather than the globus pallidus.

There is limited data about the long-term effects of each approach. Brain surgery for dystonia is an evolving science, and investigators are continually collecting information.

Chapter 51

Plasmapheresis May Be Used to Treat Movement Disorders

Plasmapheresis and Autoimmune Disease

Many diseases, including myasthenia gravis, Lambert-Eaton syndrome, Guillain-Barré syndrome and others, are caused by a so-called autoimmune, or self-immune, process. In autoimmune conditions, the body's immune system mistakenly turns against itself, attacking its own tissues. Some of the specialized cells involved in this process can attack tissues directly, while others can produce substances known as antibodies that circulate in the blood and carry out the attack. Antibodies produced against the body's own tissues are known as autoantibodies.

Treatment with medications that suppress the activities of the immune system and/or reduce inflammation of tissues has been the most common approach to autoimmune disease for more than 30 years. Many new immunosuppressants have become available since the 1960s, but all the medications used to treat autoimmune disease have serious side effects when taken in high doses for months or years.

In the 1970s, with the support of the Muscular Dystrophy Association, researchers developed a new approach to the treatment of autoimmune conditions. Instead of trying to change the immune system with medication alone, they thought that it might be possible to mechanically remove autoantibodies from the bloodstream in a process

"Facts About Plasmapheresis," © 2005. Reprinted with permission of the Muscular Dystrophy Association [MDA] of the United States.

similar to that used in an "artificial kidney," or dialysis, treatment. The procedure became known as plasmapheresis, meaning plasma separation. It's also known as plasma exchange.

Medications that suppress the immune system or reduce inflammation are often combined with plasmapheresis, but they can usually be given in lower doses than when used alone.

Today, plasmapheresis is widely accepted for the treatment of myasthenia gravis, Lambert-Eaton syndrome, Guillain-Barré syndrome, and chronic demyelinating polyneuropathy. Its effectiveness in other conditions, such as multiple sclerosis, polymyositis, and dermatomyositis, is not as well established.

What is plasmapheresis?

Plasmapheresis is a process in which the fluid part of the blood, called plasma, is removed from blood cells by a device known as a cell separator. The separator works either by spinning the blood at high speed to separate the cells from the fluid or by passing the blood through a membrane with pores so small that only the fluid part of the blood can pass through. The cells are returned to the person undergoing treatment, while the plasma, which contains the antibodies, is discarded and replaced with other fluids. Medication to keep the blood from clotting (an anticoagulant) is given through a vein during the procedure.

What's involved in a plasmapheresis treatment?

A plasmapheresis treatment takes several hours and can be done on an outpatient basis. It can be uncomfortable but is normally not painful. The number of treatments needed varies greatly depending on the particular disease and the person's general condition. An average course of plasma exchanges is six to 10 treatments over 2 to 10 weeks. In some centers, treatments are performed once a week, while in others, more than one weekly treatment is done.

A person undergoing plasmapheresis can lie in bed or sit in a reclining chair. A small, thin tube (catheter) is placed in a large vein, usually the one in the crook of the arm, and another tube is placed in the opposite hand or foot (so that at least one arm can move freely during the procedure). Blood is taken to the separator from one tube, while the separated blood cells, combined with replacement fluids, are returned to the patient through the other tube.

The amount of blood outside the body at any one time is much less than the amount ordinarily donated in a blood bank.

Are there risks associated with plasmapheresis?

Yes, but most can be controlled. Any unusual symptoms should be immediately reported to the doctor or the person in charge of the procedure. Symptoms that may seem trivial sometimes herald the onset of a serious complication.

The most common problem is a drop in blood pressure, which can be experienced as faintness, dizziness, blurred vision, coldness, sweating, or abdominal cramps. A drop in blood pressure is remedied by lowering the patient's head, raising the legs and giving intravenous fluid.

Bleeding can occasionally occur because of the medications used to keep the blood from clotting during the procedure. Some of these medications can cause other adverse reactions, which begin with tingling around the mouth or in the limbs, muscle cramps, or a metallic taste in the mouth. If allowed to progress, these reactions can lead to an irregular heartbeat or seizures.

An allergic reaction to the solutions used to replace the plasma or to the sterilizing agents used for the tubing can be a true emergency. This type of reaction usually begins with itching, wheezing, or a rash. The plasma exchange must be stopped and the person treated with intravenous medications.

Excessive suppression of the immune system can temporarily occur with plasmapheresis, since the procedure isn't selective about which antibodies it removes. In time, the body can replenish its supply of needed antibodies, but some physicians give these intravenously after each plasmapheresis treatment. Outpatients may have to take special precautions against infection.

Medication dosages need careful observation and adjustment in people being treated with plasmapheresis because some drugs can be removed from the blood or changed by the procedure.

How long does it take to see improvement?

Improvement can sometimes occur within days, especially in myasthenia gravis. In other conditions, especially where there is extensive tissue damage, improvement is slower but can still occur within weeks.

Does MDA pay for plasmapheresis?

MDA supported pioneering research to develop plasmapheresis. However, payment for this procedure is not among the many services included in MDA's program. A number of health insurance plans do cover the procedure.

Where are plasmapheresis treatments offered?

Plasmapheresis is performed at many major medical centers across the country. MDA clinic directors can offer advice about the availability of this treatment and its use for specific conditions.

Chapter 52

Physical Strategies for Improving Movement Disorder Symptoms

Chapter Contents

Section 52.1

Why Exercise Helps People with Movement Disorders

Fallik, D. "Why Exercise Helps People with Movement Disorders," *Neurology Now* January/February 2007; 3(1): 34. © 2007 American Academy of Neurology. Reprinted by permission of Lippincott Williams and Wilkins.

Julie Robichaud, Ph.D., a research assistant professor at the department of movement sciences at the University of Illinois, knows that her Parkinson's study subjects feel better after they exercise and that their symptoms subside.

In a recent study she completed involving strength conditioning, their balance improved, walking velocity increased, and the ability to release a contraction improved by 30 percent. But she just doesn't know why.

"We know that in rats exercise stimulates dopamine production," she says. "Is that happening in humans when they exercise? We just can't measure that yet."

Generally, neurologists and other brain-disorder specialists believe that exercise of any form can do no harm, as long as it is approved and monitored by a health professional.

There's no such thing as overdosing from exercise, if patients do it at their own pace, says Howard Hurtig, M.D., chair of neurology at Pennsylvania Hospital in Philadelphia. Those with balance issues or whose disease is simply too advanced might have more difficulties, but they could benefit from trying.

The mystical side is how it affects their attitude—they get revved up, become much less depressed, and feel like they're in better control of their destiny.

Would a stroke patient respond as well to a dance class as someone living with Parkinson's disease? It's unclear. But researchers suspect that a better understanding of brain plasticity may help answer that question.

The plasticity of the brain allows it to heal and rewire after an injury, and exercise may play a role in that, says Chen Daofen Chen,

Ph.D., program director for sensorimotor integration at the National Institute of Neurological Disorders and Stroke.

With stroke patients, it's a use it or lose it factor, he said. "We know that when animals are engaged in voluntary exercise that it increases new neuronal survival, but does it bring new neurons into functional structure or new neurons?"

There is a window of vulnerability where the movement therapy could have a maladaptive effect, he says. If you do it too early, the nervous system may not be ready to accommodate those increased behaviors, and it may adapt in a way that would not help future recovery.

Ivan Bodis-Wollner, M.D., the director of the Parkinson's Disease and Related Disorders Clinic Center of Excellence at the State University of New York at the Downstate Medical Center, believes that dance therapy helps because it works the body as a whole, not as an isolated muscle group. In addition to feeling support from the group and from feeling better from doing exercise—which in itself produces dopamine, Dr. Bodis-Wollner says—there's another benefit as well.

There's an enormous internal reward as well to dancing, he says. You move your arm and it looks good and you're satisfied. The quintessential neural transmitter in the reward system is dopamine, so part of how dance therapy works is that it's stimulating that dopamine and other transmitters.

Parkinson's patients have a tendency to freeze when they walk or when they turn, and some patients say if they listen to the music and walk to the beat, they walk much better and have less freezing, he says.

By repeating the thought over and over, patients create a new map in their heads—not exactly rewiring the neurons, but theoretically reprogramming the brain to find alternate pathways to successful movement.

So when Parkinson's patients experience bradykinesia, a general slowing of movement, that new pathway can get them back into step—literally. That internal ignition that makes the hand pick up the coffee cup slows and sometimes stops. But doing it to music, or even thinking about doing it to music, causes a shift in thinking.

Part of the ways dance teachers accomplish this is by doing the same movement over and over, reinforcing a toe-heel step instead of walking, a sideways grapevine, not a turn. That way, when a patient gets stuck, they can think of another movement and take that different map to get them to the same place.

Dr. Bodis-Wollner tells stroke patients who have lost ability in a particular limb to imagine that it is moving in a specific way. See your hand pick up the coffee cup, the toothbrush, the newspaper, he says.

"We know that imagining things creates brain activity, there's more blow flow going to a certain area of the brain," he says. "I don't know if it recircuits the brain, but maybe it reorganizes."

The conundrum for neurologists is saying 'it helps to do exercise' but not knowing exactly what kind of exercise to prescribe, Dr. Robichaud says. "We have to figure out what works, and then figure out what's best for different types of people."

Section 52.2

Dance Therapy for Better Movement Control

Fallik, D. "Finding New Life through Movement," *Neurology Now* January/February 2007; 3(1): 30–33. © 2007 American Academy of Neurology. Reprinted by permission of Lippincott Williams and Wilkins.

A lawyer, a social worker, and a teacher walk into a sunshine-filled studio, and break out into a grapevine to the sounds of "Whatever Lola Wants, Lola Gets."

It sounds almost like the beginning of a joke, but Carroll Neesemann isn't laughing. Ever since Parkinson's disease affected his career in litigation more than a decade ago, he's found new life as a dancer here on a Brooklyn corner.

For the past 5 years, Neesemann, 66, has come to the Mark Morris Dance Group headquarters for a dance class designed for people with Parkinson's disease. Taught by company members and filled with as many as three-dozen participants, it's a combination support group, workout, and brain exercise.

It's nice not to be clumsy, says Neesemann. "It's wonderful to be in control and be somewhat graceful again."

Across the country, those living with brain disorders, from Parkinson's to stroke to traumatic brain injuries, are finding ease doing the tango or tap or even a bit of modern dance choreography. Patients say the classes help loosen tight joints, improve overall movement, and generally lift spirits in a way other forms of therapy do not, and researchers are trying to find out why.

Dance therapy began more than a half-century ago, when Marian Chace began offering dance classes to psychiatric patients at St. Elizabeth's Hospital in Washington, D.C. Now there are more than 1,200 dance therapists in the country, according to the American Dance Therapy Association.

There is no standard class or specific moves, says Sally Totenbier, a spokeswoman for the dance association. It's about the movement and the rhythm and the shape.

Not all teachers are formally trained therapists, and not all classes are taught by formally trained dancers.

The class at Mark Morris started out as a whim. Olie Westheimer was just helping out her husband, Ivan Bodis-Wollner, M.D., a neurologist and director of the Parkinson's Disease Center of Excellence in Brooklyn, N.Y. She was running a Parkinson's support group and listening to participants express their frustrations that their bodies didn't move like they used to.

"I don't have a medical background at all," she says. "But I knew that dancers use all the tricks in the book to get their bodies to do difficult things. That was my gamble—that it would be beneficial."

She saw a newspaper article on the dance company's new building in the Fort Greene section of Brooklyn, and there was a quote saying that they wanted to connect to the community. Westheimer called up cold and said she had an idea for a dance class; they told her to come on in.

"I said I can bring my record player and the woman at the dance company said, 'We have an accompanist.' I said I don't know who is going to come and she asked, 'Well, would one person come?'" says Westheimer. "And I thought that was the nicest, most understanding thing. So I said yes, one person will come."

Before the class could begin, they needed a teacher. John Heginbotham, one of the company members, stepped forward. He had taught dance classes before, but nothing geared to a particular group.

The first day of class, a family member got sick. Another member, David Leventhal, stepped in. The two have been teaching the class ever since, with faculty member Misty Owens taking over during tour time.

The dancers approached the class as they would any other basic level—with combinations and repetition—but with the focus on grace and personal success, not group memorization. At the beginning, there was a little too much emphasis on strict modern dance movement, but now the teachers say the class has taught them to lighten up.

Parkinson's is so much in the forefront of their lives, says Leventhal. "This is a chance to put it on the back burner—it's just a dance class, we don't look at it like a therapy class."

At first the class met once a month, then twice, now it's every Wednesday afternoon for 75 minutes, with a separate group meeting on their own on Mondays. Both patients and caretakers come, hanging canes on the ballet barres and parking walkers in the lobby.

It begins with everyone seated. As Pachelbel's "Canon in D Major" floats in the background, Owens starts with a sun salutation, arms stretched to the ceiling, palms together, up and over and down to the floor.

Then Heginbotham takes over, demonstrating a series of poses known as the embracing phrase in the Mark Morris repertoire. The teachers often steal bits and pieces from the dances they do and modify them for the class.

"We have some 'greatest hits' of exercises that we do that we've learned have worked for the students," says Heginbotham. "Strong and sharp versus light and airy, sustained versus staccato."

The point of certain movements is to work on specific problems Parkinson's patients have, like mobility freeze or doing two things at once, such as reaching the arm one way and the leg another.

Much like people who stutter who don't do so when singing, the thought is that by reinforcing walking or reaching or moving to music, that the brain will reinforce the pathways, or simply create new ones, says Owens, who is writing a master's thesis on dance therapy and Parkinson's.

"I started including a lot of tap steps because it's sharp and you're striking the floor, spanking the floor—it's clean and clear and direct," she says. "I have seen major improvement, even in just lifting the toes up and down. It activates both mirror neurons and the muscle memory."

Beth Kaplan Westbrook, Ph.D., a former dancer turned clinical psychologist in Oregon who published a study on dance movement therapy and Parkinson's in the *American Journal of Dance Therapy*, says it's beneficial to other groups as well, not just for the exercise, but also for mood.

"People with stroke and MS and other disorders, when they moved, they began to see a great benefit because often they couldn't fully express themselves verbally," she says. "It's fascinating that a nonverbal approach can make such a difference."

Teachers at Mark Morris watch the students to see how the exercises are being accepted. If it's too complicated or too difficult, or perhaps needs to be repeated, they adapt.

Dr. Westbrook says that's the way she led her classes as well. "From my own experience, you let the class evolve from the patients," she says.

As the Mark Morris class moves into its sixth year, Westheimer, who started it all, now has a $15,000 grant from the National Parkinson Foundation to tape the classes, in the hopes of inspiring other dance companies, teachers, and therapists across the country.

On a recent Wednesday, as a cameraman strolled around the class, focusing on hand gestures and body movement, Judy Rosenblatt noticed only the music.

A retired social worker who was diagnosed in 2004, she says the class brings back memories of folk dancing. She found the Brooklyn gathering while looking for a support group a year ago.

During the class, the 64-year-old moved easily, even lightly. By the end of the class, students sidestepped across the floors as "We Will (We Will) Rock You" by Queen became the Jewish folk dance "Hava Nagila," and she said she felt free.

"It's a pleasure," Rosenblatt says. "It's easier to move when you hear the music, when you feel the music."

Neesemann, the litigator, says his medications are not working for him much anymore, and the class gives him some respite from the symptoms. So when other patients ask him why he goes to class, why dancing?

"I tell them it takes my symptoms away."

Dawn Fallik's work has appeared in *The Philadelphia Inquirer, The St. Louis Post-Dispatch*, and The Associated Press.

Section 52.3

Battling Fatigue with Yoga

Lindsey, H. "Battling MS Fatigue with Yoga," *Neurology Now* Fall 2005; 1(3):22–23. © 2005 American Academy of Neurology. Reprinted by permission of Lippincott Williams and Wilkins.

Deborah Jacobs has lived with multiple sclerosis (MS) for 25 years, so she has tried lots of strategies to ease her symptoms over the years. Of late, however, she has discovered that yoga helps her combat the fatigue related to the disease.

"Yoga makes me feel calm and energized," says Jacobs, 54, who has taken a weekly yoga class especially for people with MS since September. "I would normally be exhausted this time of day if I wasn't taking the class," she adds.

Recent research confirms her experience. A June 2004 study in the journal *Neurology* found that taking a weekly yoga class, along with home practice, lessens the fatigue that accompanies MS. In the 6-month study, 69 volunteers with MS were divided into three groups: one-third practiced yoga, one-third performed regular aerobic exercise, and one-third did neither. Previous surveys found yoga to be beneficial, but this was the first study that compared yoga to aerobic exercise and to no exercise at all.

The improvement in fatigue was clearly noticeable, says Barry Oken, M.D., the lead author of the study, who is medical director of Clinical Neurophysiology at Oregon Health & Science University in Portland and a professor of Neurology and Behavioral Neuroscience there. The study wasn't limited to yoga. It also found that aerobic exercise, riding a stationary bike, had a similar effect. It's important for MS patients to engage in some sort of physical activity, says Dr. Oken. It could be either a stationary bike or yoga. It really depends on patient preference.

Jack Burks, M.D., a clinical professor of Medicine in the department of Neurology at the University of Nevada School of Medicine in Reno, has recommended yoga to his MS patients for the past 25 years.

Yoga does not cure people, but they tend to feel better when doing it, he says.

It's encouraging to see study results that document the improvement in patients, he adds. While the research found that patients experienced improvements in fatigue, it did not find that their mood or thinking clarity improved. However, the number of participants in the study may have been too small to measure such benefits, he explains.

Other Potential Benefits

The study may not have documented that yoga improves mood, but engaging in yoga and aerobic exercise classes does seem to be have this effect, possibly because people get to socialize, says Dr. Burks. Jacobs agrees. "Meeting with a group of people during yoga class affects me in a positive way," she says.

Yoga has also made her stronger and improved her posture, she says, adding that she also sleeps better on nights after taking her yoga class.

One potential benefit of yoga, says Dr. Oken, is improved flexibility, which could theoretically help with spasticity (the muscle tightness that affects people with MS). And it is also an excellent way to reduce stress. But, Dr. Oken notes, these potential benefits for MS patients have not yet been studied.

How often patients should exercise depends on what they can do. Exercising for a half hour, three times a week, works for some people, while others may be able to handle more or less, says Dr. Burks. "I don't recommend exercising to the point of extreme fatigue," he notes.

Dr. Oken recommends doing yoga and exercise at home as much as possible. He noted that everyone's needs are different, and that people with neurological problems should discuss their exercise plan with their doctor.

Special MS Yoga Classes

Yoga has become so popular that there are now special classes for people with MS, and these are a wise choice for patients, says Dr. Oken. The classes are designed for people in wheelchairs or those with limited mobility, he explains. In Jacobs' class, for instance, some of the typical standing yoga poses are adapted so they can be done while seated. Despite such adaptations, Jacobs is impressed by the abilities her classmates demonstrate. She was astonished when she learned that one of her substitute yoga instructors uses a wheelchair outside of class. "I was amazed at what she was able to do," says Jacobs.

The class has given her confidence in her physical abilities. "When I first saw someone do a shoulder stand, I thought, 'Oh my God, I'm not going to do that,' but the class has given me courage to do it. I can do a shoulder stand now."

Chapter 53

Vocal Cord Paralysis and Its Treatment

What is vocal cord paralysis?

Vocal cord paralysis is a voice disorder that occurs when one or both of the vocal cords (or vocal folds) do not open or close properly. Vocal cord paralysis is a common disorder, and symptoms can range from mild to life threatening.

The vocal cords are two elastic bands of muscle tissue located in the larynx (voice box) directly above the trachea (windpipe). The vocal cords produce voice when air held in the lungs is released and passed through the closed vocal cords, causing them to vibrate. When a person is not speaking, the vocal cords remain apart to allow the person to breathe.

Someone who has vocal cord paralysis often has difficulty swallowing and coughing because food or liquids slip into the trachea and lungs. This happens because the paralyzed cord or cords remain open, leaving the airway passage and the lungs unprotected.

What causes vocal cord paralysis?

Vocal cord paralysis may be caused by head trauma, a neurologic insult such as a stroke, a neck injury, lung or thyroid cancer, a tumor

"Vocal Cord Paralysis," from the National Institute on Deafness and Other Communication Disorders (NIDCD, www.nidcd.nih.gov), part of the National Institutes of Health, June 1999. Reviewed by David A. Cooke, M.D., August 26, 2008.

481

pressing on a nerve, or a viral infection. In older people, vocal cord paralysis is a common problem affecting voice production. People with certain neurologic conditions, such as multiple sclerosis or Parkinson disease, or people who have had a stroke may experience vocal cord paralysis. In many cases, however, the cause is unknown.

What are the symptoms?

People who have vocal cord paralysis experience abnormal voice changes, changes in voice quality, and discomfort from vocal straining. For example, if only one vocal cord is damaged, the voice is usually hoarse or breathy. Changes in voice quality, such as loss of volume or pitch, may also be noticeable. Damage to both vocal cords, although rare, usually causes people to have difficulty breathing because the air passage to the trachea is blocked.

How is vocal cord paralysis diagnosed?

Vocal cord paralysis is usually diagnosed by an otolaryngologist— a doctor who specializes in ear, nose, and throat disorders. Noting the symptoms the patient has experienced, the otolaryngologist will ask how and when the voice problems started in order to help determine their cause. Next, the otolaryngologist listens carefully to the patient's voice to identify breathiness or harshness. Then, using an endoscope— a tube with a light at the end—the otolaryngologist looks directly into the throat at the vocal cords. A speech-language pathologist may also use an acoustic spectrograph, an instrument that measures voice frequency and clarity, to study the patient's voice and document its strengths and weaknesses.

How is vocal cord paralysis treated?

There are several methods for treating vocal cord paralysis, among them surgery and voice therapy. In some cases, the voice returns without treatment during the first year after damage. For that reason, doctors often delay corrective surgery for at least a year to be sure the voice does not recover spontaneously. During this time, the suggested treatment is usually voice therapy, which may involve exercises to strengthen the vocal cords or improve breath control during speech. Sometimes, a speech-language pathologist must teach patients to talk in different ways. For instance, the therapist might suggest that the patient speak more slowly or consciously open the mouth wider when speaking.

Surgery involves adding bulk to the paralyzed vocal cord or changing its position. To add bulk, an otolaryngologist injects a substance, commonly Teflon, into the paralyzed cord. Other substances currently used are collagen, a structural protein; silicone, a synthetic material; and body fat. The added bulk reduces the space between the vocal cords so the nonparalyzed cord can make closer contact with the paralyzed cord and thus improve the voice.

Sometimes an operation that permanently shifts a paralyzed cord closer to the center of the airway may improve the voice. Again, this operation allows the nonparalyzed cord to make better contact with the paralyzed cord. Adding bulk to the vocal cord or shifting its position can improve both voice and swallowing. After these operations, patients may also undergo voice therapy, which often helps to fine-tune the voice.

Treating people who have two paralyzed vocal cords may involve performing a surgical procedure called a tracheotomy to help breathing. In a tracheotomy, an incision is made in the front of the patient's neck and a breathing tube (tracheotomy tube) is inserted through a hole, called a stoma, into the trachea. Rather than breathing through the nose and mouth, the patient now breathes through the tube. Following surgery, the patient may need therapy with a speech-language pathologist to learn how to care for the breathing tube properly and how to reuse the voice.

What research is being done on vocal cord paralysis?

The National Institute on Deafness and Other Communication Disorders (NIDCD) supports research studies that may help provide new clinical measurements to diagnose vocal cord paralysis. For instance, computer software is being developed that can describe important aspects of the health of a person's larynx by analyzing the sounds it produces. By measuring instabilities in the motion of the vocal cords, the software may allow scientists and treatment clinics to relate these measurements to the study of the misuse of the voice and help diagnose disorders such as muscle paralysis and tissue loss.

Currently, the treatment for patients with damage to both vocal cords involves a tracheotomy, which may, however, cause voice production problems and decrease protection of the lungs in an effort to improve the airway. Recent studies show that another feasible approach to laryngeal rehabilitation may be using an electrical stimulation device to activate the reflexes of the paralyzed muscles that open the airway during breathing.

Where can I get help?

If you notice any unexplained voice changes or discomfort, you should consult an otolaryngologist or a speech-language pathologist for evaluation and possible treatment.

Chapter 54

What the Future Holds: Stem Cell Research for Neurological and Movement Disorders

What are stem cells?

Stem cells have the remarkable potential to develop into many different cell types in the body. Serving as a sort of repair system for the body, they can theoretically divide without limit to replenish other cells as long as the person or animal is still alive. When a stem cell divides, each new cell has the potential to either remain a stem cell or become another type of cell with a more specialized function, such as a muscle cell, a red blood cell, or a brain cell.

Research on stem cells is advancing knowledge about how an organism develops from a single cell and how healthy cells replace damaged cells in adult organisms. This promising area of science is also leading scientists to investigate the possibility of cell-based therapies to treat disease, which is often referred to as regenerative or reparative medicine.

Stem cells are one of the most fascinating areas of biology today. But like many expanding fields of scientific inquiry, research on stem cells raises scientific questions as rapidly as it generates new discoveries.

Excerpted from Stem Cell Basics. In Stem Cell Information [http://stemcells.nih.gov/staticresources/info/basics/StemCellBasics.pdf]. Bethesda, MD: National Institutes of Health, U.S. Department of Health and Human Services, 2008. Available at http://stemcells.nih.gov/info/basics.

Why are stem cells important?

Stem cells have two important characteristics that distinguish them from other types of cells. First, they are unspecialized cells that renew themselves for long periods through cell division. The second is that under certain physiologic or experimental conditions, they can be induced to become cells with special functions such as the beating cells of the heart muscle or the insulin-producing cells of the pancreas.

Scientists primarily work with two kinds of stem cells from animals and humans: embryonic stem cells and adult stem cells. Scientists discovered ways to obtain or derive stem cells from early mouse embryos more than 20 years ago. Many years of detailed study of the biology of mouse stem cells led to the discovery, in 1998, of how to isolate stem cells from human embryos and grow the cells in the laboratory. These are called human embryonic stem cells. The embryos used in these studies were created for infertility purposes through in vitro fertilization procedures and when they were no longer needed for that purpose, they were donated for research with the informed consent of the donor.

Stem cells are important for living organisms for many reasons. In the 3- to 5-day-old embryo, called a blastocyst, stem cells in developing tissues give rise to the multiple specialized cell types that make up the heart, lung, skin, and other tissues. In some adult tissues, such as bone marrow, muscle, and brain, discrete populations of adult stem cells generate replacements for cells that are lost through normal wear and tear, injury, or disease.

It has been hypothesized by scientists that stem cells may, at some point in the future, become the basis for treating diseases such as Parkinson disease, diabetes, and heart disease.

Scientists want to study stem cells in the laboratory so they can learn about their essential properties and what makes them different from specialized cell types. As scientists learn more about stem cells, it may become possible to use the cells not just in cell-based therapies, but also for screening new drugs and toxins and understanding birth defects. However, as mentioned above, human embryonic stem cells have only been studied since 1998. Therefore, in order to develop such treatments scientists are intensively studying the fundamental properties of stem cells, which include:

1. determining precisely how stem cells remain unspecialized and self renewing for many years; and

2. identifying the signals that cause stem cells to become specialized cells.

What are the potential uses of human stem cells and the obstacles that must be overcome before these potential uses will be realized?

There are many ways in which human stem cells can be used in basic research and in clinical research. However, there are many technical hurdles between the promise of stem cells and the realization of these uses, which will only be overcome by continued intensive stem cell research.

Studies of human embryonic stem cells may yield information about the complex events that occur during human development. A primary goal of this work is to identify how undifferentiated stem cells become differentiated. Scientists know that turning genes on and off is central to this process. Some of the most serious medical conditions, such as cancer and birth defects, are due to abnormal cell division and differentiation. A better understanding of the genetic and molecular controls of these processes may yield information about how such diseases arise and suggest new strategies for therapy. A significant hurdle to this use and most uses of stem cells is that scientists do not yet fully understand the signals that turn specific genes on and off to influence the differentiation of the stem cell.

Human stem cells could also be used to test new drugs. For example, new medications could be tested for safety on differentiated cells generated from human pluripotent cell lines. Other kinds of cell lines are already used in this way. Cancer cell lines, for example, are used to screen potential antitumor drugs. But, the availability of pluripotent stem cells would allow drug testing in a wider range of cell types. However, to screen drugs effectively, the conditions must be identical when comparing different drugs. Therefore, scientists will have to be able to precisely control the differentiation of stem cells into the specific cell type on which drugs will be tested. Current knowledge of the signals controlling differentiation fall well short of being able to mimic these conditions precisely to consistently have identical differentiated cells for each drug being tested.

Perhaps the most important potential application of human stem cells is the generation of cells and tissues that could be used for cell-based therapies. Today, donated organs and tissues are often used to replace ailing or destroyed tissue, but the need for transplantable tissues and organs far outweighs the available supply. Stem cells, directed to differentiate into specific cell types, offer the possibility of a renewable source of replacement cells and tissues to treat diseases including Parkinson and Alzheimer diseases, spinal cord injury, stroke, burns, heart disease, diabetes, osteoarthritis, and rheumatoid arthritis.

For example, it may become possible to generate healthy heart muscle cells in the laboratory and then transplant those cells into patients with chronic heart disease. Preliminary research in mice and other animals indicates that bone marrow stem cells, transplanted into a damaged heart, can generate heart muscle cells and successfully repopulate the heart tissue. Other recent studies in cell culture systems indicate that it may be possible to direct the differentiation of embryonic stem cells or adult bone marrow cells into heart muscle cells.

In people who suffer from type I diabetes, the cells of the pancreas that normally produce insulin are destroyed by the patient's own immune system. New studies indicate that it may be possible to direct the differentiation of human embryonic stem cells in cell culture to form insulin-producing cells that eventually could be used in transplantation therapy for diabetics.

To realize the promise of novel cell-based therapies for such pervasive and debilitating diseases, scientists must be able to easily and reproducibly manipulate stem cells so that they possess the necessary characteristics for successful differentiation, transplantation, and engraftment. The following is a list of steps in successful cell-based treatments that scientists will have to learn to precisely control to bring such treatments to the clinic. To be useful for transplant purposes, stem cells must be reproducibly made to:

- proliferate extensively and generate sufficient quantities of tissue;
- differentiate into the desired cell type(s);
- survive in the recipient after transplant;
- integrate into the surrounding tissue after transplant;
- function appropriately for the duration of the recipient's life; and
- avoid harming the recipient in any way.

Also, to avoid the problem of immune rejection, scientists are experimenting with different research strategies to generate tissues that will not be rejected.

To summarize, the promise of stem cell therapies is an exciting one, but significant technical hurdles remain that will only be overcome through years of intensive research.

How could stem cells be used for the future treatment of Parkinson disease?

Parkinson disease (PD) is a very common neurodegenerative disorder that affects more than 2% of the population over 65 years of age. PD is caused by a progressive degeneration and loss of dopamine (DA)-producing neurons, which leads to tremor, rigidity, and hypokinesia (abnormally decreased mobility). It is thought that PD may be the first disease to be amenable to treatment using stem cell transplantation. Factors that support this notion include the knowledge of the specific cell type (DA neurons) needed to relieve the symptoms of the disease. In addition, several laboratories have been successful in developing methods to induce embryonic stem cells to differentiate into cells with many of the functions of DA neurons.

In a recent study, scientists directed mouse embryonic stem cells to differentiate into DA neurons by introducing the gene Nurr1. When transplanted into the brains of a rat model of PD, these stem cell-derived DA neurons reinnervated the brains of the rat Parkinson model, released dopamine and improved motor function.

Regarding human stem cell therapy, scientists are developing a number of strategies for producing dopamine neurons from human stem cells in the laboratory for transplantation into humans with Parkinson disease. The successful generation of an unlimited supply of dopamine neurons could make neurotransplantation widely available for Parkinson patients at some point in the future.

Part Six

Living with Movement Disorders

Chapter 55

Making Choices about Everyday Care

Understanding Long-Term Care: Definitions and Risks

Long-term care is a variety of services and supports to meet health or personal care needs over an extended period of time. Most long-term care is non-skilled personal care assistance, such as help performing everyday activities of daily living (ADLs), which are:

- bathing;
- dressing;
- using the toilet;
- transferring (to or from bed or chair);
- caring for incontinence; and
- eating.

The goal of long-term care services is to help you maximize your independence and functioning at a time when you are unable to be fully independent.

This chapter includes information from "Understanding Long-Term Care: Definitions and Risks," "Understanding Long-Term Care: Services and Providers," and "Understanding Long-Term Care: Costs and Paying," by the National Clearinghouse for Long-Term Care Information (www.longtermcare.gov), U.S. Department of Health and Human Services, 2008.

Who Needs Long-Term Care?

Long-term care is needed when you have a chronic illness or disability that causes you to need assistance with activities of daily living. Your illness or disability could include a problem with memory loss, confusion, or disorientation. (This is called cognitive impairment and can result from conditions such as Alzheimer disease.)

This year, about 9 million Americans over the age of 65 will need long-term care services. By 2020, that number will increase to 12 million. While most people who need long-term care are age 65 or older, a person can need long-term care services at any age. Forty (40) percent of people currently receiving long-term care are adults 18 to 64 years old.

What Are My Risks of Needing Long-Term Care?

About 70 percent of individuals over age 65 will require at least some type of long-term care services during their lifetime. Over 40 percent will need care in a nursing home for some period of time. Factors that increase your risk of needing long-term care are:

- Age: The risk generally increases as you get older.
- Marital status: Single people are more likely to need care from a paid provider.
- Gender: Women are at a higher risk than men, primarily because they tend to live longer.
- Lifestyle: Poor diet and exercise habits can increase your risk.
- Health and family history: These factors also impact your risk.

How Much Care Might I Need?

It is difficult to predict how much or what type of care any one person might need. On average, someone age 65 today will need some long-term care services for 3 years. Service and support needs vary from one person to the next and often change over time. Women need care for longer (on average 3.7 years) than do men (on average 2.2 years). While about one third of today's 65-year-olds may never need long-term care services, 20 percent of them will need care for more than 5 years. If you need long-term care, you may need one or more of the following:

- care or assistance with activities of daily living in your home from an unpaid caregiver who can be a family member or friend;

- services at your home from a nurse, home health/home care aide, therapist, or homemaker;
- care in the community; and/or
- care in any of a variety of long-term facilities.

Generally, services provided by caregivers who are family or friends are unpaid. This is sometimes called informal care. Paid services are sometimes referred to as formal services. Paid services often supplement the services provided by family and friends.

How Do Care Needs Change over Time?

Many people who need long-term care develop the need for care gradually. They may begin needing care only a few times a week or one or two times a day, for example, help with bathing or dressing. Care needs often progress as you age or as your chronic illness or disability become more debilitating, causing you to need care on a more continual basis—for example, help using the toilet or ongoing supervision because of a progressive condition such as Alzheimer disease.

Some people need long-term care in a facility for a relatively short period of time while they are recovering from a sudden illness or injury, and then may be able to be cared for at home. Others may need long-term care services on an ongoing basis—for example, someone who is disabled from a severe stroke. Some people may need to move to a nursing home or other type of facility-based setting for more extensive care or supervision if their needs can no longer be met at home.

Understanding Long-Term Care: Services and Providers

Where Is Long-Term Care Provided?

Long-term care, often associated with institutional care, is provided in many different settings. But, most long-term care is actually provided at home—either in the home of the person receiving care or at a family member's home. It's estimated that individuals currently turning 65 may need 3 years of long-term care in their lifetime, with almost 2 years of that care provided at home. The majority of care that is provided at home—about 80%—is provided by unpaid caregivers.

There is also an increasing amount of long-term care available in the community through programs such as adult day service centers, transportation services, and home care agencies that often supplement care at home or provide respite for family caregivers.

For people who cannot stay at home, but who do not need the level of care provided in a nursing home, there are a variety of residential care settings, such as assisted living, board and care homes, and continuing care retirement communities (CCRCs). Nursing homes provide long-term care to people who need more extensive care, particularly those whose needs include nursing care or 24-hour supervision in addition to their personal care needs.

Caregivers

A caregiver is a family member, partner, friend, or neighbor who helps care for an elderly individual or person with a disability who lives at home. In 2004, there were more than 44 million caregivers age 18 or older in the United States—about 21% of the adult population—providing care for an adult family member or friend. Approximately 60% of caregivers are women. Thirteen percent (13%) of caregivers caring for older adults are themselves aged 65 or over. The typical caregiver is a 46-year-old woman who is married and employed, and is caring for her widowed mother who does not live with her.

Caregivers provide a vast array of emotional, financial, nursing, social, homemaking, and other services on a daily or intermittent basis. A 2006 study of caregivers found that on average caregivers spend 21 hours a week giving care. Half of them have intensive caregiving responsibilities, performing at least one activity of daily living, such as bathing and feeding, for their care recipients. Twenty-six percent (26%) perform three or more of these activities. Eighty percent (80%) of caregivers perform activities like fixing meals, doing housework, and providing transportation to medical appointments.

Home and Community-Based Services

Home and community-based services (HCBS) describe a range of personal, support, and health services provided to individuals in their homes or communities to help them stay at home and live as independently as possible. Most people who receive long-term care at home generally require additional help either from family or friends to supplement services from paid providers. This is because so much of the care needed is personal care: help with activities such as bathing and dressing, help managing medications, or supervision for someone with a condition such as Alzheimer disease.

Some of the most common home and community services are:

Adult day service (ADS) programs, designed to meet the needs of adults with cognitive or functional impairments, as well as adults needing social interaction and a place to go when their family caregivers are at work. They provide a variety of health, social, and other support services in a protective setting during part of the day. Adult day centers typically operate programs during normal business hours 5 days a week; some have evening and weekend hours. These programs do not provide 24-hour care.

Case managers/geriatric care managers, health care professionals (typically nurses or social workers) who specialize in assisting you and your family with your long-term care needs. This includes, but is not limited to assisting, coordinating, and managing long-term care services; developing a plan of care; and monitoring your long-term care needs over extended periods of time.

Emergency response systems, which provide an automatic response to a medical or other emergency via electronic monitors. If you live alone, you wear a signaling device that you activate when you need assistance.

Friendly visitor/companion services, which are typically staffed by volunteers who regularly pay short visits (under two hours) to someone who is frail or living alone.

Home health care/home care are two different services, which may be provided by a single agency or separate agencies. Home health care typically includes skilled, short-term services such as nursing, physical, or other therapies ordered by a physician for a specific condition. Home care services are most often limited to personal care services such as bathing and dressing, and often also include homemaker services such as help with meal preparation or household chores.

Homemaker/chore services can help you with general household activities such as meal preparation, routine household care, and heavy household chores such as washing floors, windows, or shoveling snow.

Meals programs, which include both home-delivered meals (so called "Meals-on-Wheels") or congregate meals, which are provided in a variety of community settings.

Respite care, which gives families temporary relief from the responsibility of caring for family members who are unable to care for themselves. Respite care is provided in a variety of settings including in the home, at an adult day center, or in a nursing home.

Senior centers, which provide a variety of services including nutrition, recreation, social and educational services, and comprehensive information and referral to help people find the care and services they might need; and

Transportation services that can help you get to and from medical appointments, shopping centers, and access a variety of community services and resources.

Facility-Based Long-Term Care Services

There are numerous types of facility-based programs that provide a range of long-term care services. Some facilities provide only housing and related housekeeping, but many also include help managing medications, assistance with personal care, supervision and special programs for individuals with Alzheimer disease, or 24-hour nursing care. The services available in each facility are often regulated by the state in which the facility operates (for example, some states do not allow some types of facilities to include residents who are wheelchair bound or who cannot exit the facility on their own in an emergency). Facility-based care is known by a wide variety of names, including board and care, assisted living, adult foster care, continuing care retirement communities (CCRCs), and nursing homes.

Facility-based service providers include the following.

Adult foster care: Adult foster care can be provided for individuals or for small groups of adults who need help functioning or who cannot live safely on their own. The foster family provides room and board, 24-hour availability, help managing medications, and assistance with activities of daily living. Licensure requirements and the terminology used for this type of facility vary greatly from state to state.

Board and care homes: Board and care homes, also called residential care facilities or group homes, are smaller private facilities, usually with 20 or fewer residents. Most board and care homes accept six or fewer residents. Rooms may be private or residents may share rooms. Residents receive meals, personal care, and have staff available 24 hours a day. Nursing and medical attention are usually not provided on the premises. State licensure and the terminology used for this type of facility vary greatly.

Assisted living: Assisted living is designed for people who want to live in a community setting and who need or expect to need help functioning, but who do not need as much care as they would receive at a nursing home. Some assisted living facilities are quite small—with as few as 25 residents—while some can accommodate 120 or more units. Residents often live in their own apartments or rooms, but enjoy the support services that a community setting makes possible, such as:

- up to three meals a day;
- assistance with personal care;
- help with medications, housekeeping, and laundry;
- 24-hour security and onsite staff for emergencies; and
- social programs.

The cost of assisted living varies widely, depending in part upon the services needed by the resident and the amenities provided by the facility. Assisted living is regulated in all states, however, the requirements vary.

Continuing care retirement communities (CCRCs): Continuing care retirement communities (CCRCs) are also called life care communities. They offer several levels of care in one location. For example, many offer independent housing for people who need little or no care, but also have assisted living housing and a nursing facility, all on one campus, for those who need greater levels of care or supervision. In a continuing care retirement community, if you become unable to live independently, you can move to the assisted living area, or sometimes you can receive home care in your independent living unit. If necessary, you can enter the onsite or affiliated nursing home. The fee arrangements for CCRCs vary by the type of community. In addition to a monthly fee, many CCRCs also charge a one-time "entrance fee" that may be partially or completely refundable (often on the sale of the unit).

Nursing homes: Nursing homes, also called skilled nursing facilities (SNF) or convalescent care facilities, provide a wide range of

499

services, including nursing care, 24-hour supervision, assistance with activities of daily living, and rehabilitation services such as physical, occupational, and speech therapy. Some people need nursing home services for a short period of time for recovery or rehabilitation after a serious illness or operation, while others need longer stays because of chronic physical, health, or cognitive conditions that require constant care or supervision.

Families typically seek nursing home care when it is no longer possible to care for a person at home safely or when the cost of round-the-clock care at home becomes too great. Nursing homes are highly regulated. They must be licensed by state governments.

Understanding Long-Term Care: Costs and Paying

Long-term care is expensive. One year of care in a nursing home, based on the 2008 national average, costs over $68,000 for a semi-private room. One year of care at home, assuming you need periodic personal care help from a home health aide (the average is about three times a week), would cost almost $18,000 a year.

Costs for long-term care services vary greatly depending on the type and amount of care you need, the provider you use, and where you live. For example, many care facilities charge extra for services provided beyond the basic room-and-board charge, although some may have "all inclusive" fees. Home health and home care services are usually provided in 2-to-4-hour blocks of time referred to as "visits." An evening, weekend or holiday visit may cost more than a weekday visit. Some community programs, such as adult day service programs, are provided at a per-day rate, and rates may differ based on the type and variety of programs and services offered.

Who Pays for Long-Term Care?

Consumer surveys have revealed some common misunderstandings people have about which public programs pay for long-term care services. Many people believe they can rely on Medicare to pay for any long-term care services they will need. However, Medicare only pays for long-term care if you require skilled services or recuperative care for a short period of time. Medicare does not pay for what comprises the majority of long-term care services—non-skilled assistance with activities of daily living.

Medicaid is the joint federal and state program that pays for the largest share of long-term care services, but only if you meet financial and functional criteria. Other federal programs such as the Older Americans Act and Veterans Affairs pay for some long-term care services, but only for specific populations and in specific circumstances.

Most forms of employer-sponsored or private health insurance, including Health Maintenance Organizations (HMO) or managed care, follow the same general rules as Medicare. If they do cover long-term care, it is typically only for skilled, short-term, medically necessary care. Therefore most people who need long-term care end up paying for some or all of their care on their own out of their income or assets.

There are, however, an increasing number of private payment options that help to cover the costs of long-term care services. These include long-term care insurance, reverse mortgages, and other options.

It is important to understand the differences among the public programs and private financing options for long-term care services. Each public program and each private financing source has its own rules for what services it covers, eligibility requirements, co-pays, and premiums.

Chapter 56

Dressing with Ease, Style, and Comfort

Dressing and undressing are often challenging tasks for people with limited mobility. While buttoning buttons and zipping zippers are frustrating for some, others may have difficulty reaching arms through armholes or inserting legs through leg-holes. Selecting attire to meet individual needs can make dressing easier and may eliminate unnecessary aggravation and fatigue. Getting dressed everyday will boost one's self-esteem, even if one is homebound.

In general, clothing should not restrict joint motion. Lightweight or stretch-knit fabrics permit greater freedom of movement. Roomy armholes and garments that open in the front prevent the need to raise arms over the head and are easier to put on and take off. Large buttons, hooks, and snaps are fasteners that are easy to use. Velcro closures require little finger/hand coordination, can replace standard fasteners, and are concealed under the openings of shirts, blouses, dresses, and pants. Zippered fronts on tops and dresses also offer accessibility. Buttons sewn on with elastic thread make buttoning less tedious.

Fabric loops, sewn inside pants and underwear, make it simpler to pull pants up and down. Trousers with elastic waistbands or drawstrings and underpants with wide leg openings or boxer shorts make dressing easier. Leg-brace wearers should choose knit pants loose enough to pull over braces.

Wrap-around skirts go on better than skirts that fasten in the back and the style can accommodate weight changes. Wearing a wrap-around skirt (with the opening in the back), as well as drop-easy pants, are ideal when using the toilet. By wearing culottes, ladies can enjoy the look of a skirt and the convenience of pants. Pulling a slip over the head can be avoided by wearing a half-slip. Front-fastening bras or all-stretch bras permit more independence in dressing.

Some people find dressing safer and easier while lying down, especially when pulling up pants; while others prefer to sit on the edge of the bed or chair. Those with one side weaker than the other should dress the weaker side first. Dressing aids are also available to help persons dress and undress. Some devices include:

- a dressing stick with a hook on the end to assist in pulling up pants without bending over;
- buttoners to pull buttons through button holes;[1]
- zipper pulls to open and close zippers;
- stocking aids to pull on socks or stockings;
- long wooden scissors for reaching clothing;
- long-handled shoehorn to help slide the foot into the shoe.

What to wear on the feet depends on one's ability to walk. Persons with weak ankles and feet may benefit from an evaluation by a physical therapist. Lightweight, supportive shoes may be recommended for walking, and possibly for brace support. Some persons prefer smooth-soled shoes or moccasins because rubber-soled shoes may cause tripping. However, wheelchair users may prefer shoes with rubber soles to help keep the feet from slipping off wheelchair footplates.

To put laced shoes on and off with ease and without having to retie them, use elastic laces. Other types of easy-access shoes are loafers or shoes with Velcro fasteners across the top. For added convenience, women can wear thigh-high hosiery or knee socks with skirts instead of pantyhose. Wearing knee-high fashion boots or calf high leg warmers are ideas for hiding leg braces when wearing a skirt.

Persons who are sedentary should choose accessible clothing that not only feels comfortable, but also looks attractive. A flexible fabric, such as a soft cotton/polyester blend, moves with the body and provides the most comfort. Loose tops, which are worn on the outside of pants and skirts, look and feel the best. Wheelchair users find short jackets, ponchos, or capes more convenient than long coats. Men who wear suits may need to alter their suits by adding extra room in the shoulders and the seat. Many men find it helpful to use clip-on ties or ready-tied ties with a Velcro fastener. Dresses and skirts that are cut fuller in the hips prevent "riding up" when sitting.

Although outfits with fullness are comfortable, excess fullness in the sleeves, pant legs, and skirts can get caught in wheelchair spokes and cause tripping. Sitters should avoid wearing pants with heavy seams that may cause pressure areas when sitting.

The comfortableness of a fabric depends on the way it feels, the amount of heat it retains, and the manner in which it absorbs moisture. Because immobility and loss of subcutaneous fat can cause some persons to feel cold, wearing several layers of lightweight clothing retains heat and is more effective in keeping warm than wearing heavy clothing. Lightweight clothing made of terrycloth or cotton flannelette may feel comfortable both in the summer and winter.

Color and texture are important factors for dressing with ease, style, and comfort. Colorful tops add brilliance to basic slacks and skirts. Fleecewear is both functional and fashionable, and is easy to wear anytime, anywhere. The young-at-hearts who like denims will find stone-washed cotton the softest.

Slippery fabrics, such as nylon, allow the body to glide easier from one surface to another, which includes transferring from bed to the chair. Wearing nylon or satin pajamas helps a person with limited mobility to move, turn, and slide more easily in bed. Persons with breathing problems should wear loose-fitting tops or have wide-open necklines. They should also avoid hairy fabrics, like mohair, as floating filaments could be inhaled.

Dressing for success means wearing clothes that are easy to wear, attractive, and comfortable all the time. Finding solutions to dressing problems will take the stress out of dressing. And feeling your best begins by looking your best.

1. ButtonAngel. Solutions for Living LTD, www.solutionsforliving.us.

Chapter 57

Assistive Technology Can Help People with Movement Disorders Live More Independently

Introduction

Sometimes called assistive devices, independent living aids, and adaptive equipment, assistive technology (AT) can help your loved one live more independently. It may also make your job as a caregiver easier and more enjoyable.

If you're caring for someone with dementia, you may be worried about their falling, wandering, or getting lost. Certain types of AT can help. A loved one with a physical or cognitive (thinking) impairment can use AT to make the activities of daily living, such as dressing, bathing, grooming, eating, and toileting, a little easier.

This information describes different types of AT that may be helpful to you and your loved one. In addition, it addresses how to find AT, how to pay for devices, and how to decide what devices or home modifications you might need.

Definition

Assistive technology can be as simple as a hearing aid or cane, or as sophisticated as a voice-activated computer system or mechanical hoist to lift and turn someone in bed. Assistive technology devices are basically helpful products that improve a person's ability to live and function independently. Some AT is considered "low-tech"— canes, magnifiers, and pill organizers—while "high tech" assistive devices include computer applications, sensors, and smart phone systems.

AT is a rapidly growing area and is used by people with disabilities and older adults who want to stay in their communities and remain independent as long as possible. More than 15 million Americans with disabilities use some type of AT. In a 2003 AARP [American Association of Retired Persons] survey of persons over 50, one third of people reported using AT in their daily activities. The top three most popular AT devices were:

- Walker, cane, or crutches;
- Aids for bathing or toileting;
- Wheelchair or scooter.

What Kind of AT Is Right for Your Loved One?

The area of assistive technology has grown tremendously in recent years, and many manufacturers now provide a wide range of products and devices. It can be confusing, however, to determine which products might be right for your loved one. Here are a few basic tips to help you in this task:

- Focus on the actual tasks your loved one wants or needs to do when choosing devices. While this might seem obvious, it's easy to get drawn into buying a product that looks good but doesn't really address your loved one's needs.

- Generally, it is best to pick the simplest product available to meet the need. Simpler devices are often easier to use, less expensive, and easier to repair and maintain than more complex devices. For example, if someone does not have difficulty remembering to take their medications, but gets confused about which pills to take at which times, a weekly pill organizer that can be filled by a caregiver would solve the problem. Purchasing an automated pill dispenser with alarms to remind the person to take medications would be more complicated than necessary and would certainly be more expensive than the simpler pill organizer.

- Ask experts that provide care to your loved one, like rehabilitation specialists or physical and occupational therapists, about which type of technology might be best.

- Ask other people with disabilities what products they have found to be helpful.

- Ask to use the device on a trial basis to see if it is truly going to meet your loved one's needs.

- Ultimately, your loved one's opinion about a certain piece of AT is the most important. The device needs to be comfortable, attractive, and simple to use.

The following website provides comparisons of assistive devices and is a good resource for consumers trying to decide which equipment and devices to purchase:

Technology for Long-Term Care
Phone: 213-371-2354
Website: www.techforltc.org

Where Can You Buy AT?

With so many vendors and manufacturers producing AT, it can be confusing to decide which products to buy. There are a few public agencies which keep a complete list of AT products and manufacturers and can help you find the right products for your loved one. Because these agencies do not sell equipment, they are a more trustworthy source of information than contacting manufacturers directly. The following national agencies can be contacted by phone or you can browse online for products:

Center for Assistive Technology & Environmental Access
Toll-Free: 800-726-9119
Website: www.assistivetech.net

ABLEDATA
Toll-Free: 800-227-0216
Website: www.abledata.com

Project LINK, Department of Occupational Therapy, University of Florida
Phone: 877-770-7303
Website: www.hp.ufl.edu/ot/projectlink

In addition to the national programs above, every state and territory has a State Technology Assistance Project that has information about AT, financial assistance to buy equipment, and AT loan programs. ABLEDATA can connect you with someone in your state, or you can contact the following agency which oversees the State Technology Assistance projects:

Rehabilitation Engineering and Assistive Technology Society of North America (RESNA)
Phone: 703-524-6686
Website: www.resna.org/taproject/at/statecontacts.html

Paying for Aids and Equipment

Some government programs and other funding sources will help pay for some medical equipment, also called "durable medical equipment" such as canes, walkers, wheelchairs, and scooters, if prescribed by a physician or otherwise determined to be medically necessary. However, other independent living aids, like grab bars, bath mats, and dressing aids, are typically not covered. The following funding sources and agencies may help you purchase certain kinds of aids:

- Medicare
- Medicaid, particularly waiver programs
- Private health insurance plans
- Public service organizations like United Way and Easter Seals
- National Family Caregiver Support Program
- Department of Veterans Affairs

To find out which medical equipment and aids are covered by these programs, see the Resources section at the end of this chapter for contact information.

Types of AT

In this section, the most popular categories of AT are outlined. To find out more information on these products or others not listed, refer to the agencies listed in the Resources section at the end of this fact sheet. Pictures of many products and devices can be seen at the following website: StrokeCenter: Adapting the Home after a Stroke, www.strokecenter.org.

Independent Living Aids

A wide variety of products and appliances help people perform "activities of daily living"—i.e., eating, food preparation, bathing, dressing. Many of these items are available from drugstores and large retail stores:

- Kitchen items include easy-to-grip silverware, high-lipped dishes and plate guards, specialized cutting boards and utensils, self-opening scissors, reaching tools, and jar openers.

- Bedroom items include bed bars, bedside organizers, reaching tools, various orthopedic support cushions, hip pads for fall protection, bedside commode, transfer board, night lights, and large-numeral alarm clocks.

- Bathroom items include full-length tub mats, bathtub and shower seats, transfer benches, toilet riser or raised commode, night lights, long-handled scrub brushes, shampoo basins, lotion applicators, colored tape or mark for hot water controls, and handheld showerheads.

Personal Care Products

A variety of personal care products are designed to help people with physical or cognitive limitations dress, disrobe, groom, and maintain good hygiene.

- Dressing and grooming aids include dressing sticks, elastic or non-tie shoelaces, buttonhooks, zipper pulls, Velcro, easy-to-pull sock and panty hose aids, long-handled combs and brushes, pumps for soap or toothpaste, and various reaching tools.

- No-rinse shampoo, body bath, and body wash that does not require rinsing off with water, which can be helpful if your loved one has difficulty getting in and out of a bathtub.

- Adaptive clothing is designed for people who have difficulty dressing because of cognitive and/or physical disability, or who need frequent changing due to incontinence. The clothing is made to be both fashionable and convenient.

Medication Aids

People with chronic illnesses often take several prescription or non-prescription medications daily for which the following devices can help:

- Daily or weekly pill organizers can help ensure that correct dosages of medications are taken each day.

- Timers and specialized mini-alarms can remind your loved one when the next dose is due.

- Pill crushers and splitters help when swallowing is difficult. Medication aids are available in many drugstores and hospital pharmacies.

Incontinence and Toileting Supplies/Aids

Adult protective undergarments can help individuals who have problems with bladder or bowel control. Fortunately, these are now widely available at drugstores under brand names like Depends, Attends, and Dignity.

- Mattress and floor protectors, such as a plastic fitted sheet or mattress pad to repel or absorb urine before it damages the mattress, and floor runners that protect flooring.

- Antiseptic skin lotions and wipes, catheters, portable receptacles, and a host of related products for incontinence can make the affected person more comfortable and minimize difficulties for the caregiver.

To order the National Association for Continence resource guide of products and services for incontinence call 800-252-6667 or go to: www.nafc.org.

- Commodes, toilet seat modifiers, and urinals come in a variety of designs to help someone with incontinence or someone who has difficulty getting to the bathroom. Items include raised and adjustable seats, safety rails, grab bars, and portable commodes.

AT for Improving Mobility

If your loved one needs assistance walking, the following AT, which is available at most medical supply stores, may help:

- Gait belts and lift vests help facilitate transfers and can help a caregiver balance a person's center of gravity. When moving a person from one position to another the belt can help the caregiver more safely lift or shift directions of the person being transferred.

- Canes are certainly simple but effective walking aids. Designs include folding canes, adjustable canes, double-grip canes, and three- and four-pronged canes.

- Walkers provide more stability and should be tested to make sure they are sturdy, lightweight, at a sufficient height for the individual, and can be moved or rolled easily. Foldable walkers and those that double as a seat are also convenient. Many people like to attach a basket or pouch on the front to store things.

If your loved one can no longer walk safely, he or she will most likely need a wheelchair or a scooter:

- Wheelchairs come in many different varieties (both manual and electric). You may want to consider getting removable footrests and/or a collapsible wheelchair for loading into a car for added convenience. Other wheelchair accessories such as rim covers, gloves, seat covers, cushions, security pouches, and carry packs can also be handy.

  - Manual wheelchairs require the person to use some arm strength or leg strength and skill to move the chair—unless there is someone to push. A lowered wheelchair, called a "hemi-height" wheelchair allows a person's heels to touch the floor, and is recommended when a person uses their feet to move the chair.

  - Electric or "power" wheelchairs are useful for individuals who can move around on their own but lack the strength to wheel themselves. Electric wheelchairs require the ability to make decisions and maneuver the chair. They are often not recommended for someone with impaired judgment.

- Three-wheeled scooters are a great option for individuals who are able to get in and out of the chair. Scooters are popular among individuals with Multiple Sclerosis or those who can walk very short distances and get around by themselves.

FCA does not recommend ordering wheelchairs or scooters by mail or online. Purchasing a chair or scooter through a local dealer or supplier will insure that you have a convenient place to take your product if it needs to be replaced or repaired. Talk with your local Center for Independent Living to find out which dealers have a good reputation in your community.

Communication AT

Advances in computer and telephone technology have greatly helped physically disabled and frail elders to live independently while maintaining connections to family, friends, and support services.

- Modified telephones may use large buttons, headsets, speakerphone capabilities, or keyboard and visual displays to make telephones useable by disabled people.

- Computer technology can allow people to stay in contact via e-mail, while more sophisticated technology can employ modified keyboards or voice recognition software to enable disabled individuals to use computers effectively.

For people with communication difficulties due to stroke, ALS [amyotrophic lateral sclerosis], aphasia, quadriplegia, or other disorders, assistive technology can be very helpful in allowing them to communicate with others. Rapid advances in technology have resulted in products that dramatically increase the independence of people with very limited mobility, allowing them to "speak," operate lights and other controls, and remain active members of their families and communities.

- Communication boards can be simple low-tech plastic boards with graphics and a keyboard-style letter display to convey messages. Automated boards with voice input or a computer screen are also available.

- Voice- or eye-activated communication systems allow people with complex physical difficulties to operate a computer or a telephone to communicate with others.

- Speech amplification and adaptation systems are automated speech processing systems which can correct garbled speech for improved communication.

Home Modifications

Making a house safe and comfortable can allow an individual to remain at home as their abilities change. You may be able to make some simple modifications to your loved one's home with relatively little cost or assistance. For larger modifications, such as widening doorways, lowering counters, remodeling hallways, and installing lifts or elevators, you may need to hire a licensed contractor.

Two useful checklists to determine if your loved one's home needs to undergo some changes to make the house safer and more accessible can be found at the following websites: www.homemods.org and www.rebuildingtogether.org/downloads/home_safety_checklist.pdf.

The following list of independent living aids may provide easy, low-cost installation solutions to a number of problems with home design:

- Grab bars, bath seats, and transfer benches
- Hand rails for stairways
- Bathmats and skid resistant rugs
- Glow tape for hazardous furniture
- Attachable grips for turning doorknobs, lamp switches, and faucet handles
- Lever door handles

Other useful home modifications include:

- Wheelchair and threshold ramps, which come in a variety of predesigned sizes with predrilled slots for easy installation. Lightweight portable wheelchair ramps can be folded or rolled up for easy transport and storage.
- Elevators and lifts, which need to be installed by a contractor to assure that installations meet code and safety standards. Lifts and elevators are available for most inclined or vertical surfaces, including porches, balconies, and curved or straight stairs.

Home modification and repair programs may provide elderly and low-income people with loans, grants, and free or reduced services. Programs often vary from state to state and county to county. To find out about local home modification programs, contact the following organizations:

National Resource Center on Supportive Housing and Home Modification
Phone: 213-740-1364
Website: www.homemods.org

Rebuilding Together
Toll-Free: 800-4-REHAB-9
Website: www.rebuildingtogether.org

AARP: Home Design
Toll-Free: 888-687-2277
Website: www.aarp.org/life/homedesign

Vehicle Modifications and Accessible Vans

Vehicle modifications can help your loved one continue to drive or to more easily be a passenger. Most adaptive equipment can be installed in a vehicle without extensive modifications.

- Wheelchair lifts or automatic transfer seats can be installed in minivans, station wagons, and some cars.

- Accessory items such as car door openers, handles to assist with transferring, tie-down systems for wheelchairs, and portable swivel seats require little or no vehicle modification.

- Kneeler systems, which lower one corner of the vehicle for boarding, and driving controls, which mount all the vehicle's control features onto the steering wheel, are examples of more extensive vehicle modifications.

For information about adaptive equipment, accessible vehicle dealers, or funding and reimbursement programs, contact:

The National Mobility Equipment Dealers Association
Toll-Free: 800-833-0427
Website: www.nmeda.org

Several of the major auto companies offer rebates for adaptive modifications to their vehicles. Contact auto manufacturers directly to find out if they have a rebate program.

AT for Monitoring Potential Crises

Both you and your loved one can have an added degree of security by using AT which alerts you or a medical system if your loved one is in crisis. The following are examples of this type of AT:

- Personal emergency response systems (also called medical response systems) use a pendant, bracelet, or belt that your loved one wears. If he or she has an accident, fall, or other emergency when unattended, a monitor center can be alerted at the press of a button. A monitor will then call the appropriate contacts and emergency services based on the caller's medical information. This device is intended for persons who are able to activate the signal and who do not have dementia.

- Occupancy monitors may be helpful if your loved one is prone to falls. These monitors use pressure sensitive chair or bed pads that activate when your loved one moves to get up.

- Intercom systems, often called baby monitors, can be used if your loved one lives with you. The intercoms can be left on so that you can hear your loved one from another area of the house.

- Webcams and other computerized monitoring systems are more technologically-advanced methods of monitoring a loved one. Webcams are basically video cameras that can allow you to see your loved one and monitor potential problems. Other types of computerized monitoring systems are in development by a number of companies and may use motion detection or other means to monitor your loved one and continually gather and process the information at a central monitoring site which can then alert you if there is a problem.

AT for Loved Ones with Cognitive Impairment or Dementia

If your loved one is in the earlier stages of dementia, the following devices may help them to live at home more safely:

- Memory aids include jumbo analog wall clocks with daily calendar, talking clocks/wrist watches, voice-activated phone dialers, automated pill dispensers with message machine and timer, and a Find-It beeping device to keep track of small items such as car keys and glasses.

- Symbols or warning signs on doors, cabinets, and dangerous appliances can help a person with dementia maneuver more safely around the house.

If your loved one wanders or forgets where he or she is, the following can be quite helpful:

- Mobility monitors and tracking systems come in a variety of designs, though all usually require that your loved one wear a small ankle or wrist transmitter. The transmitter triggers an alert system, or a receiver which you can monitor, when your loved one passes beyond a set range or exits activated doorways.

- Medical ID bracelets have a person's diagnosis and a 24-hour hotline number inscribed on the bracelet. Such a bracelet can be helpful if your loved one is disoriented and gets lost or has an accident outside of the home. The following two programs are respected:

Medic-Alert Foundation International
Toll-Free: 800-432-5378
Website: www.medicalert.org

Alzheimer's Association Safe Return
Toll-Free: 888-572-8566
Website: www.alz.org/Services/SafeReturn.asp

Chapter 58

Coping with Chronic Illness and Depression

There are many types of chronic illness, from diabetes and AIDS [acquired immunodeficiency syndrome] to arthritis and persistent fatigue. While medical science has made great strides in developing effective treatments for the physical effects of these diseases, many victims still face a staggering challenge to their mental and emotional health.

One of the biggest fears is the uncertainty associated with a chronic illness. The condition may be sporadic, lasting only a short while. Or, it could be permanent, gradually worsening over time.

Chronic illness can force many potentially stressful lifestyle changes, such as giving up cherished activities, adapting to new physical limitations and special needs, and paying for what can be expensive medications and treatment services.

Even day-to-day living may be difficult. A study of patients suffering from chronic tension headaches experienced diminished performance in their jobs and social functioning, and were three to 15 times more likely to be diagnosed with an anxiety or mood disorder.

The Need for Emotional Endurance

Over time, these stresses and negative feelings can rob you of the emotional energy necessary to move forward with your life. Lack of progress in your recovery or worsening symptoms can trigger negative thoughts that heighten feelings of anxiety and sadness, often leading to depression.

Acting quickly to address depression is essential. In studies of patients recently diagnosed with various types of chronic illnesses, the highest risk of depressive symptoms occurred within the first two years. While these symptoms usually diminished, patients with heart disease maintain a significantly higher risk for depression as long as eight years after diagnosis. Physical limitations imposed by heart disease and other chronic illnesses such as arthritis and lung disease are also a common source of depression, particularly among older adults.

Because depression often leads to poor eating habits, lack of exercise, and inconsistent hygiene, it may actually complicate your recovery from a chronic illness and worsen your overall physical condition.

Those battling heart disease are especially at risk. Prolonged depression in patients with cardiovascular disease is a known contributor to subsequent heart attacks and strokes. And heart attack survivors suffering from major depression are three to four times more likely to die within six months.

What to Do

Coping with the mental and emotional challenges of a chronic illness requires an approach that is realistic, but also positive. Adapting to your condition or feeling good about the future may seem impossible at first, but it can be done. A recent study of kidney patients undergoing multiple dialysis treatments each week found that their perceived mood and life satisfaction was no different from a control group of healthy people.

A qualified psychologist can help you build the emotional resilience necessary to navigate the difficulties of chronic illness. Working with your physician and other specialists, the psychologist can help develop appropriate coping strategies that will not only reinforce your treatment program, but also help you find fulfillment in life regardless of any physical limitations.

Here are some other suggestions for coping with chronic illness:

- **Stay connected.** Establish and maintain quality relationships with friends and family. Many health organizations also sponsor support groups composed of other people experiencing similar challenges. These groups will not only aid your own well-being, but also provide rewarding opportunities to help others.

- **Take care of yourself.** Don't allow worries about your illness to get in the way of eating property, getting rest and exercise, and having fun.

- **Maintain a daily routine** of work, errands, household chores, and hobbies as much as possible. This will provide you with a feeling of stability amid the chaos and uncertainty of your illness.

The American Psychological Association Practice Directorate gratefully acknowledges the assistance of Rosalind Dorlen, Psy.D., ABPP, and the Council on Psychological Health of the New Jersey Psychological Health Association in developing this information.

Chapter 59

Caring for Someone with a Neurological Disorder

Chapter Contents

Section 59.1

Caring for a Loved One

"Families & Friends—Caring for a Loved One" is reprinted from The Brain Matters website (www.thebrainmatters.org) with permission of The American Academy of Neurology. © 2008 American Academy of Neurology.

Information gathering and planning are the keys to giving care to your loved one or friend. You will need to learn:

- The medical condition and how it might affect your loved one
- Other medical issues
- Legal issues

Medical Condition

Persons with neurologic disorders and their caregivers need to know the following information:

- **What is the diagnosis?** This is where you start to understand the possible causes and effects of the disorder.

- **Is the condition treatable?** You will learn what treatments are available, how they may help manage the disorder, and possible side effects. You will get a better idea of what resources you and your loved one need to help maintain quality of life.

- **How will the condition progress?** Knowing what to expect can help you decide if you have the skills and resources to be the main caregiver for your loved one.

- **What can I do to help now?** You are a vital part of the team providing care for your loved one. Plan to attend doctor appointments with your loved one. Learn as much as you can about the condition.

- **Is the treatment covered by medical insurance?** You need to know whom you might have to contact about medical coverage and what assistance may be available. There may be financial actions you and your loved one will need to take.

- **Where can I learn more about the medical condition?** The physician and nurse are excellent starting points. Bring a list of questions to the next medical appointment to help make sure that you get the information you need. Ask your neurologist's office for a list of websites, books, or brochures that they have found to be helpful.

- **Are there patient groups that can give information about coping with the disorder?** Ask the doctor's office about patient groups associated with the disorder. These groups are very helpful in providing information. They can tell you how people with neurological disorders, families, and friends have learned to live with the disorder.

Other Medical Issues

As a partner in your loved one's care you may need the following information:

- Date of his or her birth and Social Security number

- List of healthcare insurance policies and contact numbers

- Access to Medicare account numbers

- List of all doctors treating your loved one (and those who have treated him or her in the past) including name, phone number, and medical specialty

- List of all current and past medications and allergies

- Medical history; family medical history can be helpful in diagnosing disorders with genetic aspects

Legal Issues

You may be called upon to help make decisions about your loved one's care and/or to pay bills, if needed. Two documents, if available, would be most helpful:

- **A copy of your loved one's advanced healthcare directive:** The advanced healthcare directive is a written statement of how your loved one wants care to be provided. This is used if he or she is unable to communicate his or her wishes at the time care is needed.

- **Knowledge of your loved one's durable power of attorney:** This document names the person who has the legal authority to pay bills, deposit checks, and handle day-to-day matters.

If your loved one does not have these documents, the two of you may wish to meet with an attorney to discuss how to best handle the situation.

Section 59.2

Support for Spouses of People with Neurological Disorders

Haupt, J. "United Front," *Neurology Now* July/August 2007; 3(4):26–29.
© 2007 American Academy of Neurology. Reprinted by permission of
Lippincott Williams and Wilkins.

Jennifer and Jason Elsenbroek have been married for 12 years, but there are still times when communication is difficult because of her traumatic brain injury (TBI). That's why they do whatever they can to face her illness together, including attending a TBI support group. Jennifer started the group through her church in Chatham, MI, two years ago, and Jason has become a frequent face by her side.

Even little things like a cookie tin scraping across a table top or the sound of someone chewing can be like nails on a chalkboard for TBI patients, and that can be very difficult for spouses to understand, explains the 35-year-old stay-at-home mother, who has dealt with TBI since a car accident at age 16. "It really helps us when Jason comes to the support group meetings and sees that it's not just me who is irritated by these things. Knowing that it's part of the disease helps him to be more understanding with me at home."

There is growing concern among the health care community about providing emotional and practical support for the spouses of people suffering from Alzheimer's disease, multiple sclerosis (MS), stroke,

Parkinson's disease, and other neurological disorders—especially as the numbers of people living with these conditions is expected to increase dramatically. While the benefits of caregiver support groups are widely recognized, providing support for patients and spouses as a couple is also becoming an important part of the equation.

Facing Illness Together

"Traditionally, we take the caregiver and talk to them in one room, and talk to the patient in another room," explains Mary Mittelman, Dr. P.H., director of psychosocial and support programs at the Silberstein Aging and Dementia Research Center at New York University (NYU) School of Medicine. She is currently leading a 3-year clinical trial to determine the efficacy of couples therapy for marriages in which one partner has Alzheimer's.

The next logical step is to teach couples to open up to each other and take those skills home, into their marriage. Open communication is the best way to ward off the resentment, guilt, and other hidden feelings that both the ill spouse and the caregiving spouse can have difficulty expressing, says Dr. Mittelman.

A study conducted by Purdue University in Indiana examined how the perceived burdens of caregiving spouses influenced how well people with Parkinson's disease managed their condition. As the caregiver's worries about their own health, social life, and financial status increased, so did the negative impact on how the patient managed their illness. The study concluded that sharing these concerns as a couple with a trained counselor and educator was helpful for both spouses. Sharing perceived burdens and dealing with them together seems to be the key to success. Corinne Samios McCrosky, age 69, has been a caregiver for her husband John, age 76, since his stroke in 1995. Two years ago, when John began showing signs of Alzheimer's, the couple participated in six weekly therapy sessions at NYU for 2 months (the duration of counseling in Dr. Mittelman's study). "John has been a very private person for the 40 years I've known him, and I'd hear things from him during our sessions that that I wouldn't otherwise know," Corinne says. "The couples therapy gave John a safe space to tell me things that he wouldn't normally say because he didn't want to hurt my feelings. And sometimes he'd just think about things we talked about with the therapist and bring them up to me alone later."

One issue that came up for John and Corinne was that he didn't want her helping him all the time and doting over him. At the same time, there were many instances where he really did need his wife's help: to get in and out of the tub, remind him to take his medications, and a host of other safety issues and daily practicalities. "We talked a lot with the counselor about when it was okay to help John, and when I needed to let him try things on his own," Corinne recalls. "I had to learn how to give him enough rope but also be there just in case he needed me."

Learning to Be an Advocate

For patients with neurological conditions that affect their ability to communicate, such as Alzheimer's, Parkinson's, and TBI, the benefits of improving the level of understanding with their spouse may reach far beyond the marriage. Many times, these patients rely on their partner to be their advocate in the world. For example, while it's been nearly 20 years since the car accident that left Jennifer Elsenbroek with TBI, she still often talks slowly, deliberately searching for words.

"One of the long term effects of the brain injury is that it makes it difficult to explain myself; and the more frustrated I become, the harder it is," Jennifer explains. "Luckily, my husband has learned to be my advocate when I'm overwhelmed or think I'm articulating something well and the other person is just not getting it. This happens all the time—at the doctor's office, the dentist, or even at the mall. Jason knows me so well that he can interpret things for me."

In their TBI support group, which has about 20 members—two or three of which are spouses—the Elsenbroeks set an example for how to advocate tactfully. Jason will take over for Jennifer if she's struggling to tell the group something, and other couples have begun to do the same thing. Sometimes, there's a fear of interrupting your spouse, Jennifer says. But people see that there's a polite and gentle way to take over, and it's really a relief for the TBI patient to have a partner who knows when they need help.

Sticking with It

A 2005 study from the Karolinska Institute in Stockholm concluded that educational support groups for couples may improve the quality of life for spouses of stroke patients if they attend at least five times during a 6-month period. Both spouses reported feeling a significant decrease in negative feelings and an improvement in quality of life over time. The Karolinska study suggests that support groups work best when they are ongoing and consistent. Like just about everything else in life, hard work pays off.

Dr. Mittelman admits that the 2-month therapy sessions that her study permits may be only a starting point for some couples. The good news is that most of the couples who attended all six therapy sessions reported positive changes in the quality of their communication and their marriage.

For Corinne Samios McCrosky, the couples therapy sessions she attended with her husband 2 years ago have led her to seek consistent support for herself. "It seems like different issues are coming up as the illness progresses, so I find that I need ongoing support on a weekly basis," says Corinne, who goes to individual counseling as well as a Thursday morning support group with 13 other Alzheimer's caregivers. As far as couples therapy goes, however, she says that while it was helpful during the early states of John's illness, he no longer has the mental alertness or retention to benefit from it.

Support Groups as Extended Family

For many, attending a support group on a consistent basis becomes as much a social outlet as an educational resource.

The Parkinson's support group that Pat and Marge Moylan belong to in Herkimer, NY, is the mainstay of their social life. Thirty-five couples belong to the group of 133 members, and the Moylans have known some of them for the past 15 years. They've had Saturday brunch bunches for people who couldn't get to the monthly meetings and a big picnic in July. Their connection, though, goes way beyond social gatherings.

"We have a wonderful support system in place, and we all call members who are having trouble to see how they're getting along," says Marge, 63, who was diagnosed with MS in 1984 and then Parkinson's in 1986. "When someone dies, one of our members calls everyone on the roster to make sure that they know. That kind of support means a lot to the spouses—sometimes, they keep coming to our meetings for months or even years after their husband or wife dies."

For Denise Ellis, 42, of Port St. Lucie, Florida, the MS support group she started through her church in 2003 is like a family, so it just makes sense for spouses to join in. At first, only a few spouses would attend the monthly meetings because they were driving, says Ellis, who encouraged more members to bring their husband or wife, and now there are eight couples among the 25 members. The truth is that MS doesn't just affect the patient, it affects the spouse and the entire family. The best thing that you can do to combat the disease is to face it with your spouse, as a united team.

Ellis says that the close-knit nature of the group helps her to bring up intimate issues, like sexual dysfunction and the fatigue that can leave MS patients feeling like they don't have the energy for romance or much of anything else. "I heard one gentleman say that he just thought his wife was being lazy, not wanting to do anything," Ellis recalls. When he came to the group, he began to see she wasn't the only one dealing with the fatigue.

Couples Therapy or Support Group?

The function of couples therapy is different from being in a larger group with other couples and individuals who are dealing with a common neurological illness. Which one is right for you depends partially on the illness you or your spouse is facing and partially on your personal preference.

One of the benefits of couples therapy is that spouses deal with each other directly in the session in the supportive presence of a third party, says Ursula Auclair, C.S.W., a licensed social worker who is one of the counselors in the NYU study with Alzheimer's patients and their spouses, and has also led support groups. "They're able to replicate their home life and then adjust their interactions with suggestions from the therapist."

According to Auclair, Alzheimer's patients don't do well with lots of stimuli, especially when dealing with emotion-laden issues. So for them, couples therapy is less stressful than group therapy. On the other hand, Denise Ellis says that there can be power in numbers.

"I've seen a real look of relief on the faces of spouses and MS patients alike as we talk about some of the issues they are afraid to discuss one-on-one," Ellis says. "They are so concerned with hurting each other's feelings that things just don't get brought up. We'll bring up their fears about the MS patient winding up blind and in a wheelchair, for example, and, assure them that this doesn't have to happen. That's the beauty of support groups—everyone is going through the same issues, together."

Support-Group 101

Marge and Pat Moylan have been so successful in bolstering their Parkinson's support group to 133 members, including 35 couples, that they were recently asked to help folks in a neighboring town start their own support group. Here are some of their tips for success:

- **Bring in speakers:** Make sure they address the needs of spouses as well as patients.

- **Spread the word:** People want to know they aren't the only one—talk up your group at your church, your book club, wherever you go, says Pat.

- **Publish:** Put out a quarterly newsletter.

- **Have fun:** Arrange social gatherings outside the weekly meetings.

- **Couple up:** Encourage folks to bring their spouses. Sometimes, people just don't know they are allowed to bring a spouse—and they're happy to do so, says Pat.

Jennifer Haupt frequently writes health and lifestyle articles for Woman's Day, AARP: The Magazine, Cure, and Reader's Digest.

Chapter 60

Parenting a Child with a Movement Disorder: Special Concerns

Chapter Contents

Section 60.1

How to Care for a Seriously Ill Child

Taking care of a chronically ill child is one of the most draining and difficult tasks a parent can face. Beyond handling physical challenges and medical needs, you'll have to deal with the emotional needs your child may have and the emotional impact that the prolonged illness can have on the entire family.

Luckily, this tough balancing act doesn't have to be done alone: support groups, social workers, and family friends often can lend a helping hand.

Explaining Long-Term Illness to a Child

Honest communication is crucial to helping a child adjust to a serious medical condition. It's important for a child to know that he or she is sick and will be getting lots of care. The hospital and the medicine may feel frightening, but they're part of helping your child feel better.

As you explain the illness and its treatment, give clear and honest answers to all questions in a way your child can understand. It's also important to accurately explain and prepare your child for any treatments—and possible discomfort that might go with along with those treatments.

Avoid saying "This won't hurt" if the procedure is likely to be painful. Instead, be honest if a procedure may cause some discomfort, pain, pressure, or stinging, but then reassure your child that it will be temporary and that you'll be there to offer support while or after it's done.

Many hospitals give parents the option to speak to their child about a long-term diagnosis alone, or with the doctor or the entire medical team (doctors, social workers, nurses, etc.) present. Your doctor or other medical professional probably can offer advice on how to talk to your child about the illness.

Tackling Tough Emotions

Your child will have many feelings about the changes affecting his or her body, and should be encouraged and given opportunities to express any feelings, concerns, and fears. Ask what your child is experiencing and listen to the answers before bringing up your own feelings or explanations.

This kind of communication doesn't always have to be verbal.

Music, drawing, or writing can often help kids living with a life-threatening disease express their emotions and escape through a fantasy world of their own design.

Kids may also need reminders that they're not responsible for the illness. It's common for them to fear that they brought their sickness on by something they thought, said, or did. Reassure your child that this is not the case, and explain in simple terms what caused the illness. (You may also want to reassure your other kids that nothing they said or did caused their sibling's illness.)

For many questions, there won't be easy answers. And you can't always promise that everything is going to be fine. But you can help your child feel better by listening, saying it's OK and completely understandable to have those feelings, and explaining that you and your family will make him or her as comfortable as possible.

If a child asks "why me?" it's OK to offer an honest "I don't know." Explain that even though no one knows why the illness occurred, the doctors do have treatments for it (if that's the case). If your child says "it's not fair that I'm sick," acknowledge that your child is right. It's important for kids to know it's OK to feel angry about the illness.

Your child may ask "am I going to die?" How you answer will depend on your child's age and maturity level. It's important to know, if possible, what specific fears or concerns your child has and to address them specifically. For example, your child actually may be worried about being in pain.

If it is reassuring to your child, you may refer to your religious, spiritual, and cultural beliefs about death. You might want to stay away from euphemisms for death such as "going to sleep." Saying that may cause your child and siblings to fear going to sleep.

Regardless of their age, it's important for kids to know that there are people who love them and will be there for them, and that they'll be kept comfortable.

Just like any adult, a child will need time to adjust to the diagnosis and the physical changes and is likely to feel sad, depressed, angry, afraid, or even denial. Think about getting professional counseling if you see signs that these feelings are interfering with daily function, or your child seems withdrawn, depressed, and shows radical changes in eating and sleeping habits unrelated to the physical illness.

Behavioral Issues

Kids with chronic illnesses certainly require extra "TLC," but also need the routines of childhood. The foremost—and perhaps trickiest—task for worried parents is to treat a sick child as normally as possible.

Despite the circumstances, this means setting limits on unacceptable behavior, sticking to normal routines, and avoiding overindulgence. This may seem impossible, particularly if you have feelings of guilt or an intense need to protect your sick child. But spoiling or coddling can only make it harder for a child to return to daily activities.

When your child leaves the hospital for home, normalcy is the goal. Your child may want to visit or stay in touch with friends through visits, if possible, or through e-mail, the phone, or letters.

Dealing with Siblings

Family dynamics can be severely tested when a child is sick. Clinic visits, surgical procedures, and frequent checkups can throw big kinks into everyone's schedules and take an emotional toll on the entire family.

To ease the pressure, seek help to keep the family routines as close to normal as possible. Friends and family members may be able to help handle errands, carpools, and meals. Siblings should continue to attend school and their usual recreational activities; the family should strive for normalcy and time for everyone to be together.

Flexibility is key. The old "normal" may have been the entire family around the table for a home-cooked meal at 6:00, while the new "normal" may be takeout pizza on clinic nights.

Also, consider talking with your other kids' teachers or school counselors and let them know that a sibling in the family is ill. They can keep an eye out for behavioral changes or signs of stress among your kids.

It's common for siblings of a chronically ill child to become angry, sullen, resentful, fearful, or withdrawn. They may pick fights or fall behind in schoolwork. In all cases, parents should pay close attention, so that the kids don't feel pushed aside by the demands of their sick brother or sister.

It may also help them to be included in the treatment process when possible. Depending on their ages and maturity level, visiting the hospital, meeting the nursing and physician staffs, or accompanying their sick sibling to the clinic for treatments can also help make the situation less frightening and more understandable.

What they imagine about the illness and hospital visits are often worse than the reality. When they come to the hospital, they can develop a more realistic picture and see that, while unpleasant things may be part of the treatment, there are people who care about their sibling and do their best to help.

Lightening Your Load

The stress involved in caring for a child with a long-term illness is considerable, but these tips might ease the strain:

- Break problems into manageable parts. If your child's treatment is expected to be given over an extended time, view it in more manageable time blocks. Planning a week or a month at a time may be less overwhelming.

- Attend to your own needs. Get appropriate rest and food. To the extent possible, pay attention to your relationship with your spouse, hobbies, and friendships.

- Depend on friends. Let them carpool siblings to soccer or theater practice. Permit others—relatives, friends—to share responsibilities of caring for your child. Remember that you can't do it all.

- Ask for help in managing the financial aspects of your child's illness.

- Recognize that everyone handles stress differently. If you and your spouse have distinct worrying styles, talk about them and try to accommodate them. Don't pretend that they don't exist.

- Develop collaborative working relationships with health care professionals. Realize you are all part of the team. Ask questions and learn all you can about your child's illness.

- Consult other parents in support groups at your care center or hospital. They can offer information and understanding.

- Explore support groups for parents who have children with the same or similar illness.

- Keep a journal.

- Utilize support staff offered at the treating hospital.

Section 60.2

Helping Children Deal with Bullies

"Helping Kids Deal with Bullies," June 2007, reprinted with permission from www.kidshealth.org. Copyright © 2007 The Nemours Foundation. This information was provided by KidsHealth, one of the largest resources online for medically reviewed health information written for parents, kids, and teens. For more articles like this one, visit www.KidsHealth.org, or www.TeensHealth.org.

Each day, 10-year-old Seth asked his mom for more and more lunch money. Yet he seemed skinnier than ever and came home from school hungry. It turned out that Seth was handing his lunch money to a fifth-grader, who was threatening to beat him up if he didn't pay.

Kayla, 13, thought things were going well at her new school, since all the popular girls were being so nice to her. But then she found out that one of them had posted mean rumors about her on a website. Kayla cried herself to sleep that night and started going to the nurse's office complaining of a stomachache to avoid the girls in study hall.

Unfortunately, the kind of bullying that Seth and Kayla experienced is widespread. In national surveys, most kids and teens say that bullying happens at school.

A bully can turn something like going to the bus stop or recess into a nightmare for kids. Bullying can leave deep emotional scars that last for life. And in extreme situations, it can culminate in violent threats, property damage, or someone getting seriously hurt.

If your child is being bullied, there are ways to help him or her cope with it on a day-to-day basis and lessen its lasting impact. And even if bullying isn't an issue right in your house right now, it's important to discuss it so your kids will be prepared if it does happen.

What Is Bullying?

Most kids have been teased by a sibling or a friend at some point. And it's not usually harmful when done in a playful, friendly, and mutual way, and both kids find it funny. But when teasing becomes hurtful, unkind, and constant, it crosses the line into bullying and needs to stop.

Bullying is intentional tormenting in physical, verbal, or psychological ways. It can range from hitting, shoving, name-calling, threats, and mocking to extorting money and treasured possessions. Some kids bully by shunning others and spreading rumors about them. Others use e-mail, chat rooms, instant messages, social networking websites, and text messages to taunt others or hurt their feelings.

It's important to take bullying seriously and not just brush it off as something that kids have to "tough out." The effects can be serious and affect kids' sense of self-worth and future relationships. In severe cases, bullying has contributed to tragedies, such as school shootings.

Why Do Kids Bully?

Kids bully for a variety of reasons. Sometimes they pick on kids because they need a victim—someone who seems emotionally or physically weaker, or just acts or appears different in some way—to feel more important, popular, or in control. Although some bullies are bigger or stronger than their victims, that's not always the case.

Sometimes kids torment others because that's the way they've been treated. They may think their behavior is normal because they come from families or other settings where everyone regularly gets angry, shouts, or calls names. Some popular TV shows even seem to promote meanness—people are "voted off," shunned, or ridiculed for their appearance or lack of talent.

Signs of Bullying

Unless your child tells you about bullying—or has visible bruises or injuries—it can be difficult to figure out if it's happening.

But there are some warning signs. You might notice your child acting differently or seeming anxious, or not eating, sleeping well, or doing the things that he or she usually enjoys. When kids seem moodier or more easily upset than usual, or when they start avoiding certain situations, like taking the bus to school, it may be because of a bully.

If you suspect bullying but your child is reluctant to open up, find opportunities to bring up the issue in a more roundabout way. For instance, you might see a situation on a TV show and use it as a conversation starter, asking "What do you think of this?" or "What do you think that person should have done?" This might lead to questions like: "Have you ever seen this happen?" or "Have you ever experienced this?" You might want to talk about any experiences you or another family member had at that age.

Let your child know that if he or she is being bullied—or sees it happening to someone else—it's important to talk to someone about it, whether it's you, another adult (a teacher, school counselor, or family friend), or a sibling.

Helping Kids

If your child tells you about a bully, focus on offering comfort and support, no matter how upset you are. Kids are often reluctant to tell adults about bullying. They feel embarrassed and ashamed that it's happening. They worry that their parents will be disappointed.

Sometimes kids feel like it's their own fault, that if they looked or acted differently it wouldn't be happening. Sometimes they're scared that if the bully finds out that they told, it will get worse. Others are worried that their parents won't believe them or do anything about it. Or kids worry that their parents will urge them to fight back when they're scared to.

Praise your child for being brave enough to talk about it. Remind your child that he or she isn't alone—a lot of people get bullied at some point. Emphasize that it's the bully who is behaving badly—not your child. Reassure your child that you will figure out what to do about it together.

Sometimes an older sibling or friend can help deal with the situation. It may help your daughter to hear how the older sister she idolizes was teased about her braces and how she dealt with it. An older sibling or friend may also be able to give you some perspective on what's happening at school, or wherever the bullying is happening, and help you figure out the best solution.

Take it seriously if you hear that the bullying will get worse if the bully finds out that your child told. Sometimes it's useful to approach the bully's parents. In other cases, teachers or counselors are the best ones to contact first. If you've tried those methods and still want to speak to the bullying child's parents, it's best to do so in a context where a school official, such as a counselor, can mediate.

Many states have bullying laws and policies. Find out about the laws in your community. In certain cases, if you have serious concerns about your child's safety, you may need to contact legal authorities.

Advice for Kids

The key to helping kids is providing strategies that deal with bullying on an everyday basis and also help restore their self-esteem and regain a sense of dignity.

It may be tempting to tell a kid to fight back. After all, you're angry that your child is suffering and maybe you were told to "stand up for yourself" when you were young. And you may worry that your child will continue to suffer at the hands of the bully.

But it's important to advise kids not to respond to bullying by fighting or bullying back. It can quickly escalate into violence, trouble, and someone getting injured. Instead, it's best to walk away from the situation, hang out with others, and tell an adult.

Here are some other strategies to discuss with kids that can help improve the situation and make them feel better:

- **Avoid the bully and use the buddy system:** Use a different bathroom if a bully is nearby and don't go to your locker when there is nobody around. Make sure you have someone with you so that you're not alone with the bully. Buddy up with a friend on the bus, in the hallways, or at recess—wherever the bully is. Offer to do the same for a friend.

- **Hold the anger:** It's natural to get upset by the bully, but that's what bullies thrive on. It makes them feel more powerful. Practice not reacting by crying or looking red or upset. It takes a lot of practice, but it's a useful skill for keeping off of a bully's radar. Sometimes kids find it useful to practice "cool down" strategies such as counting to 10, writing down their angry words, taking deep breaths or walking away. Sometimes the best thing to do is to teach kids to wear a "poker face" until they are clear of any danger (smiling or laughing may provoke the bully).

- **Act brave, walk away, and ignore the bully:** Firmly and clearly tell the bully to stop, then walk away. Practice ways to ignore the hurtful remarks, like acting uninterested or texting someone on your cell phone. By ignoring the bully, you're showing that you don't care. Eventually, the bully will probably get bored with trying to bother you.

- **Tell an adult:** Teachers, principals, parents, and lunchroom personnel at school can all help stop bullying.

- **Talk about it:** Talk to someone you trust, such as a guidance counselor, teacher, sibling, or friend. They may offer some helpful suggestions, and even if they can't fix the situation, it may help you feel a little less alone.

- **Remove the incentives:** If the bully is demanding your lunch money, start bringing your lunch. If he's trying to get your music player, don't bring it to school.

Reaching Out

At home you can lessen the impact of the bullying. Encourage your kids to get together with friends that help build their confidence. Help them meet other kids by joining clubs or sports programs. And find activities that can help a child feel confident and strong. Maybe it's a self-defense class like karate or a movement or other gym class.

And just remember: As upsetting as bullying can be for you and your family, lots of people and resources are available to help.

Chapter 61

Social Security Benefits for People with Disabilities

Disability is something most people do not like to think about. But the chances that you will become disabled probably are greater than you realize. Studies show that a 20-year-old worker has a 3 in 10 chance of becoming disabled before reaching retirement age.

This chapter provides basic information on Social Security disability benefits and is not intended to answer all questions. For specific information about your situation, you should talk with a Social Security representative.

We pay disability benefits through two programs: the Social Security disability insurance program and the Supplemental Security Income (SSI) program. This chapter is about the Social Security disability program. For information about the SSI disability program for adults, go to www.socialsecurity.gov.

Who can get Social Security disability benefits?

Social Security pays benefits to people who cannot work because they have a medical condition that is expected to last at least 1 year or result in death. Federal law requires this very strict definition of disability. While some programs give money to people with partial disability or short-term disability, Social Security does not.

Certain family members of disabled workers also can receive money from Social Security.

Excerpted from "Disability Benefits," by the Social Security Administration (SSA, www.ssa.gov), Publication No. 05-10029, June 2008.

How do I meet the earnings requirement for disability benefits?

In general, to get disability benefits, you must meet two different earnings tests:

1. A "recent work" test based on your age at the time you became disabled; and

2. A "duration of work" test to show that you worked long enough under Social Security.

Certain blind workers have to meet only the "duration of work" test.

How do I apply for disability benefits?

There are two ways that you can apply for disability benefits. You can:

1. Apply online at www.socialsecurity.gov; or

2. Call our toll-free number, 800-772-1213, to make an appointment to file a disability claim at your local Social Security office or to set up an appointment for someone to take your claim over the telephone. The disability claims interview lasts about 1 hour. If you are deaf or hard of hearing, you may call our toll-free TTY number, 800-325-0778, between 7 a.m. and 7 p.m. on business days. If you schedule an appointment, a Disability Starter Kit will be mailed to you. The Disability Starter Kit will help you get ready for your disability claims interview. If you apply online, the Disability Starter Kit is available at www.socialsecurity.gov/disability.

When should I apply and what information do I need?

You should apply for disability benefits as soon as you become disabled. It can take a long time to process an application for disability benefits (3 to 5 months).To apply for disability benefits, you will need to complete an application for Social Security Benefits and the Disability Report. You can complete the Disability Report online at www.socialsecurity.gov/disability/3368. You can also print the Disability Report, complete it and return it to your local Social Security office. We may be able to process your application faster if you help us by getting any other information we need.

The information we need includes:

- Your Social Security number;

- Your birth or baptismal certificate;

- Names, addresses, and phone numbers of the doctors, caseworkers, hospitals, and clinics that took care of you and dates of your visits;

- Names and dosage of all the medicine you take;

- Medical records from your doctors, therapists, hospitals, clinics, and caseworkers that you already have in your possession;

- Laboratory and test results;

- A summary of where you worked and the kind of work you did; and

- A copy of your most recent W-2 Form (Wage and Tax Statement) or, if you are self-employed, your federal tax return for the past year.

In addition to the basic application for disability benefits, there are other forms you will need to fill out. One form collects information about your medical condition and how it affects your ability to work. Other forms give doctors, hospitals, and other health care professionals who have treated you permission to send us information about your medical condition.

Do not delay applying for benefits if you cannot get all of this information together quickly. We will help you get it.

Who decides if I am disabled?

We will review your application to make sure you meet some basic requirements for disability benefits. We will check whether you worked enough years to qualify. Also, we will evaluate any current work activities. If you meet these requirements, we will send your application to the Disability Determination Services office in your state.

This state agency completes the disability decision for us. Doctors and disability specialists in the state agency ask your doctors for information about your condition. They will consider all the facts in your case. They will use the medical evidence from your doctors and hospitals, clinics, or institutions where you have been treated and all other information. They will ask your doctors:

- What your medical condition is;
- When your medical condition began;
- How your medical condition limits your activities;
- What the medical tests have shown; and
- What treatment you have received.

They also will ask the doctors for information about your ability to do work-related activities, such as walking, sitting, lifting, carrying, and remembering instructions. Your doctors are not asked to decide if you are disabled.

The state agency staff may need more medical information before they can decide if you are disabled. If more information is not available from your current medical sources, the state agency may ask you to go for a special examination. We prefer to ask your own doctor, but sometimes the exam may have to be done by someone else. Social Security will pay for the exam and for some of the related travel costs.

How do we make the decision?

We use a five-step process to decide if you are disabled.

1. Are you working? If you are working and your earnings average more than a certain amount each month, we generally will not consider you disabled. The amount changes each year.

If you are not working, or your monthly earnings average the current amount or less, the state agency then looks at your medical condition.

2. Is your medical condition "severe"? For the state agency to decide that you are disabled, your medical condition must significantly limit your ability to do basic work activities—such as walking, sitting, and remembering—for at least 1 year. If your medical condition is not that severe, the state agency will not consider you disabled. If your condition is that severe, the state agency goes on to step three.

3. Is your medical condition on the List of Impairments? The state agency has a List of Impairments that describes medical conditions that are considered so severe that they automatically mean that you are disabled as defined by law. If your condition (or combination of medical conditions) is not on this list, the state agency looks to see if your condition is as severe as a condition that is on the list. If the severity of your medical condition meets or equals that of a listed impairment, the state agency will decide that you are disabled. If it does not, the state agency goes on to step four.

4. Can you do the work you did before? At this step, the state agency decides if your medical condition prevents you from being able to do the work you did before. If it does not, the state agency will decide that you are not disabled. If it does, the state agency goes on to step five.

5. Can you do any other type of work? If you cannot do the work you did in the past, the state agency looks to see if you would be able to do other work. It evaluates your medical condition, your age, education, past work experience, and any skills you may have that could be used to do other work. If you cannot do other work, the state agency will decide that you are disabled. If you can do other work, the state agency will decide that you are not disabled.

How will you tell me your decision?

When the state agency reaches a decision on your case, we will send you a letter. If your application is approved, the letter will show the amount of your benefit and when your payments start. If your application is not approved, the letter will explain why and tell you how to appeal the decision if you do not agree with it.

What if I disagree?

If you disagree with a decision made on your claim, you can appeal it. The steps you can take are explained in The Appeals Process (Publication No. 05-10041), which is available from Social Security.

You have the right to be represented by an attorney or other qualified person of your choice when you do business with Social Security. More information is in Your Right To Representation (Publication No. 05-10075), which is also available from Social Security.

Chapter 62

Legal Issues in Planning for Incapacity

We like to think that we will always be healthy and able to make decisions for ourselves. But if you develop a sudden illness or serious condition or are involved in an accident, you might not be able to make decisions for yourself.

Making your wishes known while you are still healthy is a good idea. Sharing your healthcare decisions with others is the best way to make sure they are respected.

Your family and loved ones will benefit from your advance planning. Knowing your wishes will help ease their burden and reduce their uncertainty if they ever have to make medical decisions on your behalf.

In this text, you will learn about the types of decisions you can make ahead of time and how to let others know what you want.

Your Advance Directive for Health Care

An advance directive is a written or spoken statement about your future medical care. The advance directive lets your doctor, family, and others know how you want to be treated if you are unable to tell them. The two main types of advance directives are the "Living Will" and the "Power of Attorney for Health Care."

"Advance Care Planning: Making Choices Known," © 2004 Center on Aging, University of Hawaii at Manoa (www.hawaii.edu/aging). Reprinted with permission.

Planning in advance for health care decisions is the best way to make sure your voice is heard and your wishes are respected.

In your advance directive you may share your wishes about:

- The kind of medical treatment you want or don't want

- The person you want to make health care decisions for you when you cannot

- What you wish to have for comfort care (care that focuses on reducing pain and suffering when a cure is no longer possible)

- Ethical, religious, and spiritual instructions

- Anything else about your health care preferences that you want your loved ones and your health care providers to know

Benefits of Advance Directives

They help people know what to do: Your written advance directive is a gift to your family and friends. By documenting your wishes, others won't have to guess what you want if you can no longer speak for yourself. If your family has to guess, they may disagree and argue. That makes it hard for the doctor to honor your wishes. An advance directive is the best way to make sure that your wishes are carried out. Even if you currently have a living will, new laws enacted in your state may be more comprehensive and may give you more choices.

Health care decisions will not be left to chance: You make choices every day about your work, your home, and your life. Why leave health care decisions to chance? Now is the time to decide about the kind of care you want. Now is the time to share your thoughts.

They let others know your values: Advanced technology makes it possible for patients with little or no hope of recovery to be kept alive for months or even years. This makes it even more important for you to think and talk about what kind of care you would want if you were unable to make your own decisions.

Talking about It

Talking now is a gift you give to those close to you: In the event you become so ill that you can no longer speak for yourself, advance planning will help those close to you make the decisions you would want. Surviving family members of people who died without advance directives tell us that they struggled over their decisions and always wondered if they did the right thing.

Use an example of someone you know: Many people, including some doctors, are uncomfortable talking about care at the end of life. You can start the discussion by talking about someone else's experience. For example, you could ask: Do you remember when our neighbor was in the hospital before she died? What did you think about the treatment she received? Then describe what you would want if you were ever in this condition. Or ask your family members what they would want. Enlist the help of your family or loved ones in making sure that, if this happens to you, they will respect your wishes. It also is important to discuss your concerns and wishes with your doctor.

Getting help: Sometimes you may need the help of a friend, counselor, social worker, or clergy person to start talking with your family about the end of life. There are people from all walks of life and religious groups who have the experience to help.

Understanding Life-Sustaining Treatments

The following are examples of some of the common medical treatments used to extend or sustain life in terminal conditions. It is good to become familiar with them, as you may be asked to consider them for yourself or a loved one.

Always discuss the risks and benefits of all surgeries and other medical treatment decisions with your doctor.

Nutrition (food) and hydration (fluids): Advance directives commonly include instructions to carry out or to stop life-sustaining treatments such as artificial nutrition (food) and hydration (fluids). People in a terminal condition will generally receive artificial nutrition and hydration, unless they have stated their wishes against this means of prolonging life.

Forcing food when a person is dying and not hungry can increase pain, cause the person to choke (aspirate), and worsen the condition. Forcing fluids may also aggravate the situation. Even intravenous feeding (IVs) at this time can cause complications, such as swelling and congestive heart failure.

Blood transfusion: This includes whole blood or blood products. Some people do not want whole blood, but will accept plasma. There comes a point at which blood transfusions no longer improve the quality of the terminally ill person's life.

Surgery: Before a surgery is considered, you should understand the risks and benefits of the surgery. Will it provide comfort and relieve suffering, or merely extend life? In terminal conditions, some surgical procedures are performed to reduce pain and increase comfort and are not meant to be curative. Are there other, less invasive procedures that can increase comfort and reduce pain?

Cardiopulmonary resuscitation (CPR): Normally, when someone suffers a heart attack, also known as a cardiac arrest, a "code" is called and cardiopulmonary resuscitation (CPR) is initiated. An attempt is made to "jump-start" the heart with an electrical impulse, and manual compressions are applied to the chest in an effort to restore the heart to its normal rhythm. In specific medical crises, CPR can help to save a person's life. However, in persons with terminal or life-limiting illnesses, CPR is rarely helpful. In a hospital or health care facility, unless there is a written order not to resuscitate, CPR will be given. If cardiac arrest occurs and 911 is called, CPR will always be initiated unless the person is terminally ill and wearing a "comfort care only" bracelet or necklace ordered by a doctor. Comfort Care bracelets or necklaces, however, may not be available in all states. Those who receive CPR are often put on mechanical ventilators, or breathing machines.

Mechanical ventilation: When people can no longer breathe on their own and wish to have their lives prolonged, they are "vented" or placed on mechanical ventilators. These are machines that breathe for them, forcing air into the lungs. In emergency situations, such as cardiac arrest, mechanical ventilation is common. Persons who are "brain dead" can no longer breathe on their own, and they can be kept physically alive only through mechanical ventilation. Once it has begun, withdrawing mechanical ventilation is usually a difficult decision for family members, as they may feel responsible for the death. Be assured that the dying process that began before mechanical ventilation is now being allowed to take its natural course.

Antibiotics: Antibiotics have become a cornerstone of modern medicine. They are commonly given to treat many different infections.

However, the use of antibiotics should be carefully considered in terminal conditions. For example, pneumonia used to be called "the old person's friend." Today, it can be effectively treated. But if a person is close to death, is the use of antibiotics the best thing to do? For persons nearing the end of life, symptoms of an infection may be effectively managed without the use of antibiotics.

Documenting Your Wishes

Think about the kind of care you would want (or not want) if you were seriously ill, and talk about it with your loved ones and your health care provider.

Even though oral (spoken) instructions regarding your health care are considered legal, it is best to write down your wishes in an advance directive.

In the United States, every state has a law about how advance directives can be completed. These laws also require doctors and health care facilities to honor advance directives.

Advance directive forms often are available from your health care provider or local legal aid society. Advance directive forms are also available on the internet.

State-specific forms may be downloaded from www.partnershipfor caring.org (800-658-8898).

Most advance directives allow you to document your answers to these questions:

1. What kind of care do I want if I can no longer make decisions for myself and I have little or no chance of recovery?

You can specify whether or not you want your life prolonged indefinitely, if you want to be fed through tubes if you can not feed yourself, and if you want treatment for pain. This information can be documented on a "living will," also called a health care directive.

2. Who will make decisions for me if I can't make them for myself?

You can specify someone as your "agent" to make health care decisions for you if you are unable. This type of directive is called a "Power of Attorney for Health Care" in most states. Your agent can be your spouse, an adult child, a friend, or any other trusted person but cannot be an employee of a health care facility where you are receiving care (unless related to you by blood or marriage).

3. Do I want to donate my organs or tissues after my death?

Anyone over the age of 18 can become an organ and tissue donor. Those under 18 years of age need parental consent. Donor cards and additional information may be obtained from www.organdonor.gov or by calling 800-DONORS-1.

Most states allow you to indicate on your driver's license if you are an organ donor. Some states also allow you to indicate your decision in your advance directive. Find out more at www.donatelife.net.

4. Do I want to donate my body to medical science?

Some states allow you to donate your body to medical science. For rules about body donation in your state, visit www.med.ufl.edu/anatbd/usprograms.html

5. Does my advance directive need to be notarized?

Your state may require that your advance directive be witnessed or notarized. The witnesses cannot be the same people listed as your agent(s). One of them cannot be related to you by blood, marriage, or adoption.

Once you have completed your advance directive, give copies to your family members, your doctor, and your clergy person or temple leader. Bring a copy with you if you are hospitalized. Do not leave copies in a safe deposit box where they will be found too late to do any good.

Checklist

- Talk with your spouse, adult children, family, friends, spiritual advisors, and doctors about the type of care that is important to you.

- Ask someone you trust to be your health care agent. Discuss your wishes with this person.

- Complete an advance directive. State-specific advance directive documents and instructions may be downloaded free of charge by visiting www.partnershipforcaring.org. A printed set of documents may be ordered by calling 800-658-8898.

- Finalize your advance directive. You must comply with your state's witness and signature requirements. All states require you to date your advance directive. All states require that your signature be witnessed by at least one adult not related by blood, marriage, or adoption. Some states require two witnesses. Advance directives may also be notarized. Most states give you the right to revoke or change your advance directive at any time, orally or in writing.

- Tell your family, friends, and doctors that you have an advance directive. Keep them informed about your current wishes.

Part Seven

Additional Help
and Information

Chapter 63

Glossary of Terms Related to Movement Disorders

acquired cerebral palsy: A condition that occurs as a result of injury to the brain after birth or during early childhood.

agonist: A drug capable of combining with a receptor and initiating action.

akinesia: Trouble initiating or carrying out movements.

amyotrophic lateral sclerosis (ALS): Sometimes called Lou Gehrig disease, ALS is a rapidly progressive, invariably fatal neurological disease that attacks the nerve cells (neurons) responsible for controlling voluntary muscles.

antagonist: A drug that opposes the effects of another by physiological or chemical action or by a competitive mechanism.

anticholinergic drugs: Drugs that interfere with production or uptake of the neurotransmitter acetylcholine.

apoptosis: Also called programmed cell death. A form of cell death in which a programmed sequence of events leads to the elimination of old, unnecessary, and unhealthy cells.

This glossary contains terms excerpted from publications by the National Institute of Neurological Disorders and Stroke (NINDS, www.ninds.nih.gov), part of the National Institutes of Health, October 27, 2008.

arrhythmia: An abnormal heart rhythm. The heartbeats may be too slow, too rapid, too irregular, or too early.

asphyxia: A lack of oxygen due to trouble with breathing or poor oxygen supply in the air.

ataxia (ataxic): The loss of muscle control.

ataxia-telangiectasia: A rare, childhood neurological disorder that causes degeneration in the part of the brain that controls motor movements and speech.

athetoid: Making slow, sinuous, involuntary, writhing movements, especially with the hands.

atrophy: A decrease in size or wasting away of a body part or tissue.

autonomic dysreflexia: A potentially dangerous complication of spinal cord injury in which blood pressure rises to dangerous levels. If not treated, autonomic dysreflexia can lead to stroke and possibly death.

axial traction: The application of a mechanical force to stretch the spine; used to relieve pressure by separating vertebral surfaces and stretching soft tissues.

axon: The long, thin extension of a nerve cell that conducts impulses away from the cell body.

basal ganglia: A region located at the base of the brain composed of four clusters of neurons, or nerve cells. This area is responsible for body movement and coordination.

benign essential blepharospasm: A progressive neurological disorder characterized by involuntary muscle contractions and spasms of the eyelid muscles.

biopsy: A procedure in which tissue or other material is removed from the body and studied for signs of disease.

bisphosphonates: A family of drugs that strengthen bones and reduce the risk of bone fracture in elderly adults.

botulinum toxin: A drug commonly used to relax spastic muscles; it blocks the release of acetylcholine, a neurotransmitter that energizes muscle tissue.

bradykinesia: A gradual loss of spontaneous movement.

cardiomyopathy: Heart muscle weakness that interferes with the heart's ability to pump blood.

caudate nuclei: Part of the striatum in the basal ganglia.

cerebral dysgenesis: Defective brain development.

cerebral: Relating to the two hemispheres of the human brain.

cervical: The part of the spine in the neck region.

chemodenervation: A treatment that relaxes spastic muscles by interrupting nerve impulse pathways via a drug, such as botulinum toxin, which prevents communication between neurons and muscle tissue.

chorea: Chorea is an abnormal voluntary movement disorder, one of a group of neurological disorders called dyskinesias, which are caused by overactivity of the neurotransmitter dopamine in the areas of the brain that control movement.

choreoathetoid: A condition characterized by aimless muscle movements and involuntary motions.

chromosomes: Genetic structures that contain deoxyribonucleic acid.

coccygeal: The part of the spine at the bottom of the spinal column, above the buttocks.

computed tomography (CT): A technique used for diagnosing brain disorders. CT uses a computer to produce a high-quality image of brain structures.

congenital cerebral palsy: Cerebral palsy that is present at birth from causes that have occurred during fetal development.

contracture: Chronic shortening of a muscle or tendon that limits movement of a bony joint, such as the elbow.

corpus striatum: A part of the brain that helps regulate motor activities.

cortex: Part of the brain responsible for thought, perception, and memory. HD affects the basal ganglia and cortex.

corticobasal degeneration: A progressive neurological disorder characterized by nerve cell loss and atrophy (shrinkage) of multiple areas of the brain including the cerebral cortex and the basal ganglia.

creatine kinase: A protein needed for the chemical reactions that produce energy for muscle contractions; high levels in the blood indicate muscle damage.

cytokine: A small protein released by immune cells that has a specific effect on the interactions between cells, or communications between cells, or on the behavior of cells.

deep brain stimulation: A treatment that uses an electrode implanted into part of the brain to stimulate it in a way that temporarily inactivates some of the signals it produces.

dementia: Loss of intellectual abilities.

dendrite: A short arm-like protuberance from a neuron. Dendrite is from the Greek for "branched like a tree."

deoxyribonucleic acid (DNA): The substance of heredity containing the genetic information necessary for cells to divide and produce proteins. DNA carries the code for every inherited characteristic of an organism.

developmental delay: Behind schedule in reaching the milestones of early childhood development.

disk: Shortened terminology for an intervertebral disk, a disk-shaped piece of specialized tissue that separates the bones of the spinal column.

disuse atrophy: Muscle wasting caused by the inability to flex and exercise muscles.

dopamine: A chemical messenger, deficient in the brains of Parkinson disease patients, that transmits impulses from one nerve cell to another.

dyskinesias: Abnormal involuntary twisting and writhing movements that can result from long-term use of high doses of levodopa.

dysphagia: Difficulty swallowing.

dystonias: Movement disorders in which sustained muscle contractions cause twisting and repetitive movements or abnormal postures.

dystrophin: A protein that helps maintain the shape and structure of muscle fibers.

electroencephalogram: A technique for recording the pattern of electrical currents inside the brain.

electromyography: A special recording technique that detects muscle activity.

embryonic stem cells: Undifferentiated cells from the embryo that have the potential to become a wide variety of specialized cell types.

excitotoxicity: A neurological process that is the result of the release of excessive amounts of the neurotransmitter glutamate.

festination: A symptom characterized by small, quick, forward steps.

focal (partial) seizure: A brief and temporary alteration in movement, sensation, or autonomic nerve function caused by abnormal electrical activity in a localized area of the brain.

Friedreich ataxia: An inherited disease that causes progressive damage to the nervous system resulting in symptoms ranging from muscle weakness and speech problems to heart disease.

functional electrical stimulation: The therapeutic use of low-level electrical current to stimulate muscle movement and restore useful movements such as standing or stepping; also called functional neuromuscular stimulation.

gait analysis: A technique that uses cameras, force plates, electromyography, and computer analysis to objectively measure an individual's pattern of walking.

gastrostomy: A surgical procedure that creates an artificial opening in the stomach for the insertion of a feeding tube.

gene: The basic unit of heredity, composed of a segment of DNA containing the code for a specific trait.

gestation: The period of fetal development from the time of conception until birth.

hemiparesis: Paralysis affecting only one side of the body.

homonymous: Having the same description, name, or term.

Huntington disease: A progressively disabling movement disorder that affects the individual's judgment, memory, and other cognitive functions.

hypertonia: Increased muscle tone.

hypothermia: Abnormally low body temperature.

hypotonia: Decreased muscle tone.

hypoxic-ischemic encephalopathy: Brain damage caused by poor blood flow or insufficient oxygen supply to the brain.

intracranial hemorrhage: Bleeding in the brain.

intrathecal baclofen: Baclofen that is injected into the cerebrospinal fluid of the spinal cord to reduce spasticity.

intubation: The process of putting a tube into a hollow organ or passageway, often into the airway.

kindred: A group of related persons, such as a family or clan.

levodopa: A drug used in the treatment of Parkinson disease.

ligament: A tough band of connective tissue that connects various structures such as two bones.

linkage studies: Tests conducted among family members to determine how a genetic trait is passed on through generations.

lumbar: The part of the spine in the middle back, below the thoracic vertebrae and above the sacral vertebrae.

macrophage: A type of white blood cell that engulfs foreign material. Macrophages are key players in the immune response to foreign invaders such as infectious microorganisms.

magnetic resonance imaging (MRI): An imaging technique that uses radio waves, magnetic fields, and computer analysis to create a picture of body tissues and structures.

merosin: A protein found in the connective tissue that surrounds muscle fibers.

methylprednisolone: A steroid drug used to improve recovery from spinal cord injury.

mitochondria: Microscopic, energy-producing bodies within cells that are the cells' "power plants."

monocyte: A white blood cell that has a single nucleus and can engulf foreign material. Monocytes emigrate from blood into the tissues of the body and evolve into macrophages.

mutation: In genetics, any defect in a gene.

myasthenia gravis: A chronic autoimmune neuromuscular disease characterized by varying degrees of weakness of the skeletal (voluntary) muscles of the body.

myelin: A structure of cell membranes that forms a sheath around axons, insulating them and speeding conduction of nerve impulses.

myelotomy: A surgical procedure that cuts into the spinal cord.

myoclonus: A condition in which muscles or portions of muscles contract involuntarily in a jerky fashion.

myoglobin: An oxygen-binding protein in muscle cells that generates energy by turning glucose into carbon dioxide and water.

myopathy: Any disorder of muscle tissue or muscles.

myotonia: An inability to relax muscles following a sudden contraction.

nerve entrapment: Repeated or prolonged pressure on a nerve root or peripheral nerve.

neural prostheses: Prosthetic devices that can respond to signals from the brain.

neuroacanthocytosis: A rare movement disorder marked by progressive muscle weakness and atrophy, progressive cognitive loss, chorea, and acanthocytosis.

neurogenic pain: Generalized pain that results from nervous system malfunction.

neuromodulation: A series of techniques employing electrical stimulation or the administration of medication by means of devices implanted in the body. These techniques allow the treatment of a range of disorders including certain forms of pain, spasticity, tremor, and urinary problems.

neuron: Also known as a nerve cell; the structural and functional unit of the nervous system. A neuron consists of a cell body and its processes: an axon and one or more dendrites.

neuroprotective: Describes substances that protect nervous system cells from damage or death.

neurostimulation: The act of stimulating neurons with electrical impulses delivered via electrodes attached to the brain.

neurotransmitter: A chemical released from neurons that transmits an impulse to another neuron, muscle, organ, or other tissue.

neurotrophic factors: Proteins responsible for the growth and survival of neurons.

neurotrophins: A family of molecules that encourage survival of nervous system cells.

neutrophil: A type of white blood cell that engulfs, kills, and digests microorganisms.

on-off effect: A change in the patient's condition, with sometimes rapid fluctuations between uncontrolled movements and normal movement, usually occurring after long-term use of levodopa and probably caused by changes in the ability to respond to this drug.

orthostatic hypotension: A sudden drop in blood pressure when a person stands up from a lying-down position. It may cause dizziness, lightheadedness, and, in extreme cases, loss of balance or fainting.

orthotic devices: Special devices, such as splints or braces, used to treat posture problems involving the muscles, ligaments, or bones.

osteopenia: Reduced density and mass of the bones.

overuse syndrome: A condition in which repetitive movements or constrained posture cause nerve and muscle damage, which results in discomfort or persistent pain in muscles, tendons, and other soft tissues.

pallidotomy: A surgical procedure in which a part of the brain called the globus pallidus is lesioned in order to improve symptoms of tremor, rigidity, and bradykinesia.

pallidum: Part of the basal ganglia of the brain. The pallidum is composed of the globus pallidus and the ventral pallidum.

palsy: Paralysis, or the lack of control over voluntary movement.

paralysis: The inability to control movement of a part of the body.

paraplegia: A condition involving complete paralysis of the legs.

parkinsonian gait: A characteristic way of walking that includes a tendency to lean forward; small, quick steps as if hurrying forward (called festination); and reduced swinging of the arms.

parkinsonism: A term referring to a group of conditions that are characterized by four typical symptoms: tremor, rigidity, postural instability, and bradykinesia.

Parkinson-plus syndromes: A group of diseases that includes corticobasal degeneration, progressive supranuclear palsy, and multiple system atrophy. These diseases cause symptoms like those of Parkinson disease in addition to other symptoms.

periodic limb movement disorder: A disorder characterized by repetitive stereotyped movements of the limbs, primarily the legs, during sleep.

positron emission tomography (PET): A tool used to diagnose brain functions and disorders. PET produces three-dimensional, colored images of chemicals or substances functioning within the body.

post-impairment syndrome: A combination of pain, fatigue, and weakness due to muscle abnormalities, bone deformities, overuse syndromes, or arthritis.

postural instability: Impaired balance that causes a tendency to lean forward or backward and to fall easily.

pressure sore: A reddened area or open sore caused by unrelieved pressure on the skin over bony areas such as the hip-bone or tailbone.

prevalence: The number of cases of a disease that are present in a particular population at a given time.

pseudohypertrophy: A condition in which muscles may be enlarged by an accumulation of fat and connective tissue, causing them to look larger and healthier than they actually are.

ptosis: An abnormal drooping of the eyelids.

quadriplegia: Paralysis of both the arms and legs.

receptor: A structure on the surface or interior of a cell that selectively receives and binds to a specific substance.

recessive: A trait that is apparent only when the gene or genes for it are inherited from both parents.

regeneration: Repair, regrowth, or restoration of tissues; opposite of degeneration.

respite care: Rest or relief from caretaking obligations.

restless legs syndrome: A neurological disorder characterized by unpleasant sensations in the legs and an uncontrollable urge to move them for relief.

Rett syndrome: A childhood neurodevelopmental disorder that affects females almost exclusively. Loss of muscle tone is usually the first symptom.

Rh incompatibility: A blood condition in which antibodies in a pregnant woman's blood attack fetal blood cells and impair an unborn baby's supply of oxygen and nutrients.

rhizotomy: An operation to disconnect specific nerve roots in order to stop severe spasticity.

rigidity: A symptom of the disease in which muscles feel stiff and display resistance to movement even when another person tries to move the affected part of the body, such as an arm.

rubella: A viral infection that can damage the nervous system of an unborn baby if a mother contracts the disease during pregnancy.

sacral: Refers to the part of the spine in the hip area.

secondary parkinsonism: Any condition with symptoms that resemble those of Parkinson disease but which result from other causes.

selective dorsal rhizotomy: A surgical procedure in which selected nerves are severed to reduce spasticity in the legs.

selective vulnerability: A term that describes why some neurons are more vulnerable than others to particular diseases or conditions.

spastic (or spasticity): Describes stiff muscles and awkward movements.

spastic diplegia (or diparesis): A form of cerebral palsy in which spasticity affects both legs, but the arms are relatively or completely spared.

spastic hemiplegia (or hemiparesis): A form of cerebral palsy in which spasticity affects an arm and leg on one side of the body.

spastic quadriplegia (or quadriparesis): A form of cerebral palsy in which all four limbs are paralyzed or weakened equally.

spina bifida: A neural tube defect (a disorder involving incomplete development of the brain, spinal cord, and/or their protective coverings) caused by the failure of the fetus's spine to close properly during the first month of pregnancy.

spinal muscular atrophy: A group of hereditary diseases that cause weakness and wasting of the voluntary muscles in the arms and legs of infants and children.

spinal shock: A temporary physiological state that can occur after a spinal cord injury in which all sensory, motor, and sympathetic functions of the nervous system are lost below the level of injury.

stem cell: Special cells that have the ability to grow into any one of the body's more than 200 cell types.

stereognosia: Difficulty perceiving and identifying objects using the sense of touch.

striatum: Part of the basal ganglia of the brain. The striatum is composed of the caudate nucleus, putamen, and ventral striatum.

substantia nigra: Movement-control center in the brain where loss of dopamine-producing nerve cells triggers the symptoms of Parkinson disease; substantia nigra means "black substance," so called because the cells in this area are dark.

synapse: A specialized junction between two nerve cells. At the synapse, a neuron releases neurotransmitters that diffuse across the gap and activate receptors situated on the target cell.

T-cell: An immune system cell that produces substances called cytokines, which stimulate the immune response.

tardive dyskinesia: A neurological syndrome caused by the long-term use of neuroleptic drugs. It is characterized by repetitive, involuntary, purposeless movements.

thalamotomy: A procedure in which a portion of the brain's thalamus is surgically destroyed, usually reducing tremors.

thoracic: The part of the spine at the upper-back to mid-back level.

tonic-clonic seizure: A type of seizure that results in loss of consciousness, generalized convulsions, loss of bladder control, and tongue biting followed by confusion and lethargy when the convulsions end.

Tourette syndrome: A neurological disorder characterized by repetitive, stereotyped, involuntary movements and vocalizations called tics.

trait: Any genetically determined characteristic.

tremor: An involuntary trembling or quivering.

ultrasound: A technique that bounces sound waves off tissue and bone and uses the pattern of echoes to form an image, called a sonogram.

ventricles: Cavities within the brain that are filled with cerebrospinal fluid.

vertebrae: The 33 hollow bones that make up the spine.

wearing-off effect: The tendency, following long-term levodopa treatment, for each dose of the drug to be effective for shorter and shorter periods.

Wilson disease: A rare inherited disorder in which excessive amounts of copper accumulate in the body.

Chapter 64

Directory of Agencies That Provide Information about Movement Disorders

Government Agencies That Provide Information about Movement Disorders

Administration on Aging
Washington, DC 20201
Toll-Free: 800-677-1116
(Eldercare Locator)
Phone: 202-619-0724
Website: www.aoa.gov
E-mail: aoainfo@aoa.hhs.gov

Agency for Healthcare Research and Quality
Office of Communications and Knowledge Transfer
540 Gaither Road, Suite 2000
Rockville, MD 20850
Phone: 301-427-1364
Fax: 301-427-1430
Website: www.ahrq.gov

Centers for Disease Control and Prevention
1600 Clifton Road
Atlanta, GA 30333
Toll-Free: 800-311-3435
Phone: 404-639-3311
Website: www.cdc.gov
E-mail: cdcinfo@cdc.gov

Clearinghouse on Disability Information
Special Education & Rehabilitative Services Communications & Customer Service Team
400 Maryland Ave., SW
Washington, DC 20202-7100
Phone: 202-245-7468
Phone: 202-245-7307
TTD: 202-205-5637
Website: www.ed.gov/about/offices/list/osers/index.html

Resources in this chapter were compiled from several sources deemed reliable; all contact information was verified and updated in October 2008.

571

Healthfinder®
National Health Information
Center
P.O. Box 1133
Washington, DC 20013-1133
Toll-Free: 800-336-4797
Phone: 301-565-4167
Fax: 301-984-4256
Website: www.healthfinder.gov
E-mail: healthfinder@nhic.org

National Cancer Institute
Cancer Information Service
6116 Executive Boulevard
Room 3036A
Bethesda, MD 20892-8322
Toll-Free: 800-4-CANCER
(422-6237)
TTY Toll-Free: 800-332-8615
Website: www.cancer.gov
E mail:
cancergovstaff@mail.nih.gov

National Eye Institute
Information Office
31 Center Drive MSC 2510
Bethesda, MD 20892-2510
Phone: 301-496-5248
Website: www.nei.nih.gov
E-mail: 2020@nei.nih.gov

**National Human Genome
Research Institute**
National Institutes of Health
Building 31, Room 4B09
31 Center Drive, MSC 2152
9000 Rockville Pike
Bethesda, MD 20892-2152
Phone: 301-402-0911
Fax: 301-402-2218
Website: www.genome.gov

**National Institute of Arthritis and Musculoskeletal and
Skin Diseases**
National Institutes of Health
1 AMS Circle
Bethesda, MD 20892-3675
Toll-Free: 877-22-NIAMS
(226-4267)
Phone: 301-495-4484
Fax: 301-718-6366
Website: www.niams.nih.gov
E-mail:
NIAMSinfo@mail.nih.gov

**National Institute of
Child Health and Human
Development**
P.O. Box 3006
Rockville, MD 20847
Toll-Free: 800-370-2943
Phone: 800-370-2943
TTY: 888-320-6942
Fax: 301-984-1473
Website: www.nichd.nih.gov
E-mail: NICHDInformation
ResourceCenter@mail.nih.gov

**National Institute of
Diabetes and Digestive
and Kidney Diseases**
National Institutes of Health,
DHHS
Building 31, Room 9A06
31 Center Drive, MSC 2560
Bethesda, MD 20892-2560
Phone: 301-496-3583
Website: www.niddk.nih.gov

National Institute of Mental Health

National Institutes of Health, DHHS
6001 Executive Blvd. Rm. 8184
MSC 9663
Bethesda, MD 20892-9663
Toll-Free: 866-615-NIMH (6464)
Phone: 301-443-4513
TTY: 301-443-8431 (TTY)
Fax: 301-443-4279
Website: www.nimh.nih.gov
E-mail: nimhinfo@nih.gov

National Institute of Neurological Disorders and Stroke

NIH Neurological Institute
P.O. Box 5801
Bethesda, MD 20824
Toll-Free: 800-352-9424
Phone: 301-496-5751
TTY: 301-468-5981
Website: www.ninds.nih.gov
E-mail: braininfo@ninds.nih.gov

National Institute on Aging

Building 31, Room 5C27
31 Center Drive, MSC 2292
Bethesda, MD 20892
Publications Toll-Free:
800-222-2225
Phone: 301-496-1752
TTY: 800-222-4225
Fax: 301-496-1072
Websites: www.nia.nih.gov
Publications Website:
www.niapublications.org
E-mail: niainfo@nia.nih.gov

National Institute on Deafness and Communication Disorders

31 Center Drive, MSC 2320
Bethesda, MD 20892-2320
Toll-Free: 800-241-1044
TTY: 800-241-1055
Website: www.nidcd.nih.gov
E-mail: nidcdinfo@nidcd.nih.gov

National Institute on Disability and Rehabilitation Research

U.S. Department of Education
Office of Special Education and
Rehabilitative Services
400 Maryland Ave., S.W.
Mailstop PCP-6038
Washington, DC 20202-7100
TTY: 202-245-7316
Website: www.ed.gov/about/
offices/list/osers/nidrr

National Institute on Drug Abuse

6001 Executive Boulevard,
Room 5213
Bethesda, MD 20892-9561
Phone: 301-443-1124
Website: www.nida.nih.gov
E-mail:
information@nida.nih.gov

National Institutes of Health

9000 Rockville Pike
Bethesda, MD 20892
Phone: 301-496-4000
TTY: 301-402-9612
Website: www.nih.gov
E-mail: NIHinfo@od.nih.gov

National Women's Health Information Center
8270 Willow Oaks Corporate Dr.
Fairfax, VA 22031
Toll-Free: 800-994-9662
Website: www.4women.gov

Social Security Administration
Windsor Park Building
6401 Security Boulevard
Baltimore, MD 21235
Toll-Free: 800-772-1213
TTY: 800-325-0778
Website: www.ssa.gov

U.S. Department of Health and Human Services
200 Independent Avenue, SW
Washington, DC 20201
Toll-Free: 877-696-6775
Phone: 202-619-0257
Website: www.hhs.gov

U.S. Food and Drug Administration
5600 Fishers Lane
Rockville, MD 20857-0001
Toll-Free: 888-463-6332
Website: www.fda.gov

U.S. National Library of Medicine
8600 Rockville Pike
Bethesda, MD 20894
Toll-Free: 888-346-3656
Phone: 301-594-5983
TDD: 800-735-2258
Website: www.nlm.nih.gov
E-mail: custserv@nlm.nih.gov

Private Agencies That Provide Information about Movement Disorders

American Academy of Neurology
1080 Montreal Avenue
Saint Paul, MN 55116
Toll-Free: 800-879-1960
Phone: 651-695-2717
Fax: 651-695-2791
Website: www.aan.com

American Academy of Pediatrics
141 Northwest Point Boulevard
Elk Grove Village, IL, 60007
Phone: 847-434-4000
Fax: 847-434-8000
Website: www.aap.org
E-mail: kidsdocs@aap.org

American Association of Neurological Surgeons
5550 Meadowbrook Drive
Rolling Meadows, IL 60008
Toll-Free: 888-566-AANS
(566-2267)
Phone: 847-378-0500
Fax: 847-378-0600
Website: www.aans.org
E-mail: info@aans.org

American Heart Association
National Center
7272 Greenville Avenue
Dallas, TX 75231
Toll-Free: 800-AHA-USA-1
(242-8721)
Website:
www.americanheart.org

American Liver Foundation
75 Maiden Lane, Suite 603
New York, NY 10038-4810
Toll-Free: 800-GO LIVER
(465-4837)
Phone: 212-668-1000
Fax: 212-483-8179
Website: www.liverfoundation
.org
E-mail: info@liverfoundation.org

American Medical Association/Medem
100 Pine Street, 3rd Floor
San Francisco, CA 94111
Toll-Free: 877-926-3336
Phone: 415-644-3800
Fax: 415-644-3950
Website: www.medem.com
E-mail: info@medem.com

American Parkinson Disease Association
135 Parkinson Avenue
Staten Island, NY 10305-1425
Toll-Free: 800-223-2732
Phone: 718-981-8001
Fax: 718-981-4399
Website: www.apdaparkinson
.org
E-mail: apda@apdaparkinson
.org

American Psychological Association
750 First Street, NE
Washington, DC 20002-4242
Toll-Free: 800-374-2721
Phone: 202-336-5500
Website: www.apa.org

Amyotrophic Lateral Sclerosis (ALS) Association
27001 Agoura Road
Suite 250
Calabasas Hills, CA 91301-5104
Toll-Free: 800-782-4747
Phone: 818-880-9007
Fax: 818-880-9006
Website: www.alsa.org
E-mail:
alsinfo@alsa-national.org

ALS Therapy Development Institute
215 First Street
Cambridge, MA 02142
Phone: 617-441-7200
Fax: 617-441-7299
Website: www.als.net
E-mail: info@als.net

A-T (Ataxia-Telangiectasia) Children's Project
668 South Military Trail
Deerfield Beach, FL 33442-3023
Toll-Free: 800-5-HELP-A-T
(543-5728)
Phone: 954-481-6611
Fax: 954-725-1153
Website: www.communityatcp
.org
E-mail: info@atcp.org

575

Bachmann-Strauss
Dystonia and Parkinson
Foundation
Fred French Building
551 Fifth Avenue
Suite 520
New York, NY 10176
Phone: 212-682-9900
Fax: 212-682-6156
Website:
www.dystonia-parkinsons.org
E-mail: Bachmann.Strauss
@mssm.edu

Benign Essential
Blepharospasm Research
Foundation
637 North 7th Street
Suite 102
P.O. Box 12468
Beaumont, TX 77726-2468
Phone: 409-832-0788
Fax: 409-832-0890
Website:
www.blepharospasm.org
E-mail:
bebrf@blepharospasm.org

Children's Hemiplegia and
Stroke Association (CHASA)
4101 West Green Oaks Blvd.
Suite 305
PMB 149
Arlington, TX 76016
Phone: 817-492-4325
Website: www.hemi-kids.org
E-mail: info437@chasa.org

Children's Neurobiological
Solutions (CNS) Foundation
1826 State Street
Santa Barbara, CA 93101
Phone: 866-CNS-5580
(267-5580)
Phone: 805-898-4442
Website: www.cnsfoundation.org
E-mail: info@cnsfoundation.org

Cleveland Clinic
9500 Euclid Avenue
Cleveland, OH 44195
Toll-Free: 800-223-2273
Phone: 216-444-2200
TTY: 216-444-0261
Website: www.clevelandclinic.org

CUREPSP (Society for
Progressive Supranuclear
Palsy)
Executive Plaza III
11350 McCormick Road
Suite 906
Hunt Valley, MD 21031
Toll-Free: 800-457-4777
Phone: 410-785-7004
Fax: 410-785-7009
Website: www.curepsp.org
E-mail: info@curepsp.org

Disabled Sports USA
451 Hungerford Drive
Suite 100
Rockville, MD 20850
Phone: 301-217-0960
Fax: 301-217-0968
Website: www.dsusa.org
E-mail: dsusa@dsusa.org

Dystonia Medical Research Foundation

1 East Wacker Drive, Suite 2810
Chicago, IL 60601-1905
Toll-Free: 800-377-DYST (3978)
Phone: 312-755-0198
Fax: 312-803-0138
Website:
www.dystonia-foundation.org
E-mail: dystonia
@dystonia-foundation.org

Dystonia Society

Camelford House
89 Albert Embankment
London SE1 7TP
United Kingdom
Phone: +44 0845 458 6211
Helpline: +44 0845 458 6322
Website: www.dystonia.org.uk
E-mail: info@dystonia.org.uk

Easter Seals

230 West Monroe Street
Suite 1800
Chicago, IL 60606-4802
Toll-Free: 800-221-6827
Phone: 312-726-6200
TTY: 312-726-4258
Fax: 312-726-1494
Website: www.easterseals.com
E-mail: info@easterseals.com

Facioscapulohumeral Muscular Dystrophy (FSHD) Society

64 Grove Street
Watertown, MA 02472
Phone: 617-658-7878
Fax: 617-658-7879
Website: www.fshsociety.org
E-mail: info@fshsociety.org

Family Caregiver Alliance

180 Montgomery Street
Suite 1100
San Francisco, CA 94104
Toll-Free: 800-445-8106
Phone: 415-434-3388
Website: www.caregiver.org
E-mail: info@caregiver.org

Michael J. Fox Foundation for Parkinson's Research

Church Street Station
P.O. Box 780
New York, NY 10008-0780
Toll-Free: 800-708-7644
Phone: 212-509-0995
Website: www.michaeljfox.org

Friedreich's Ataxia Research Alliance (FARA)

102 Pickering Way
Suite 200
Exton, PA 19341
Phone: 484-875-3015
Fax: 610-363-1506
Website: www.CureFA.org
E-mail: fara@CureFA.org

Hereditary Disease Foundation

3960 Broadway, 6th Floor
New York, NY 10032
Phone: 212-928-2121
Fax: 212-928-2172
Website: www.hdfoundation.org
E-mail: cures@hdfoundation.org

**Huntington's Disease
Society of America**
505 Eighth Avenue, Suite 902
New York, NY 10018
Toll-Free: 800-345-HDSA
(345-4372)
Phone: 212-242-1968
Fax: 212-239-3430
Website: www.hdsa.org
E-mail: hdsainfo@hdsa.org

**International Essential
Tremor Foundation**
P.O. Box 14005
Lenexa, KS 66285-4005
Toll-Free: 888-387-3667
Phone: 913-341-3880
Fax: 913-341-1296
Website: www.essentialtremor.org
E-mail: staff@essentialtremor.org

**International Joseph
Disease Foundation, Inc.**
P.O. Box 994268
Redding, CA 96099-4268
Website: www.ijdf.net
E-mail: MJD@ijdf.net

**International Myotonic
Dystrophy Organization**
P.O. Box 1121
Sunland, CA 91041-1121
Toll-Free: 866-679-7954
Phone: 818-951-2311
Website:
www.myotonicdystrophy.org
E-mail: info@myotonicdystrophy
.org

**International Radiosurgery
Association**
3002 N. 2nd Street
Harrisburg, PA 17110
Phone: 717-260-9808
Website: www.irsa.org

**International Rett
Syndrome Foundation**
4600 Devitt Drive
Cincinnati, OH 45246
Phone: 513-874-3020
Fax: 513-874-2520
Website: www.rettsyndrome.org
E-mail: mgriffin@rettsyndrome
.org

March of Dimes Foundation
1275 Mamaroneck Avenue
White Plains, NY 10605
Toll-Free: 888-MODIMES
(663-4637)
Phone: 914-428-7100
Fax: 914-428-8203
Website:
www.marchofdimes.com
E-mail: askus@marchofdimes
.com

**Muscular Dystrophy
Association**
3300 E. Sunrise Drive
Tucson, AZ 85718
Toll-Free: 800-572-1717
Phone: 520-529-2000
Fax: 520-529-5300
Website: www.mda.org
E-mail: mda@mdausa.org

Muscular Dystrophy Family Foundation
3951 N. Meridian Street
Suite 100
Indianapolis, IN 46208-4062
Toll-Free: 800-544-1213
Phone: 317-923-6333 (MDFF)
Fax: 317-923-6334
Website: www.mdff.org
E-mail: mdff@mdff.org

Myasthenia Gravis Foundation of America
1821 University Avenue W.
Suite S256
St. Paul, MN 55104
Toll-Free: 800-541-5454
Phone: 651-917-6256
Fax: 651-917-1835
Website: www.myasthenia.org
This organization will be moving to 15th Floor 355 Lexington Avenue, New York, NY 10017 in January 2009.

National Alliance on Mental Illness
Colonial Place Three
2107 Wilson Boulevard
Suite 300
Arlington, VA 22201-3042
Toll-Free: 800-950-NAMI (6264)
Phone: 703-524-7600
Fax: 703-524-9094
Website: www.nami.org

National Ataxia Foundation (NAF)
2600 Fernbrook Lane North
Suite 119
Minneapolis, MN 55447-4752
Phone: 763-553-0020
Fax: 763-553-0167
Website: www.ataxia.org
E-mail: naf@ataxia.org

National Dysautonomia Research Foundation
P.O. Box 301
Red Wing, MN 55066-0301
Phone: 651-267-0525
Fax: 651-267-0524
Website: www.ndrf.org
E-mail: ndrf@ndrf.org

National Multiple Sclerosis Society
733 3rd Avenue, 3rd Floor
New York, NY 101107
Toll-Free: 800-344-4867
Website:
www.nationalmssociety.org

National Organization for Rare Disorders (NORD)
P.O. Box 1968
55 Kenosia Avenue
Danbury, CT 06813-1968
Toll-Free: 800-999-NORD
(999-6673)
Phone: 203-744-0100
TDD: 203-797-9590
Fax: 203-798-2291
Website: www.rarediseases.org
E-mail: orphan@rarediseases.org

National Parkinson Foundation

1501 N.W. 9th Avenue
Bob Hope Road
Miami, FL 33136-1494
Toll-Free: 800-327-4545
Phone: 305-243-6666
Fax: 305-243-5595
Website: www.parkinson.org
E-mail: contact@parkinson.org

National Rehabilitation Information Center (NARIC)

8201 Corporate Drive, Suite 600
Landover, MD 20785
Toll-Free: 800-346-2742
Phone: 301-459-5900
TTY: 301-459-5984
Fax: 301-459-4263
Website: www.naric.com
E-mail: naricinfo
@heitechservices.com

National Spasmodic Torticollis Association

9920 Talbert Avenue
Fountain Valley, CA 92708
Toll-Free: 800-HURTFUL
(487-8385)
Phone: 714-378-9837
Website: www.torticollis.org
E-mail: NSTAmail@aol.com

National Spinal Cord Injury Association

1 Church Street, #600
Rockville, MD 20850
Toll-Free: 800-962-9629
Fax: 301-963-1265
Website: www.spinalcord.org
E-mail: info@spinalcord.org

Nemours Foundation Center for Children's Health Media

1600 Rockland Road
Wilmington, DE 19803
Phone: 302-651-4000
Fax: 302-651-4055
Website: www.kidshealth.org
E-mail: info@kidshealth.org

Neurology Now

Website: www.neurologynow.com

Paralyzed Veterans of America (PVA)

801 18th Street, NW
Washington, DC 20006-3517
Toll-Free: 800-424-8200
Health Care Hotline:
800-232-1782
Donor Service Line:
800-555-9140
Phone: 202-USA-1300
(872-1300)
TTY: 800-795-4327
Fax: 202-785-4452
Website: www.pva.org
E-mail: info@pva.org

Parent Project Muscular Dystrophy (PPMD)

158 Linwood Plaza
Suite 220
Fort Lee, NJ 07024
Toll-Free: 800-714-KIDS
(714-5437)
Phone: 201-944-9985
Fax: 201-944-9987
Website: www.parentprojectmd
.org
E-mail: info@parentprojectmd.org

Parkinson Alliance
P.O. Box 308
Kingston, NJ 08528-0308
Toll-Free: 800-579-8440
Fax: 609-688-0875
Website: www.parkinsonalliance
.org
E-mail: admin
@parkinsonalliance.org

Parkinson's Action Network (PAN)
1025 Vermont Ave., NW
Suite 1120
Washington, DC 20005
Toll-Free: 800-850-4726
Phone: 202-638-4101
Fax: 202-638-7257
Website: www.parkinsonsaction
.org
E-mail: info@parkinsonsaction
.org

Parkinson's Disease Foundation (PDF)
1359 Broadway, Suite 1509
New York, NY 10018
Toll-Free: 800-457-6676
Phone: 212-923-4700
Fax: 212-923-4778
Website: www.pdf.org
E-mail: info@pdf.org

Parkinson's Institute
675 Almanor Avenue
Sunnyvale, CA 94085-2935
Toll-Free: 800-655-2273
Phone: 408-734-2800
Fax: 408-734-9208
Website: www.thepi.org
E-mail: info@thepi.org

Parkinson's Resource Organization
74-090 El Paseo Drive, Suite 102
Palm Desert, CA 92260-4135
Toll-Free: 877-775-4111
Phone: 760-773-5628
Fax: 760-773-9803
Website:
www.parkinsonsresource.org
E-mail:
info@parkinsonsresource.org

Pathways Awareness Foundation [For Children With Movement Difficulties]
150 N. Michigan Avenue
Suite 2100
Chicago, IL 60601
Toll-Free: 800-955-CHILD
(955-2445)
Phone: 312-893-6620
Fax: 312-893-6621
Website:
www.pathwaysawareness.org
E-mail:
friends@pathwaysawareness.org

Project ALS
900 Broadway, Suite 901
New York, NY 10003
Toll-Free: 800-603-0270
Phone: 212-420-7382
Fax: 212-420-7387
Website: www.projectals.org
E-mail: info@projectals.org

Christopher and Dana Reeve Foundation
636 Morris Turnpike, Suite 3A
Short Hills, NJ 07078
Toll-Free: 800-225-0292
Phone: 973-379-2690
Fax: 973-912-9433
Website: www.christopherreeve.org
E-mail: info@christopherreeve.org

Rehabilitation Institute of Chicago
345 E. Superior Street, Floor 1
Chicago, IL 60611
Toll-Free: 800-354-REHAB (354-7342)
Phone: 312-238-1000
Website: www.ric.org

Shy-Drager/Multiple System Atrophy Support Group, Inc.
P.O. Box 279
Coupland, TX 78615
Phone: 866-SDS-4999 (737-4999)
Fax: 512-251-3315
Website: www.shy-drager.org

Spasmodic Torticollis Dystonia/ST Dystonia
P.O. Box 28
Mukwonago, WI 53149
Toll-Free: 888-445-4588
Phone: 262-560-9534
Fax: 262-560-9535
Website: www.spasmodictorticollis.org
E-mail: info@spasmodictorticollis.org

Spastic Paraplegia Foundation
7700 Leesburg Pike, Suite 123
Falls Church, VA 22043
Toll-Free: 877-773-4483
Website: www.sp-foundation.org
E-mail: information@sp-foundation.org

Spina Bifida Association of America
4590 MacArthur Blvd. NW, Suite 250
Washington, DC 20007-4266
Toll-Free: 800-621-3141
Phone: 202-944-3285
Fax: 202-944-3295
Website: www.spinabifidaassociation.org
E-mail: sbaa@sbaa.org

Spinal Cord Society
19051 County Highway 1
Fergus Falls, MN 56537
Phone: 218-739-5252
Fax: 218-739-5262
Website: members.aol.com/scsweb

Tremor Action Network
P.O. Box 5013
Pleasanton, CA 94566-5013
Phone: 510-681-6565
Fax: 925-369-0485
Website: www.tremoraction.org
E-mail: info@tremoraction.org

Tourette Syndrome Association
42-40 Bell Boulevard, Suite 205
Bayside, NY 11361-2820
Toll-Free: 888-4-TOURET
(486-8738)
Phone: 718-224-2999
Fax: 718-279-9596
Website: tsa-usa.org
E-mail: ts@tsa-usa.org

Les Turner ALS Foundation
5550 W. Touhy Avenue, Suite 302
Skokie, IL 60077-3254
Toll-Free: 888-ALS-1107
Phone: 847-679-3311
Fax: 847-679-9109
Website: www.lesturnerals.org
E-mail: info@lesturnerals.org

United Cerebral Palsy (UCP)
1660 L Street, NW, Suite 700
Washington, DC 20036
Toll-Free: 800-USA-5UCP
(872-5827)
Phone: 202-776-0406
Fax: 202-776-0414
Website: www.ucp.org
E-mail: national@ucp.org

WE MOVE (Worldwide Education & Awareness for Movement Disorders)
204 West 84th Street
New York, NY 10024
Phone: 212-875-8312
Fax: 212-875-8389
Website: www.wemove.org
E-mail: wemove@wemove.org

Wilson's Disease Association International
1802 Brookside Drive
Wooster, OH 44691
Toll-Free: 888-264-1450
Phone: 330-264-1450
Fax: 330-264-0974
Website: www.wilsonsdisease.org
E-mail: info@wilsonsdisease.org

Index

Index

Page numbers followed by 'n' indicate a footnote. Page numbers in *italics* indicate a table or illustration.

Health Reference Series

COMPLETE CATALOG

List price $87 per volume. **School and library price $78 per volume.**

Adolescent Health Sourcebook, 2nd Edition

Basic Consumer Health Information about the Physical, Mental, and Emotional Growth and Development of Adolescents, Including Medical Care, Nutritional and Physical Activity Requirements, Puberty, Sexual Activity, Acne, Tanning, Body Piercing, Common Physical Illnesses and Disorders, Eating Disorders, Attention Deficit Hyperactivity Disorder, Depression, Bullying, Hazing, and Adolescent Injuries Related to Sports, Driving, and Work

Along with Substance Abuse Information about Nicotine, Alcohol, and Drug Use, a Glossary, and Directory of Additional Resources

Edited by Joyce Brennfleck Shannon. 683 pages. 2006. 978-0-7808-0943-7.

"It is written in clear, nontechnical language aimed at general readers. . . . Recommended for public libraries, community colleges, and other agencies serving health care consumers."
— *American Reference Books Annual, 2003*

"Recommended for school and public libraries. Parents and professionals dealing with teens will appreciate the easy-to-follow format and the clearly written text. This could become a 'must have' for every high school teacher." — *E-Streams, Jan '03*

"A good starting point for information related to common medical, mental, and emotional concerns of adolescents." — *School Library Journal, Nov '02*

"This book provides accurate information in an easy to access format. It addresses topics that parents and caregivers might not be aware of and provides practical, useable information."
— *Doody's Health Sciences Book Review Journal, Sep-Oct '02*

"Recommended reference source."
— *Booklist, American Library Association, Sep '02*

AIDS Sourcebook, 3rd Edition

Basic Consumer Health Information about Acquired Immune Deficiency Syndrome (AIDS) and Human Immunodeficiency Virus (HIV) Infection, Including Facts about Transmission, Prevention, Diagnosis, Treatment, Opportunistic Infections, and Other Complications, with a Section for Women and Children, Including Details about Associated Gynecological Concerns, Pregnancy, and Pediatric Care

Along with Updated Statistical Information, Reports on Current Research Initiatives, a Glossary, and Directories of Internet, Hotline, and Other Resources

Edited by Dawn D. Matthews. 664 pages. 2003. 978-0-7808-0631-3.

"The 3rd edition of the *AIDS Sourcebook*, part of Omnigraphics' *Health Reference Series*, is a welcome update. . . . This resource is highly recommended for academic and public libraries."
— *American Reference Books Annual, 2004*

"Excellent sourcebook. This continues to be a highly recommended book. There is no other book that provides as much information as this book provides."
— *AIDS Book Review Journal, Dec-Jan '00*

"Recommended reference source."
— *Booklist, American Library Association, Dec '99*

Alcoholism Sourcebook, 2nd Edition

Basic Consumer Health Information about Alcohol Use, Abuse, and Dependence, Featuring Facts about the Physical, Mental, and Social Health Effects of Alcohol Addiction, Including Alcoholic Liver Disease, Pancreatic Disease, Cardiovascular Disease, Neurological Disorders, and the Effects of Drinking during Pregnancy

Along with Information about Alcohol Treatment, Medications, and Recovery Programs, in Addition to Tips for Reducing the Prevalence of Underage Drinking, Statistics about Alcohol Use, a Glossary of Related Terms, and Directories of Resources for More Help and Information

Edited by Amy L. Sutton. 653 pages. 2006. 978-0-7808-0942-0.

"This title is one of the few reference works on alcoholism for general readers. For some readers this will be a welcome complement to the many self-help books on the market. Recommended for collections serving general readers and consumer health collections."
— *E-Streams, Mar '01*

"This book is an excellent choice for public and academic libraries."
— *American Reference Books Annual, 2001*

"Recommended reference source."
— *Booklist, American Library Association, Dec '00*

"Presents a wealth of information on alcohol use and abuse and its effects on the body and mind, treatment, and prevention." — *SciTech Book News, Dec '00*

"Important new health guide which packs in the latest consumer information about the problems of alcoholism." — *Reviewer's Bookwatch, Nov '00*

SEE ALSO Drug Abuse Sourcebook

Allergies Sourcebook, 3rd Edition

Basic Consumer Health Information about Allergic Disorders, Such as Anaphylaxis, Hives, Eczema, Rhinitis, Sinusitis, and Conjunctivitis, and Their Triggers, Including Pollen, Mold, Dust Mites, Animal Dander, Insects, Chemicals, Food, Food Additives, and Medications;

Along with Advice about the Diagnosis and Treatment of Allergy Symptoms, a Glossary of Related Terms, a Directory of Resources for Help and Information, and Suggestions for Additional Reading

Edited by Amy L. Sutton. 598 pages. 2007. 978-0-7808-0950-5.

"This book brings a great deal of useful material together.... This is an excellent addition to public and consumer health library collections."
— *American Reference Books Annual, 2003*

"This second edition would be useful to laypersons with little or advanced knowledge of the subject matter. This book would also serve as a resource for nursing and other health care professions students. It would be useful in public, academic, and hospital libraries with consumer health collections." — *E-Streams, Jul '02*

■

Alternative Medicine Sourcebook

SEE Complementary & Alternative Medicine Sourcebook

■

Alzheimer's Disease Sourcebook, 3rd Edition

Basic Consumer Health Information about Alzheimer's Disease, Other Dementias, and Related Disorders, Including Multi-Infarct Dementia, AIDS Dementia Complex, Dementia with Lewy Bodies, Huntington's Disease, Wernicke-Korsakoff Syndrome (Alcohol-Related Dementia), Delirium, and Confusional States

Along with Information for People Newly Diagnosed with Alzheimer's Disease and Caregivers, Reports Detailing Current Research Efforts in Prevention, Diagnosis, and Treatment, Facts about Long-Term Care Issues, and Listings of Sources for Additional Information

Edited by Karen Bellenir. 645 pages. 2003. 978-0-7808-0666-5.

"This very informative and valuable tool will be a great addition to any library serving consumers, students and health care workers."
— *American Reference Books Annual, 2004*

"This is a valuable resource for people affected by dementias such as Alzheimer's. It is easy to navigate and includes important information and resources."
— *Doody's Review Service, Feb '04*

"Recommended reference source."
— *Booklist, American Library Association, Oct '99*

SEE ALSO *Brain Disorders Sourcebook*

Arthritis Sourcebook, 2nd Edition

Basic Consumer Health Information about Osteoarthritis, Rheumatoid Arthritis, Other Rheumatic Disorders, Infectious Forms of Arthritis, and Diseases with Symptoms Linked to Arthritis, Featuring Facts about Diagnosis, Pain Management, and Surgical Therapies

Along with Coping Strategies, Research Updates, a Glossary, and Resources for Additional Help and Information

Edited by Amy L. Sutton. 593 pages. 2004. 978-0-7808-0667-2.

"This easy-to-read volume is recommended for consumer health collections within public or academic libraries." — *E-Streams, May '05*

"As expected, this updated edition continues the excellent reputation of this series in providing sound, usable health information.... Highly recommended."
— *American Reference Books Annual, 2005*

"Excellent reference." — *The Bookwatch, Jan '05*

■

Asthma Sourcebook, 2nd Edition

Basic Consumer Health Information about the Causes, Symptoms, Diagnosis, and Treatment of Asthma in Infants, Children, Teenagers, and Adults, Including Facts about Different Types of Asthma, Common Co-Occurring Conditions, Asthma Management Plans, Triggers, Medications, and Medication Delivery Devices

Along with Asthma Statistics, Research Updates, a Glossary, a Directory of Asthma-Related Resources, and More

Edited by Karen Bellenir. 609 pages. 2006. 978-0-7808-0866-9.

"A worthwhile reference acquisition for public libraries and academic medical libraries whose readers desire a quick introduction to the wide range of asthma information." — *Choice, Association of College & Research Libraries, Jun '01*

"Recommended reference source."
— *Booklist, American Library Association, Feb '01*

"Highly recommended." — *The Bookwatch, Jan '01*

"There is much good information for patients and their families who deal with asthma daily."
— *American Medical Writers Association Journal, Winter '01*

"This informative text is recommended for consumer health collections in public, secondary school, and community college libraries and the libraries of universities with a large undergraduate population."
— *American Reference Books Annual, 2001*

■

Attention Deficit Disorder Sourcebook

Basic Consumer Health Information about Attention Deficit/Hyperactivity Disorder in Children and Adults,

Including Facts about Causes, Symptoms, Diagnostic Criteria, and Treatment Options Such as Medications, Behavior Therapy, Coaching, and Homeopathy

Along with Reports on Current Research Initiatives, Legal Issues, and Government Regulations, and Featuring a Glossary of Related Terms, Internet Resources, and a List of Additional Reading Material

Edited by Dawn D. Matthews. 470 pages. 2002. 978-0-7808-0624-5.

"Recommended reference source."
— Booklist, American Library Association, Jan '03

"This book is recommended for all school libraries and the reference or consumer health sections of public libraries." — American Reference Books Annual, 2003

Back & Neck Sourcebook, 2nd Edition

Basic Consumer Health Information about Spinal Pain, Spinal Cord Injuries, and Related Disorders, Such as Degenerative Disk Disease, Osteoarthritis, Scoliosis, Sciatica, Spina Bifida, and Spinal Stenosis, and Featuring Facts about Maintaining Spinal Health, Self-Care, Pain Management, Rehabilitative Care, Chiropractic Care, Spinal Surgeries, and Complementary Therapies

Along with Suggestions for Preventing Back and Neck Pain, a Glossary of Related Terms, and a Directory of Resources

Edited by Amy L. Sutton. 633 pages. 2004. 978-0-7808-0738-9.

"Recommended . . . an easy to use, comprehensive medical reference book." — E-Streams, Sep '05

"The strength of this work is its basic, easy-to-read format. Recommended." — Reference and User Services Quarterly, American Library Association, Winter '97

Blood & Circulatory Disorders Sourcebook, 2nd Edition

Basic Consumer Health Information about the Blood and Circulatory System and Related Disorders, Such as Anemia and Other Hemoglobin Diseases, Cancer of the Blood and Associated Bone Marrow Disorders, Clotting and Bleeding Problems, and Conditions That Affect the Veins, Blood Vessels, and Arteries, Including Facts about the Donation and Transplantation of Bone Marrow, Stem Cells, and Blood and Tips for Keeping the Blood and Circulatory System Healthy

Along with a Glossary of Related Terms and Resources for Additional Help and Information

Edited by Amy L. Sutton. 659 pages. 2005. 978-0-7808-0746-4.

"Highly recommended pick for basic consumer health reference holdings at all levels."
— The Bookwatch, Aug '05

"Recommended reference source."
— Booklist, American Library Association, Feb '99

"An important reference sourcebook written in simple language for everyday, non-technical users. "
— Reviewer's Bookwatch, Jan '99

Brain Disorders Sourcebook, 2nd Edition

Basic Consumer Health Information about Acquired and Traumatic Brain Injuries, Infections of the Brain, Epilepsy and Seizure Disorders, Cerebral Palsy, and Degenerative Neurological Disorders, Including Amyotrophic Lateral Sclerosis (ALS), Dementias, Multiple Sclerosis, and More

Along with Information on the Brain's Structure and Function, Treatment and Rehabilitation Options, Reports on Current Research Initiatives, a Glossary of Terms Related to Brain Disorders and Injuries, and a Directory of Sources for Further Help and Information

Edited by Sandra J. Judd. 625 pages. 2005. 978-0-7808-0744-0.

"Highly recommended pick for basic consumer health reference holdings at all levels."
— The Bookwatch, Aug '05

"Belongs on the shelves of any library with a consumer health collection." — E-Streams, Mar '00

"Recommended reference source."
— Booklist, American Library Association, Oct '99

SEE ALSO Alzheimer's Disease Sourcebook

Breast Cancer Sourcebook, 2nd Edition

Basic Consumer Health Information about Breast Cancer, Including Facts about Risk Factors, Prevention, Screening and Diagnostic Methods, Treatment Options, Complementary and Alternative Therapies, Post-Treatment Concerns, Clinical Trials, Special Risk Populations, and New Developments in Breast Cancer Research

Along with Breast Cancer Statistics, a Glossary of Related Terms, and a Directory of Resources for Additional Help and Information

Edited by Sandra J. Judd. 595 pages. 2004. 978-0-7808-0668-9.

"This book will be an excellent addition to public, community college, medical, and academic libraries."
— American Reference Books Annual, 2006

"It would be a useful reference book in a library or on loan to women in a support group."
— Cancer Forum, Mar '03

"Recommended reference source."
— Booklist, American Library Association, Jan '02

"This reference source is highly recommended. It is quite informative, comprehensive and detailed in nature, and yet it offers practical advice in easy-to-read language. It could be thought of as the 'bible' of breast cancer for the consumer." — *E-Streams, Jan '02*

"From the pros and cons of different screening methods and results to treatment options, *Breast Cancer Sourcebook* provides the latest information on the subject."
— *Library Bookwatch, Dec '01*

"This thoroughgoing, very readable reference covers all aspects of breast health and cancer. . . . Readers will find much to consider here. Recommended for all public and patient health collections."
— *Library Journal, Sep '01*

SEE ALSO Cancer Sourcebook for Women, Women's Health Concerns Sourcebook

■

Breastfeeding Sourcebook

Basic Consumer Health Information about the Benefits of Breastmilk, Preparing to Breastfeed, Breastfeeding as a Baby Grows, Nutrition, and More, Including Information on Special Situations and Concerns Such as Mastitis, Illness, Medications, Allergies, Multiple Births, Prematurity, Special Needs, and Adoption

Along with a Glossary and Resources for Additional Help and Information

Edited by Jenni Lynn Colson. 388 pages. 2002. 978-0-7808-0332-9.

"Particularly useful is the information about professional lactation services and chapters on breastfeeding when returning to work. . . . *Breastfeeding Sourcebook* will be useful for public libraries, consumer health libraries, and technical schools offering nurse assistant training, especially in areas where Internet access is problematic."
— *American Reference Books Annual, 2003*

SEE ALSO Pregnancy & Birth Sourcebook

■

Burns Sourcebook

Basic Consumer Health Information about Various Types of Burns and Scalds, Including Flame, Heat, Cold, Electrical, Chemical, and Sun Burns

Along with Information on Short-Term and Long-Term Treatments, Tissue Reconstruction, Plastic Surgery, Prevention Suggestions, and First Aid

Edited by Allan R. Cook. 604 pages. 1999. 978-0-7808-0204-9.

"This is an exceptional addition to the series and is highly recommended for all consumer health collections, hospital libraries, and academic medical centers."
— *E-Streams, Mar '00*

"This key reference guide is an invaluable addition to all health care and public libraries in confronting this ongoing health issue."
— *American Reference Books Annual, 2000*

"Recommended reference source."
— *Booklist, American Library Association, Dec '99*

SEE ALSO Dermatological Disorders Sourcebook

Cancer Sourcebook, 5th Edition

Basic Consumer Health Information about Major Forms and Stages of Cancer, Featuring Facts about Head and Neck Cancers, Lung Cancers, Gastrointestinal Cancers, Genitourinary Cancers, Lymphomas, Blood Cell Cancers, Endocrine Cancers, Skin Cancers, Bone Cancers, Metastatic Cancers, and More

Along with Facts about Cancer Treatments, Cancer Risks and Prevention, a Glossary of Related Terms, Statistical Data, and a Directory of Resources for Additional Information

Edited by Karen Bellenir. 1,133 pages. 2007. 978-0-7808-0947-5.

"With cancer being the second leading cause of death for Americans, a prodigious work such as this one, which locates centrally so much cancer-related information, is clearly an asset to this nation's citizens and others."
— *Journal of the National Medical Association, 2004*

"This title is recommended for health sciences and public libraries with consumer health collections."
— *E-Streams, Feb '01*

". . . can be effectively used by cancer patients and their families who are looking for answers in a language they can understand. Public and hospital libraries should have it on their shelves."
— *American Reference Books Annual, 2001*

"Recommended reference source."
— *Booklist, American Library Association, Dec '00*

SEE ALSO Breast Cancer Sourcebook, Cancer Sourcebook for Women, Pediatric Cancer Sourcebook, Prostate Cancer Sourcebook

■

Cancer Sourcebook for Women, 3rd Edition

Basic Consumer Health Information about Leading Causes of Cancer in Women, Featuring Facts about Gynecologic Cancers and Related Concerns, Such as Breast Cancer, Cervical Cancer, Endometrial Cancer, Uterine Sarcoma, Vaginal Cancer, Vulvar Cancer, and Common Non-Cancerous Gynecologic Conditions, in Addition to Facts about Lung Cancer, Colorectal Cancer, and Thyroid Cancer in Women

Along with Information about Cancer Risk Factors, Screening and Prevention, Treatment Options, and Tips on Coping with Life after Cancer Treatment, a Glossary of Cancer Terms, and a Directory of Resources for Additional Help and Information

Edited by Amy L. Sutton. 715 pages. 2006. 978-0-7808-0867-6.

"An excellent addition to collections in public, consumer health, and women's health libraries."
— *American Reference Books Annual, 2003*

"Overall, the information is excellent, and complex topics are clearly explained. As a reference book for the consumer it is a valuable resource to assist them to make informed decisions about cancer and its treatments."
— *Cancer Forum, Nov '02*

"Highly recommended for academic and medical reference collections." — *Library Bookwatch, Sep '02*

"This is a highly recommended book for any public or consumer library, being reader friendly and containing accurate and helpful information." — *E-Streams, Aug '02*

"Recommended reference source." —*Booklist, American Library Association, Jul '02*

SEE ALSO *Breast Cancer Sourcebook, Women's Health Concerns Sourcebook*

Cancer Survivorship Sourcebook

Basic Consumer Health Information about the Physical, Educational, Emotional, Social, and Financial Needs of Cancer Patients from Diagnosis, through Cancer Treatment, and Beyond, Including Facts about Researching Specific Types of Cancer and Learning about Clinical Trials and Treatment Options, and Featuring Tips for Coping with the Side Effects of Cancer Treatments and Adjusting to Life after Cancer Treatment Concludes

Along with Suggestions for Caregivers, Friends, and Family Members of Cancer Patients, a Glossary of Cancer Care Terms, and Directories of Related Resources

Edited by Karen Bellenir. 6561 pages. 2007. 978-0-7808-0985-7.

Cardiovascular Diseases & Disorders Sourcebook, 3rd Edition

Basic Consumer Health Information about Heart and Vascular Diseases and Disorders, Such as Angina, Heart Attacks, Arrhythmias, Cardiomyopathy, Valve Disease, Atherosclerosis, and Aneurysms, with Information about Managing Cardiovascular Risk Factors and Maintaining Heart Health, Medications and Procedures Used to Treat Cardiovascular Disorders, and Concerns of Special Significance to Women

Along with Reports on Current Research Initiatives, a Glossary of Related Medical Terms, and a Directory of Sources for Further Help and Information

Edited by Sandra J. Judd. 713 pages. 2005. 978-0-7808-0739-6.

"This updated sourcebook is still the best first stop for comprehensive introductory information on cardiovascular diseases." — *American Reference Books Annual, 2006*

"Recommended for public libraries and libraries supporting health care professionals." — *E-Streams, Sep '05*

"This should be a standard health library reference." —*The Bookwatch, Jun '05*

"Recommended reference source." —*Booklist, American Library Association, Dec '00*

"... comprehensive format provides an extensive overview on this subject." —*Choice, Association of College & Research Libraries*

Caregiving Sourcebook

Basic Consumer Health Information for Caregivers, Including a Profile of Caregivers, Caregiving Responsibilities and Concerns, Tips for Specific Conditions, Care Environments, and the Effects of Caregiving

Along with Facts about Legal Issues, Financial Information, and Future Planning, a Glossary, and a Listing of Additional Resources

Edited by Joyce Brennfleck Shannon. 600 pages. 2001. 978-0-7808-0331-2.

"Essential for most collections." —*Library Journal, Apr 1, 2002*

"An ideal addition to the reference collection of any public library. Health sciences information professionals may also want to acquire the *Caregiving Sourcebook* for their hospital or academic library for use as a ready reference tool by health care workers interested in aging and caregiving." —*E-Streams, Jan '02*

"Recommended reference source." —*Booklist, American Library Association, Oct '01*

Child Abuse Sourcebook

Basic Consumer Health Information about the Physical, Sexual, and Emotional Abuse of Children, with Additional Facts about Neglect, Munchausen Syndrome by Proxy (MSBP), Shaken Baby Syndrome, and Controversial Issues Related to Child Abuse, Such as Withholding Medical Care, Corporal Punishment, and Child Maltreatment in Youth Sports, and Featuring Facts about Child Protective Services, Foster Care, Adoption, Parenting Challenges, and Other Abuse Prevention Efforts

Along with a Glossary of Related Terms and Resources for Additional Help and Information

Edited by Dawn D. Matthews. 620 pages. 2004. 978-0-7808-0705-1.

"A valuable and highly recommended resource for school, academic and public libraries whether used on its own or as a starting point for more in-depth research." —*E-Streams, Apr '05*

"Every week the news brings cases of child abuse or neglect, so it is useful to have a source that supplies so much helpful information. . . . Recommended. Public and academic libraries, and child welfare offices." —*Choice, Association of College & Research Libraries, Mar '05*

"Packed with insights on all kinds of issues, from foster care and adoption to parenting and abuse prevention." —*The Bookwatch, Nov '04*

SEE ALSO: *Domestic Violence Sourcebook*

Childhood Diseases & Disorders Sourcebook

Basic Consumer Health Information about Medical Problems Often Encountered in Pre-Adolescent Children, Including Respiratory Tract Ailments, Ear Infections, Sore Throats, Disorders of the Skin and Scalp, Digestive and Genitourinary Diseases, Infectious Diseases, Inflammatory Disorders, Chronic Physical and Developmental Disorders, Allergies, and More

Along with Information about Diagnostic Tests, Common Childhood Surgeries, and Frequently Used Medications, with a Glossary of Important Terms and Resource Directory

Edited by Chad T. Kimball. 662 pages. 2003. 978-0-7808-0458-6.

"This is an excellent book for new parents and should be included in all health care and public libraries."
—American Reference Books Annual, 2004

SEE ALSO: Healthy Children Sourcebook

Colds, Flu & Other Common Ailments Sourcebook

Basic Consumer Health Information about Common Ailments and Injuries, Including Colds, Coughs, the Flu, Sinus Problems, Headaches, Fever, Nausea and Vomiting, Menstrual Cramps, Diarrhea, Constipation, Hemorrhoids, Back Pain, Dandruff, Dry and Itchy Skin, Cuts, Scrapes, Sprains, Bruises, and More

Along with Information about Prevention, Self-Care, Choosing a Doctor, Over-the-Counter Medications, Folk Remedies, and Alternative Therapies, and Including a Glossary of Important Terms and a Directory of Resources for Further Help and Information

Edited by Chad T. Kimball. 638 pages. 2001. 978-0-7808-0435-7.

"A good starting point for research on common illnesses. It will be a useful addition to public and consumer health library collections."
—American Reference Books Annual, 2002

"Will prove valuable to any library seeking to maintain a current, comprehensive reference collection of health resources. . . . Excellent reference."
—The Bookwatch, Aug '01

"Recommended reference source."
—Booklist, American Library Association, Jul '01

Communication Disorders Sourcebook

Basic Information about Deafness and Hearing Loss, Speech and Language Disorders, Voice Disorders, Balance and Vestibular Disorders, and Disorders of Smell, Taste, and Touch

Edited by Linda M. Ross. 533 pages. 1996. 978-0-7808-0077-9.

"This is skillfully edited and is a welcome resource for the layperson. It should be found in every public and medical library." —Booklist Health Sciences Supplement, American Library Association, Oct '97

Complementary & Alternative Medicine Sourcebook, 3rd Edition

Basic Consumer Health Information about Complementary and Alternative Medical Therapies, Including Acupuncture, Ayurveda, Traditional Chinese Medicine, Herbal Medicine, Homeopathy, Naturopathy, Biofeedback, Hypnotherapy, Yoga, Art Therapy, Aromatherapy, Clinical Nutrition, Vitamin and Mineral Supplements, Chiropractic, Massage, Reflexology, Crystal Therapy, Therapeutic Touch, and More

Along with Facts about Alternative and Complementary Treatments for Specific Conditions Such as Cancer, Diabetes, Osteoarthritis, Chronic Pain, Menopause, Gastrointestinal Disorders, Headaches, and Mental Illness, a Glossary, and a Resource List for Additional Help and Information

Edited by Sandra J. Judd. 657 pages. 2006. 978-0-7808-0864-5.

"Recommended for public, high school, and academic libraries that have consumer health collections. Hospital libraries that also serve the public will find this to be a useful resource." —E-Streams, Feb '03

"Recommended reference source."
—Booklist, American Library Association, Jan '03

"An important alternate health reference."
—MBR Bookwatch, Oct '02

"A great addition to the reference collection of every type of library." —American Reference Books Annual, 2000

Congenital Disorders Sourcebook, 2nd Edition

Basic Consumer Health Information about Non-hereditary Birth Defects and Disorders Related to Prematurity, Gestational Injuries, Congenital Infections, and Birth Complications, Including Heart Defects, Hydrocephalus, Spina Bifida, Cleft Lip and Palate, Cerebral Palsy, and More

Along with Facts about the Prevention of Birth Defects, Fetal Surgery and Other Treatment Options, Research Initiatives, a Glossary of Related Terms, and Resources for Additional Information and Support

Edited by Sandra J. Judd. 647 pages. 2006. 978-0-7808-0945-1.

"Recommended reference source."
—Booklist, American Library Association, Oct '97

SEE ALSO Pregnancy & Birth Sourcebook

Contagious Diseases Sourcebook

Basic Consumer Health Information about Infectious Diseases Spread by Person-to-Person Contact through

Direct Touch, Airborne Transmission, Sexual Contact, or Contact with Blood or Other Body Fluids, Including Hepatitis, Herpes, Influenza, Lice, Measles, Mumps, Pinworm, Ringworm, Severe Acute Respiratory Syndrome (SARS), Streptococcal Infections, Tuberculosis, and Others

Along with Facts about Disease Transmission, Antimicrobial Resistance, and Vaccines, with a Glossary and Directories of Resources for More Information

Edited by Karen Bellenir. 643 pages. 2004. 978-0-7808-0736-5.

"This easy-to-read volume is recommended for consumer health collections within public or academic libraries." —E-Streams, May '05

"This informative book is highly recommended for public libraries, consumer health collections, and secondary schools and undergraduate libraries."
—American Reference Books Annual, 2005

"Excellent reference." —The Bookwatch, Jan '05

■

Death & Dying Sourcebook, 2nd Edition

Basic Consumer Health Information about End-of-Life Care and Related Perspectives and Ethical Issues, Including End-of-Life Symptoms and Treatments, Pain Management, Quality-of-Life Concerns, the Use of Life Support, Patients' Rights and Privacy Issues, Advance Directives, Physician-Assisted Suicide, Caregiving, Organ and Tissue Donation, Autopsies, Funeral Arrangements, and Grief

Along with Statistical Data, Information about the Leading Causes of Death, a Glossary, and Directories of Support Groups and Other Resources

Edited by Joyce Brennfleck Shannon. 653 pages. 2006. 978-0-7808-0871-3.

"Public libraries, medical libraries, and academic libraries will all find this sourcebook a useful addition to their collections."
—American Reference Books Annual, 2001

"An extremely useful resource for those concerned with death and dying in the United States."
—Respiratory Care, Nov '00

"Recommended reference source."
—Booklist, American Library Association, Aug '00

"This book is a definite must for all those involved in end-of-life care." —Doody's Review Service, 2000

■

Dental Care & Oral Health Sourcebook, 2nd Edition

Basic Consumer Health Information about Dental Care, Including Oral Hygiene, Dental Visits, Pain Management, Cavities, Crowns, Bridges, Dental Implants, and Fillings, and Other Oral Health Concerns, Such as Gum Disease, Bad Breath, Dry Mouth, Genetic and Developmental Abnormalities, Oral Cancers, Orthodontics, and Temporomandibular Disorders

Along with Updates on Current Research in Oral Health, a Glossary, a Directory of Dental and Oral Health Organizations, and Resources for People with Dental and Oral Health Disorders

Edited by Amy L. Sutton. 609 pages. 2003. 978-0-7808-0634-4.

"This book could serve as a turning point in the battle to educate consumers in issues concerning oral health."
—American Reference Books Annual, 2004

"Unique source which will fill a gap in dental sources for patients and the lay public. A valuable reference tool even in a library with thousands of books on dentistry. Comprehensive, clear, inexpensive, and easy to read and use. It fills an enormous gap in the health care literature." —Reference & User Services Quarterly, American Library Association, Summer '98

"Recommended reference source."
—Booklist, American Library Association, Dec '97

■

Depression Sourcebook

Basic Consumer Health Information about Unipolar Depression, Bipolar Disorder, Postpartum Depression, Seasonal Affective Disorder, and Other Types of Depression in Children, Adolescents, Women, Men, the Elderly, and Other Selected Populations

Along with Facts about Causes, Risk Factors, Diagnostic Criteria, Treatment Options, Coping Strategies, Suicide Prevention, a Glossary, and a Directory of Sources for Additional Help and Information

Edited by Karen Bellenir. 602 pages. 2002. 978-0-7808-0611-5.

"Depression Sourcebook is of a very high standard. Its purpose, which is to serve as a reference source to the lay reader, is very well served."
—Journal of the National Medical Association, 2004

"Invaluable reference for public and school library collections alike." —Library Bookwatch, Apr '03

"Recommended for purchase."
—American Reference Books Annual, 2003

■

Dermatological Disorders Sourcebook, 2nd Edition

Basic Consumer Health Information about Conditions and Disorders Affecting the Skin, Hair, and Nails, Such as Acne, Rosacea, Rashes, Dermatitis, Pigmentation Disorders, Birthmarks, Skin Cancer, Skin Injuries, Psoriasis, Scleroderma, and Hair Loss, Including Facts about Medications and Treatments for Dermatological Disorders and Tips for Maintaining Healthy Skin, Hair, and Nails

Along with Information about How Aging Affects the Skin, a Glossary of Related Terms, and a Directory of Resources for Additional Help and Information

Edited by Amy L. Sutton. 645 pages. 2005. 978-0-7808-0795-2.

625

"... comprehensive, easily read reference book."
—Doody's Health Sciences Book Reviews, Oct '97

SEE ALSO *Burns Sourcebook*

■

Diabetes Sourcebook, 3rd Edition

Basic Consumer Health Information about Type 1 Diabetes (Insulin-Dependent or Juvenile-Onset Diabetes), Type 2 Diabetes (Noninsulin-Dependent or Adult-Onset Diabetes), Gestational Diabetes, Impaired Glucose Tolerance (IGT), and Related Complications, Such as Amputation, Eye Disease, Gum Disease, Nerve Damage, and End-Stage Renal Disease, Including Facts about Insulin, Oral Diabetes Medications, Blood Sugar Testing, and the Role of Exercise and Nutrition in the Control of Diabetes

Along with a Glossary and Resources for Further Help and Information

Edited by Dawn D. Matthews. 622 pages. 2003. 978-0-7808-0629-0.

"This edition is even more helpful than earlier versions. . . . It is a truly valuable tool for anyone seeking readable and authoritative information on diabetes."
— American Reference Books Annual, 2004

"An invaluable reference." *— Library Journal, May '00*

Selected as one of the 250 "Best Health Sciences Books of 1999." *— Doody's Rating Service, Mar-Apr '00*

"Provides useful information for the general public."
— Healthlines, University of Michigan Health Management Research Center, Sep/Oct '99

". . . provides reliable mainstream medical information . . . belongs on the shelves of any library with a consumer health collection." *— E-Streams, Sep '99*

"Recommended reference source."
— Booklist, American Library Association, Feb '99

■

Diet & Nutrition Sourcebook, 3rd Edition

Basic Consumer Health Information about Dietary Guidelines and the Food Guidance System, Recommended Daily Nutrient Intakes, Serving Proportions, Weight Control, Vitamins and Supplements, Nutrition Issues for Different Life Stages and Lifestyles, and the Needs of People with Specific Medical Concerns, Including Cancer, Celiac Disease, Diabetes, Eating Disorders, Food Allergies, and Cardiovascular Disease

Along with Facts about Federal Nutrition Support Programs, a Glossary of Nutrition and Dietary Terms, and Directories of Additional Resources for More Information about Nutrition

Edited by Joyce Brennfleck Shannon. 633 pages. 2006. 978-0-7808-0800-3.

"This book is an excellent source of basic diet and nutrition information." *— Booklist Health Sciences Supplement, American Library Association, Dec '00*

"This reference document should be in any public library, but it would be a very good guide for beginning students in the health sciences. If the other books in this publisher's series are as good as this, they should all be in the health sciences collections."
—American Reference Books Annual, 2000

"This book is an excellent general nutrition reference for consumers who desire to take an active role in their health care for prevention. Consumers of all ages who select this book can feel confident they are receiving current and accurate information." *— Journal of Nutrition for the Elderly, Vol. 19, No. 4, 2000*

SEE ALSO *Digestive Diseases & Disorders Sourcebook, Eating Disorders Sourcebook, Gastrointestinal Diseases & Disorders Sourcebook, Vegetarian Sourcebook*

■

Digestive Diseases & Disorders Sourcebook

Basic Consumer Health Information about Diseases and Disorders that Impact the Upper and Lower Digestive System, Including Celiac Disease, Constipation, Crohn's Disease, Cyclic Vomiting Syndrome, Diarrhea, Diverticulosis and Diverticulitis, Gallstones, Heartburn, Hemorrhoids, Hernias, Indigestion (Dyspepsia), Irritable Bowel Syndrome, Lactose Intolerance, Ulcers, and More

Along with Information about Medications and Other Treatments, Tips for Maintaining a Healthy Digestive Tract, a Glossary, and Directory of Digestive Diseases Organizations

Edited by Karen Bellenir. 335 pages. 2000. 978-0-7808-0327-5.

"This title would be an excellent addition to all public or patient-research libraries."
— American Reference Books Annual, 2001

"This title is recommended for public, hospital, and health sciences libraries with consumer health collections." *— E-Streams, Jul-Aug '00*

"Recommended reference source."
— Booklist, American Library Association, May '00

SEE ALSO *Eating Disorders Sourcebook, Gastrointestinal Diseases & Disorders Sourcebook*

■

Disabilities Sourcebook

Basic Consumer Health Information about Physical and Psychiatric Disabilities, Including Descriptions of Major Causes of Disability, Assistive and Adaptive Aids, Workplace Issues, and Accessibility Concerns

Along with Information about the Americans with Disabilities Act, a Glossary, and Resources for Additional Help and Information

Edited by Dawn D. Matthews. 616 pages. 2000. 978-0-7808-0389-3.

"It is a must for libraries with a consumer health section." *— American Reference Books Annual, 2002*

"A much needed addition to the Omnigraphics *Health Reference Series.* A current reference work to provide people with disabilities, their families, caregivers or those who work with them, a broad range of information in one volume, has not been available until now. . . . It is recommended for all public and academic library reference collections." —*E-Streams, May '01*

"An excellent source book in easy-to-read format covering many current topics; highly recommended for all libraries." —*Choice, Association of College & Research Libraries, Jan '01*

"Recommended reference source." —*Booklist, American Library Association, Jul '00*

Domestic Violence Sourcebook, 2nd Edition

Basic Consumer Health Information about the Causes and Consequences of Abusive Relationships, Including Physical Violence, Sexual Assault, Battery, Stalking, and Emotional Abuse, and Facts about the Effects of Violence on Women, Men, Young Adults, and the Elderly, with Reports about Domestic Violence in Selected Populations, and Featuring Facts about Medical Care, Victim Assistance and Protection, Prevention Strategies, Mental Health Services, and Legal Issues

Along with a Glossary of Related Terms and Resources for Additional Help and Information

Edited by Dawn D. Matthews. 628 pages. 2004. 978-0-7808-0669-6.

"Educators, clergy, medical professionals, police, and victims and their families will benefit from this realistic and easy-to-understand resource." —*American Reference Books Annual, 2005*

"Recommended for all collections supporting consumer health information. It should also be considered for any collection needing general, readable information on domestic violence." —*E-Streams, Jan '05*

"This sourcebook complements other books in its field, providing a one-stop resource . . . Recommended." —*Choice, Association of College & Research Libraries, Jan '05*

"Interested lay persons should find the book extremely beneficial. . . . A copy of *Domestic Violence and Child Abuse Sourcebook* should be in every public library in the United States." —*Social Science & Medicine, No. 56, 2003*

"This is important information. The Web has many resources but this sourcebook fills an important societal need. I am not aware of any other resources of this type." —*Doody's Review Service, Sep '01*

"Recommended reference source." —*Booklist, American Library Association, Apr '01*

"Important pick for college-level health reference libraries." —*The Bookwatch, Mar '01*

"Because this problem is so widespread and because this book includes a lot of issues within one volume, this work is recommended for all public libraries." —*American Reference Books Annual, 2001*

SEE ALSO Child Abuse Sourcebook

Drug Abuse Sourcebook, 2nd Edition

Basic Consumer Health Information about Illicit Substances of Abuse and the Misuse of Prescription and Over-the-Counter Medications, Including Depressants, Hallucinogens, Inhalants, Marijuana, Stimulants, and Anabolic Steroids

Along with Facts about Related Health Risks, Treatment Programs, Prevention Programs, a Glossary of Abuse and Addiction Terms, a Glossary of Drug-Related Street Terms, and a Directory of Resources for More Information

Edited by Catherine Ginther. 607 pages. 2004. 978-0-7808-0740-2.

"Commendable for organizing useful, normally scattered government and association-produced data into a logical sequence." —*American Reference Books Annual, 2006*

"This easy-to-read volume is recommended for consumer health collections within public or academic libraries." —*E-Streams, Sep '05*

"An excellent library reference." —*The Bookwatch, May '05*

"Containing a wealth of information, this book will be useful to the college student just beginning to explore the topic of substance abuse. This resource belongs in libraries that serve a lower-division undergraduate or community college clientele as well as the general public." —*Choice, Association of College & Research Libraries, Jun '01*

"Recommended reference source." —*Booklist, American Library Association, Feb '01*

SEE ALSO Alcoholism Sourcebook

Ear, Nose & Throat Disorders Sourcebook, 2nd Edition

Basic Consumer Health Information about Disorders of the Ears, Hearing Loss, Vestibular Disorders, Nasal and Sinus Problems, Throat and Vocal Cord Disorders, and Otolaryngologic Cancers, Including Facts about Ear Infections and Injuries, Genetic and Congenital Deafness, Sensorineural Hearing Disorders, Tinnitus, Vertigo, Ménière Disease, Rhinitis, Sinusitis, Snoring, Sore Throats, Hoarseness, and More

Along with Reports on Current Research Initiatives, a Glossary of Related Medical Terms, and a Directory of Sources for Further Help and Information

Edited by Sandra J. Judd. 659 pages. 2006. 978-0-7808-0872-0.

"Overall, this sourcebook is helpful for the consumer seeking information on ENT issues. It is recommended for public libraries."
— *American Reference Books Annual, 1999*

"Recommended reference source."
— *Booklist, American Library Association, Dec '98*

Eating Disorders Sourcebook, 2nd Edition

Basic Consumer Health Information about Anorexia Nervosa, Bulimia Nervosa, Binge Eating, Compulsive Exercise, Female Athlete Triad, and Other Eating Disorders, Including Facts about Body Image and Other Cultural and Age-Related Risk Factors, Prevention Efforts, Adverse Health Effects, Treatment Options, and the Recovery Process

Along with Guidelines for Healthy Weight Control, a Glossary, and Directories of Additional Resources

Edited by Joyce Brennfleck Shannon. 585 pages. 2007. 978-0-7808-0948-2.

"Recommended for health science libraries that are open to the public, as well as hospital libraries. This book is a good resource for the consumer who is concerned about eating disorders." — *E-Streams, Mar '02*

"This volume is another convenient collection of excerpted articles. Recommended for school and public library patrons; lower-division undergraduates; and two-year technical program students."
— *Choice, Association of College & Research Libraries, Jan '02*

"Recommended reference source."
— *Booklist, American Library Association, Oct '01*

SEE ALSO Diet & Nutrition Sourcebook, Digestive Diseases & Disorders Sourcebook, Gastrointestinal Diseases & Disorders Sourcebook

Emergency Medical Services Sourcebook

Basic Consumer Health Information about Preventing, Preparing for, and Managing Emergency Situations, When and Who to Call for Help, What to Expect in the Emergency Room, the Emergency Medical Team, Patient Issues, and Current Topics in Emergency Medicine

Along with Statistical Data, a Glossary, and Sources of Additional Help and Information

Edited by Jenni Lynn Colson. 494 pages. 2002. 978-0-7808-0420-3.

"Handy and convenient for home, public, school, and college libraries. Recommended."
— *Choice, Association of College & Research Libraries, Apr '03*

"This reference can provide the consumer with answers to most questions about emergency care in the United States, or it will direct them to a resource where the answer can be found."
— *American Reference Books Annual, 2003*

"Recommended reference source."
— *Booklist, American Library Association, Feb '03*

Endocrine & Metabolic Disorders Sourcebook

Basic Information for the Layperson about Pancreatic and Insulin-Related Disorders Such as Pancreatitis, Diabetes, and Hypoglycemia; Adrenal Gland Disorders Such as Cushing's Syndrome, Addison's Disease, and Congenital Adrenal Hyperplasia; Pituitary Gland Disorders Such as Growth Hormone Deficiency, Acromegaly, and Pituitary Tumors; Thyroid Disorders Such as Hypothyroidism, Graves' Disease, Hashimoto's Disease, and Goiter; Hyperparathyroidism; and Other Diseases and Syndromes of Hormone Imbalance or Metabolic Dysfunction

Along with Reports on Current Research Initiatives

Edited by Linda M. Shin. 574 pages. 1998. 978-0-7808-0207-0.

"Omnigraphics has produced another needed resource for health information consumers."
— *American Reference Books Annual, 2000*

"Recommended reference source."
— *Booklist, American Library Association, Dec '98*

Environmental Health Sourcebook, 2nd Edition

Basic Consumer Health Information about the Environment and Its Effect on Human Health, Including the Effects of Air Pollution, Water Pollution, Hazardous Chemicals, Food Hazards, Radiation Hazards, Biological Agents, Household Hazards, Such as Radon, Asbestos, Carbon Monoxide, and Mold, and Information about Associated Diseases and Disorders, Including Cancer, Allergies, Respiratory Problems, and Skin Disorders

Along with Information about Environmental Concerns for Specific Populations, a Glossary of Related Terms, and Resources for Further Help and Information

Edited by Dawn D. Matthews. 673 pages. 2003. 978-0-7808-0632-0.

"This recently updated edition continues the level of quality and the reputation of the numerous other volumes in Omnigraphics' *Health Reference Series.*"
— *American Reference Books Annual, 2004*

"An excellent updated edition."
— *The Bookwatch, Oct '03*

"Recommended reference source."
— *Booklist, American Library Association, Sep '98*

"This book will be a useful addition to anyone's library." — *Choice Health Sciences Supplement, Association of College & Research Libraries, May '98*

". . . a good survey of numerous environmentally induced physical disorders . . . a useful addition to anyone's library."
— *Doody's Health Sciences Book Reviews, Jan '98*

Ethnic Diseases Sourcebook

Basic Consumer Health Information for Ethnic and Racial Minority Groups in the United States, Including General Health Indicators and Behaviors, Ethnic Diseases, Genetic Testing, the Impact of Chronic Diseases, Women's Health, Mental Health Issues, and Preventive Health Care Services

Along with a Glossary and a Listing of Additional Resources

Edited by Joyce Brennfleck Shannon. 664 pages. 2001. 978-0-7808-0336-7.

"Recommended for health sciences libraries where public health programs are a priority."
— *E-Streams, Jan '02*

"Not many books have been written on this topic to date, and the *Ethnic Diseases Sourcebook* is a strong addition to the list. It will be an important introductory resource for health consumers, students, health care personnel, and social scientists. It is recommended for public, academic, and large hospital libraries."
— *American Reference Books Annual, 2002*

"Recommended reference source."
— *Booklist, American Library Association, Oct '01*

"Will prove valuable to any library seeking to maintain a current, comprehensive reference collection of health resources. . . . An excellent source of health information about genetic disorders which affect particular ethnic and racial minorities in the U.S."
— *The Bookwatch, Aug '01*

■

Eye Care Sourcebook, 2nd Edition

Basic Consumer Health Information about Eye Care and Eye Disorders, Including Facts about the Diagnosis, Prevention, and Treatment of Common Refractive Problems Such as Myopia, Hyperopia, Astigmatism, and Presbyopia, and Eye Diseases, Including Glaucoma, Cataract, Age-Related Macular Degeneration, and Diabetic Retinopathy

Along with a Section on Vision Correction and Refractive Surgeries, Including LASIK and LASEK, a Glossary, and Directories of Resources for Additional Help and Information

Edited by Amy L. Sutton. 543 pages. 2003. 978-0-7808-0635-1.

". . . a solid reference tool for eye care and a valuable addition to a collection."
— *American Reference Books Annual, 2004*

■

Family Planning Sourcebook

Basic Consumer Health Information about Planning for Pregnancy and Contraception, Including Traditional Methods, Barrier Methods, Hormonal Methods, Permanent Methods, Future Methods, Emergency Contraception, and Birth Control Choices for Women at Each Stage of Life

Along with Statistics, a Glossary, and Sources of Additional Information

Edited by Amy Marcaccio Keyzer. 520 pages. 2001. 978-0-7808-0379-4.

"Recommended for public, health, and undergraduate libraries as part of the circulating collection."
— *E-Streams, Mar '02*

"Information is presented in an unbiased, readable manner, and the sourcebook will certainly be a necessary addition to those public and high school libraries where Internet access is restricted or otherwise problematic." — *American Reference Books Annual, 2002*

"Recommended reference source."
— *Booklist, American Library Association, Oct '01*

"Will prove valuable to any library seeking to maintain a current, comprehensive reference collection of health resources. . . . Excellent reference."
— *The Bookwatch, Aug '01*

SEE ALSO Pregnancy & Birth Sourcebook

■

Fitness & Exercise Sourcebook, 3rd Edition

Basic Consumer Health Information about the Physical and Mental Benefits of Fitness, Including Cardiorespiratory Endurance, Muscular Strength, Muscular Endurance, and Flexibility, with Facts about Sports Nutrition and Exercise-Related Injuries and Tips about Physical Activity and Exercises for People of All Ages and for People with Health Concerns

Along with Advice on Selecting and Using Exercise Equipment, Maintaining Exercise Motivation, a Glossary of Related Terms, and a Directory of Resources for More Help and Information

Edited by Amy L. Sutton. 663 pages. 2007. 978-0-7808-0946-8.

"This work is recommended for all general reference collections."
— *American Reference Books Annual, 2002*

"Highly recommended for public, consumer, and school grades fourth through college." — *E-Streams, Nov '01*

"Recommended reference source."
— *Booklist, American Library Association, Oct '01*

"The information appears quite comprehensive and is considered reliable. . . . This second edition is a welcomed addition to the series."
— *Doody's Review Service, Sep '01*

■

Food Safety Sourcebook

Basic Consumer Health Information about the Safe Handling of Meat, Poultry, Seafood, Eggs, Fruit Juices, and Other Food Items, and Facts about Pesticides, Drinking Water, Food Safety Overseas, and the Onset, Duration, and Symptoms of Foodborne Illnesses, Including Types of Pathogenic Bacteria, Parasitic Protozoa, Worms, Viruses, and Natural Toxins

Along with the Role of the Consumer, the Food Handler, and the Government in Food Safety; a Glossary, and Resources for Additional Help and Information

Edited by Dawn D. Matthews. 339 pages. 1999. 978-0-7808-0326-8.

"This book is recommended for public libraries and universities with home economic and food science programs." — E-Streams, Nov '00

"Recommended reference source." — Booklist, American Library Association, May '00

"This book takes the complex issues of food safety and foodborne pathogens and presents them in an easily understood manner. [It does] an excellent job of covering a large and often confusing topic." — American Reference Books Annual, 2000

■

Forensic Medicine Sourcebook

Basic Consumer Information for the Layperson about Forensic Medicine, Including Crime Scene Investigation, Evidence Collection and Analysis, Expert Testimony, Computer-Aided Criminal Identification, Digital Imaging in the Courtroom, DNA Profiling, Accident Reconstruction, Autopsies, Ballistics, Drugs and Explosives Detection, Latent Fingerprints, Product Tampering, and Questioned Document Examination

Along with Statistical Data, a Glossary of Forensics Terminology, and Listings of Sources for Further Help and Information

Edited by Annemarie S. Muth. 574 pages. 1999. 978-0-7808-0232-2.

"Given the expected widespread interest in its content and its easy to read style, this book is recommended for most public and all college and university libraries." — E-Streams, Feb '01

"Recommended for public libraries." — Reference & User Services Quarterly, American Library Association, Spring 2000

"Recommended reference source." — Booklist, American Library Association, Feb '00

"A wealth of information, useful statistics, references are up-to-date and extremely complete. This wonderful collection of data will help students who are interested in a career in any type of forensic field. It is a great resource for attorneys who need information about types of expert witnesses needed in a particular case. It also offers useful information for fiction and nonfiction writers whose work involves a crime. A fascinating compilation. All levels." — Choice, Association of College & Research Libraries, Jan '00

"There are several items that make this book attractive to consumers who are seeking certain forensic data.... This is a useful current source for those seeking general forensic medical answers." — American Reference Books Annual, 2000

Gastrointestinal Diseases & Disorders Sourcebook, 2nd Edition

Basic Consumer Health Information about the Upper and Lower Gastrointestinal (GI) Tract, Including the Esophagus, Stomach, Intestines, Rectum, Liver, and Pancreas, with Facts about Gastroesophageal Reflux Disease, Gastritis, Hernias, Ulcers, Celiac Disease, Diverticulitis, Irritable Bowel Syndrome, Hemorrhoids, Gastrointestinal Cancers, and Other Diseases and Disorders Related to the Digestive Process

Along with Information about Commonly Used Diagnostic and Surgical Procedures, Statistics, Reports on Current Research Initiatives and Clinical Trials, a Glossary, and Resources for Additional Help and Information

Edited by Sandra J. Judd. 681 pages. 2006. 978-0-7808-0798-3.

"... very readable form. The successful editorial work that brought this material together into a useful and understandable reference makes accessible to all readers information that can help them more effectively understand and obtain help for digestive tract problems." — Choice, Association of College & Research Libraries, Feb '97

SEE ALSO Diet & Nutrition Sourcebook, Digestive Diseases & Disorders Sourcebook, Eating Disorders Sourcebook

■

Genetic Disorders Sourcebook, 3rd Edition

Basic Consumer Health Information about Hereditary Diseases and Disorders, Including Facts about the Human Genome, Genetic Inheritance Patterns, Disorders Associated with Specific Genes, Such as Sickle Cell Disease, Hemophilia, and Cystic Fibrosis, Chromosome Disorders, Such as Down Syndrome, Fragile X Syndrome, and Turner Syndrome, and Complex Diseases and Disorders Resulting from the Interaction of Environmental and Genetic Factors, Such as Allergies, Cancer, and Obesity

Along with Facts about Genetic Testing, Suggestions for Parents of Children with Special Needs, Reports on Current Research Initiatives, a Glossary of Genetic Terminology, and Resources for Additional Help and Information

Edited by Karen Bellenir. 777 pages. 2004. 978-0-7808-0742-6.

"This text is recommended for any library with an interest in providing consumer health resources." — E-Streams, Aug '05

"This is a valuable resource for anyone wishing to have an understandable description of any of the topics or disorders included. The editor succeeds in making complex genetic issues understandable." — Doody's Book Review Service, May '05

"A good acquisition for public libraries." — American Reference Books Annual, 2005

630

■

Head Trauma Sourcebook

Basic Information for the Layperson about Open-Head and Closed-Head Injuries, Treatment Advances, Recovery, and Rehabilitation

Along with Reports on Current Research Initiatives

Edited by Karen Bellenir. 414 pages. 1997. 978-0-7808-0208-7.

Headache Sourcebook

Basic Consumer Health Information about Migraine, Tension, Cluster, Rebound and Other Types of Headaches, with Facts about the Cause and Prevention of Headaches, the Effects of Stress and the Environment, Headaches during Pregnancy and Menopause, and Childhood Headaches

Along with a Glossary and Other Resources for Additional Help and Information

Edited by Dawn D. Matthews. 362 pages. 2002. 978-0-7808-0337-4.

■

Healthy Aging Sourcebook

Basic Consumer Health Information about Maintaining Health through the Aging Process, Including Advice on Nutrition, Exercise, and Sleep, Help in Making Decisions about Midlife Issues and Retirement, and Guidance Concerning Practical and Informed Choices in Health Consumerism

Along with Data Concerning the Theories of Aging, Different Experiences in Aging by Minority Groups, and Facts about Aging Now and Aging in the Future; and Featuring a Glossary, a Guide to Consumer Help, Additional Suggested Reading, and Practical Resource Directory

Edited by Jenifer Swanson. 536 pages. 1999. 978-0-7808-0390-9.

SEE ALSO *Physical & Mental Issues in Aging Sourcebook*

■

Healthy Children Sourcebook

Basic Consumer Health Information about the Physical and Mental Development of Children between the Ages of 3 and 12, Including Routine Health Care, Preventative Health Services, Safety and First Aid,

Healthy Sleep, Dental Care, Nutrition, and Fitness, and Featuring Parenting Tips on Such Topics as Bedwetting, Choosing Day Care, Monitoring TV and Other Media, and Establishing a Foundation for Substance Abuse Prevention

Along with a Glossary of Commonly Used Pediatric Terms and Resources for Additional Help and Information.

Edited by Chad T. Kimball. 647 pages. 2003. 978-0-7808-0247-6.

SEE ALSO *Childhood Diseases & Disorders Sourcebook*

■

Healthy Heart Sourcebook for Women

Basic Consumer Health Information about Cardiac Issues Specific to Women, Including Facts about Major Risk Factors and Prevention, Treatment and Control Strategies, and Important Dietary Issues

Along with a Special Section Regarding the Pros and Cons of Hormone Replacement Therapy and Its Impact on Heart Health, and Additional Help, Including Recipes, a Glossary, and a Directory of Resources

Edited by Dawn D. Matthews. 336 pages. 2000. 978-0-7808-0329-9.

SEE ALSO *Cardiovascular Diseases & Disorders Sourcebook, Women's Health Concerns Sourcebook*

■

Hepatitis Sourcebook

Basic Consumer Health Information about Hepatitis A, Hepatitis B, Hepatitis C, and Other Forms of Hepatitis, Including Autoimmune Hepatitis, Alcoholic Hepatitis, Nonalcoholic Steatohepatitis, and Toxic Hepatitis, with

Facts about Risk Factors, Screening Methods, Diagnostic Tests, and Treatment Options

Along with Information on Liver Health, Tips for People Living with Chronic Hepatitis, Reports on Current Research Initiatives, a Glossary of Terms Related to Hepatitis, and a Directory of Sources for Further Help and Information

Edited by Sandra J. Judd. 597 pages. 2005. 978-0-7808-0749-5.

"Highly recommended."
— American Reference Books Annual, 2006

Household Safety Sourcebook

Basic Consumer Health Information about Household Safety, Including Information about Poisons, Chemicals, Fire, and Water Hazards in the Home

Along with Advice about the Safe Use of Home Maintenance Equipment, Choosing Toys and Nursery Furniture, Holiday and Recreation Safety, a Glossary, and Resources for Further Help and Information

Edited by Dawn D. Matthews. 606 pages. 2002. 978-0-7808-0338-1.

"This work will be useful in public libraries with large consumer health and wellness departments."
— American Reference Books Annual, 2003

"As a sourcebook on household safety this book meets its mark. It is encyclopedic in scope and covers a wide range of safety issues that are commonly seen in the home." — E-Streams, Jul '02

Hypertension Sourcebook

Basic Consumer Health Information about the Causes, Diagnosis, and Treatment of High Blood Pressure, with Facts about Consequences, Complications, and Co-Occurring Disorders, Such as Coronary Heart Disease, Diabetes, Stroke, Kidney Disease, and Hypertensive Retinopathy, and Issues in Blood Pressure Control, Including Dietary Choices, Stress Management, and Medications

Along with Reports on Current Research Initiatives and Clinical Trials, a Glossary, and Resources for Additional Help and Information

Edited by Dawn D. Matthews and Karen Bellenir. 613 pages. 2004. 978-0-7808-0674-0.

"Academic, public, and medical libraries will want to add the *Hypertension Sourcebook* to their collections."
— E-Streams, Aug '05

"The strength of this source is the wide range of information given about hypertension."
— American Reference Books Annual, 2005

Immune System Disorders Sourcebook, 2nd Edition

Basic Consumer Health Information about Disorders of the Immune System, Including Immune System Function and Response, Diagnosis of Immune Disorders, Information about Inherited Immune Disease, Acquired Immune Disease, and Autoimmune Diseases, Including Primary Immune Deficiency, Acquired Immunodeficiency Syndrome (AIDS), Lupus, Multiple Sclerosis, Type 1 Diabetes, Rheumatoid Arthritis, and Graves' Disease

Along with Treatments, Tips for Coping with Immune Disorders, a Glossary, and a Directory of Additional Resources.

Edited by Joyce Brennfleck Shannon. 671 pages. 2005. 978-0-7808-0748-8.

"Highly recommended for academic and public libraries." — American Reference Books Annual, 2006

"The updated second edition is a 'must' for any consumer health library seeking a solid resource covering the treatments, symptoms, and options for immune disorder sufferers. . . . An excellent guide."
— MBR Bookwatch, Jan '06

Infant & Toddler Health Sourcebook

Basic Consumer Health Information about the Physical and Mental Development of Newborns, Infants, and Toddlers, Including Neonatal Concerns, Nutrition Recommendations, Immunization Schedules, Common Pediatric Disorders, Assessments and Milestones, Safety Tips, and Advice for Parents and Other Caregivers

Along with a Glossary of Terms and Resource Listings for Additional Help

Edited by Jenifer Swanson. 585 pages. 2000. 978-0-7808-0246-9.

"As a reference for the general public, this would be useful in any library." — E-Streams, May '01

"Recommended reference source."
— Booklist, American Library Association, Feb '01

"This is a good source for general use."
— American Reference Books Annual, 2001

Infectious Diseases Sourcebook

Basic Consumer Health Information about Non-Contagious Bacterial, Viral, Prion, Fungal, and Parasitic Diseases Spread by Food and Water, Insects and Animals, or Environmental Contact, Including Botulism, E. Coli, Encephalitis, Legionnaires' Disease, Lyme Disease, Malaria, Plague, Rabies, Salmonella, Tetanus, and Others, and Facts about Newly Emerging Diseases, Such as Hantavirus, Mad Cow Disease, Monkeypox, and West Nile Virus

Along with Information about Preventing Disease Transmission, the Threat of Bioterrorism, and Current Research Initiatives, with a Glossary and Directory of Resources for More Information

Edited by Karen Bellenir. 634 pages. 2004. 978-0-7808-0675-7.

"This reference continues the excellent tradition of the *Health Reference Series* in consolidating a wealth of information on a selected topic into a format that is easy to use and accessible to the general public."
— *American Reference Books Annual, 2005*

"Recommended for public and academic libraries."
— *E-Streams, Jan '05*

■

Injury & Trauma Sourcebook

Basic Consumer Health Information about the Impact of Injury, the Diagnosis and Treatment of Common and Traumatic Injuries, Emergency Care, and Specific Injuries Related to Home, Community, Workplace, Transportation, and Recreation

Along with Guidelines for Injury Prevention, a Glossary, and a Directory of Additional Resources

Edited by Joyce Brennfleck Shannon. 696 pages. 2002. 978-0-7808-0421-0.

"This publication is the most comprehensive work of its kind about injury and trauma."
— *American Reference Books Annual, 2003*

"This sourcebook provides concise, easily readable, basic health information about injuries. . . . This book is well organized and an easy to use reference resource suitable for hospital, health sciences and public libraries with consumer health collections."
— *E-Streams, Nov '02*

"Practitioners should be aware of guides such as this in order to facilitate their use by patients and their families."
— *Doody's Health Sciences Book Review Journal, Sep-Oct '02*

"Recommended reference source."
— *Booklist, American Library Association, Sep '02*

"Highly recommended for academic and medical reference collections."
— *Library Bookwatch, Sep '02*

■

Kidney & Urinary Tract Diseases & Disorders Sourcebook

SEE Urinary Tract & Kidney Diseases & Disorders Sourcebook

■

Learning Disabilities Sourcebook, 2nd Edition

Basic Consumer Health Information about Learning Disabilities, Including Dyslexia, Developmental Speech and Language Disabilities, Non-Verbal Learning Disorders, Developmental Arithmetic Disorder, Developmental Writing Disorder, and Other Conditions That Impede Learning Such as Attention Deficit/Hyperactivity Disorder, Brain Injury, Hearing Impairment, Klinefelter Syndrome, Dyspraxia, and Tourette's Syndrome

Along with Facts about Educational Issues and Assistive Technology, Coping Strategies, a Glossary of Re-

lated Terms, and Resources for Further Help and Information

Edited by Dawn D. Matthews. 621 pages. 2003. 978-0-7808-0626-9.

"The second edition of Learning Disabilities Sourcebook far surpasses the earlier edition in that it is more focused on information that will be useful as a consumer health resource."
— *American Reference Books Annual, 2004*

"Teachers as well as consumers will find this an essential guide to understanding various syndromes and their latest treatments. [An] invaluable reference for public and school library collections alike."
— *Library Bookwatch, Apr '03*

Named "Outstanding Reference Book of 1999."
— *New York Public Library, Feb '00*

"An excellent candidate for inclusion in a public library reference section. It's a great source of information. Teachers will also find the book useful. Definitely worth reading."
— *Journal of Adolescent & Adult Literacy, Feb 2000*

"Readable . . . provides a solid base of information regarding successful techniques used with individuals who have learning disabilities, as well as practical suggestions for educators and family members. Clear language, concise descriptions, and pertinent information for contacting multiple resources add to the strength of this book as a useful tool."
— *Choice, Association of College & Research Libraries, Feb '99*

"Recommended reference source."
— *Booklist, American Library Association, Sep '98*

"A useful resource for libraries and for those who don't have the time to identify and locate the individual publications."
— *Disability Resources Monthly, Sep '98*

■

Leukemia Sourcebook

Basic Consumer Health Information about Adult and Childhood Leukemias, Including Acute Lymphocytic Leukemia (ALL), Chronic Lymphocytic Leukemia (CLL), Acute Myelogenous Leukemia (AML), Chronic Myelogenous Leukemia (CML), and Hairy Cell Leukemia, and Treatments Such as Chemotherapy, Radiation Therapy, Peripheral Blood Stem Cell and Marrow Transplantation, and Immunotherapy

Along with Tips for Life During and After Treatment, a Glossary, and Directories of Additional Resources

Edited by Joyce Brennfleck Shannon. 587 pages. 2003. 978-0-7808-0627-6.

"Unlike other medical books for the layperson, . . . the language does not talk down to the reader. . . . This volume is highly recommended for all libraries."
— *American Reference Books Annual, 2004*

". . . a fine title which ranges from diagnosis to alternative treatments, staging, and tips for life during and after diagnosis."
— *The Bookwatch, Dec '03*

Liver Disorders Sourcebook

Basic Consumer Health Information about the Liver and How It Works; Liver Diseases, Including Cancer, Cirrhosis, Hepatitis, and Toxic and Drug Related Diseases; Tips for Maintaining a Healthy Liver; Laboratory Tests, Radiology Tests, and Facts about Liver Transplantation

Along with a Section on Support Groups, a Glossary, and Resource Listings

Edited by Joyce Brennfleck Shannon. 591 pages. 2000. 978-0-7808-0383-1.

"A valuable resource."
—American Reference Books Annual, 2001

"This title is recommended for health sciences and public libraries with consumer health collections."
—E-Streams, Oct '00

"Recommended reference source."
—Booklist, American Library Association, Jun '00

Lung Disorders Sourcebook

Basic Consumer Health Information about Emphysema, Pneumonia, Tuberculosis, Asthma, Cystic Fibrosis, and Other Lung Disorders, Including Facts about Diagnostic Procedures, Treatment Strategies, Disease Prevention Efforts, and Such Risk Factors as Smoking, Air Pollution, and Exposure to Asbestos, Radon, and Other Agents

Along with a Glossary and Resources for Additional Help and Information

Edited by Dawn D. Matthews. 678 pages. 2002. 978-0-7808-0339-8.

"This title is a great addition for public and school libraries because it provides concise health information on the lungs."
—American Reference Books Annual, 2003

"Highly recommended for academic and medical reference collections." *—Library Bookwatch, Sep '02*

SEE ALSO *Respiratory Diseases & Disorders Sourcebook*

Medical Tests Sourcebook, 2nd Edition

Basic Consumer Health Information about Medical Tests, Including Age-Specific Health Tests, Important Health Screenings and Exams, Home-Use Tests, Blood and Specimen Tests, Electrical Tests, Scope Tests, Genetic Testing, and Imaging Tests, Such as X-Rays, Ultrasound, Computed Tomography, Magnetic Resonance Imaging, Angiography, and Nuclear Medicine

Along with a Glossary and Directory of Additional Resources

Edited by Joyce Brennfleck Shannon. 654 pages. 2004. 978-0-7808-0670-2.

"Recommended for hospital and health sciences

libraries with consumer health collections."
—E-Streams, Mar '00

"This is an overall excellent reference with a wealth of general knowledge that may aid those who are reluctant to get vital tests performed."
—Today's Librarian, Jan '00

"A valuable reference guide."
—American Reference Books Annual, 2000

Men's Health Concerns Sourcebook, 2nd Edition

Basic Consumer Health Information about the Medical and Mental Concerns of Men, Including Theories about the Shorter Male Lifespan, the Leading Causes of Death and Disability, Physical Concerns of Special Significance to Men, Reproductive and Sexual Concerns, Sexually Transmitted Diseases, Men's Mental and Emotional Health, and Lifestyle Choices That Affect Wellness, Such as Nutrition, Fitness, and Substance Use

Along with a Glossary of Related Terms and a Directory of Organizational Resources in Men's Health

Edited by Robert Aquinas McNally. 644 pages. 2004. 978-0-7808-0671-9.

"A very accessible reference for non-specialist general readers and consumers." *—The Bookwatch, Jun '04*

"This comprehensive resource and the series are highly recommended."
—American Reference Books Annual, 2000

"Recommended reference source."
—Booklist, American Library Association, Dec '98

Mental Health Disorders Sourcebook, 3rd Edition

Basic Consumer Health Information about Mental and Emotional Health and Mental Illness, Including Facts about Depression, Bipolar Disorder, and Other Mood Disorders, Phobias, Post-Traumatic Stress Disorder (PTSD), Obsessive-Compulsive Disorder, and Other Anxiety Disorders, Impulse Control Disorders, Eating Disorders, Personality Disorders, and Psychotic Disorders, Including Schizophrenia and Dissociative Disorders

Along with Statistical Information, a Special Section Concerning Mental Health Issues in Children and Adolescents, a Glossary, and Directories of Resources for Additional Help and Information

Edited by Karen Bellenir. 661 pages. 2005. 978-0-7808-0747-1.

"Recommended for public libraries and academic libraries with an undergraduate program in psychology."
—American Reference Books Annual, 2006

"Recommended reference source."
—Booklist, American Library Association, Jun '00

Mental Retardation Sourcebook

Basic Consumer Health Information about Mental Retardation and Its Causes, Including Down Syndrome, Fetal Alcohol Syndrome, Fragile X Syndrome, Genetic Conditions, Injury, and Environmental Sources

Along with Preventive Strategies, Parenting Issues, Educational Implications, Health Care Needs, Employment and Economic Matters, Legal Issues, a Glossary, and a Resource Listing for Additional Help and Information

Edited by Joyce Brennfleck Shannon. 642 pages. 2000. 978-0-7808-0377-0.

"Public libraries will find the book useful for reference and as a beginning research point for students, parents, and caregivers."
— American Reference Books Annual, 2001

"The strength of this work is that it compiles many basic fact sheets and addresses for further information in one volume. It is intended and suitable for the general public. This sourcebook is relevant to any collection providing health information to the general public."
— E-Streams, Nov '00

"From preventing retardation to parenting and family challenges, this covers health, social and legal issues and will prove an invaluable overview."
— Reviewer's Bookwatch, Jul '00

Movement Disorders Sourcebook

Basic Consumer Health Information about Neurological Movement Disorders, Including Essential Tremor, Parkinson's Disease, Dystonia, Cerebral Palsy, Huntington's Disease, Myasthenia Gravis, Multiple Sclerosis, and Other Early-Onset and Adult-Onset Movement Disorders, Their Symptoms and Causes, Diagnostic Tests, and Treatments

Along with Mobility and Assistive Technology Information, a Glossary, and a Directory of Additional Resources

Edited by Joyce Brennfleck Shannon. 655 pages. 2003. 978-0-7808-0628-3.

". . . a good resource for consumers and recommended for public, community college and undergraduate libraries." *— American Reference Books Annual, 2004*

Muscular Dystrophy Sourcebook

Basic Consumer Health Information about Congenital, Childhood-Onset, and Adult-Onset Forms of Muscular Dystrophy, Such as Duchenne, Becker, Emery-Dreifuss, Distal, Limb-Girdle, Facioscapulohumeral (FSHD), Myotonic, and Ophthalmoplegic Muscular Dystrophies, Including Facts about Diagnostic Tests, Medical and Physical Therapies, Management of Co-Occurring Conditions, and Parenting Guidelines

Along with Practical Tips for Home Care, a Glossary, and Directories of Additional Resources

Edited by Joyce Brennfleck Shannon. 577 pages. 2004. 978-0-7808-0676-4.

"This book is highly recommended for public and academic libraries as well as health care offices that support the information needs of patients and their families."
— E-Streams, Apr '05

"Excellent reference." *— The Bookwatch, Jan '05*

Obesity Sourcebook

Basic Consumer Health Information about Diseases and Other Problems Associated with Obesity, and Including Facts about Risk Factors, Prevention Issues, and Management Approaches

Along with Statistical and Demographic Data, Information about Special Populations, Research Updates, a Glossary, and Source Listings for Further Help and Information

Edited by Wilma Caldwell and Chad T. Kimball. 376 pages. 2001. 978-0-7808-0333-6.

"The book synthesizes the reliable medical literature on obesity into one easy-to-read and useful resource for the general public."
— American Reference Books Annual, 2002

"This is a very useful resource book for the lay public."
— Doody's Review Service, Nov '01

"Well suited for the health reference collection of a public library or an academic health science library that serves the general population." *— E-Streams, Sep '01*

"Recommended reference source."
— Booklist, American Library Association, Apr '01

"Recommended pick both for specialty health library collections and any general consumer health reference collection." *— The Bookwatch, Apr '01*

Oral Health Sourcebook

SEE Dental Care & Oral Health Sourcebook

Osteoporosis Sourcebook

Basic Consumer Health Information about Primary and Secondary Osteoporosis and Juvenile Osteoporosis and Related Conditions, Including Fibrous Dysplasia, Gaucher Disease, Hyperthyroidism, Hypophosphatasia, Myeloma, Osteopetrosis, Osteogenesis Imperfecta, and Paget's Disease

Along with Information about Risk Factors, Treatments, Traditional and Non-Traditional Pain Management, a Glossary of Related Terms, and a Directory of Resources

Edited by Allan R. Cook. 584 pages. 2001. 978-0-7808-0239-1.

"This would be a book to be kept in a staff or patient library. The targeted audience is the layperson, but the therapist who needs a quick bit of information on a particular topic will also find the book useful."
— Physical Therapy, Jan '02

"This resource is recommended as a great reference source for public, health, and academic libraries, and is another triumph for the editors of Omnigraphics."
— *American Reference Books Annual, 2002*

"Recommended for all public libraries and general health collections, especially those supporting patient education or consumer health programs."
— *E-Streams, Nov '01*

"Will prove valuable to any library seeking to maintain a current, comprehensive reference collection of health resources. . . . From prevention to treatment and associated conditions, this provides an excellent survey."
— *The Bookwatch, Aug '01*

"Recommended reference source."
— *Booklist, American Library Association, Jul '01*

SEE ALSO *Healthy Aging Sourcebook, Physical & Mental Issues in Aging Sourcebook, Women's Health Concerns Sourcebook*

■

Pain Sourcebook, 2nd Edition

Basic Consumer Health Information about Specific Forms of Acute and Chronic Pain, Including Muscle and Skeletal Pain, Nerve Pain, Cancer Pain, and Disorders Characterized by Pain, Such as Fibromyalgia, Shingles, Angina, Arthritis, and Headaches

Along with Information about Pain Medications and Management Techniques, Complementary and Alternative Pain Relief Options, Tips for People Living with Chronic Pain, a Glossary, and a Directory of Sources for Further Information

Edited by Karen Bellenir. 670 pages. 2002. 978-0-7808-0612-2.

"A source of valuable information. . . . This book offers help to nonmedical people who need information about pain and pain management. It is also an excellent reference for those who participate in patient education."
— *Doody's Review Service, Sep '02*

"Highly recommended for academic and medical reference collections."
— *Library Bookwatch, Sep '02*

"The text is readable, easily understood, and well indexed. This excellent volume belongs in all patient education libraries, consumer health sections of public libraries, and many personal collections."
— *American Reference Books Annual, 1999*

"The information is basic in terms of scholarship and is appropriate for general readers. Written in journalistic style . . . intended for non-professionals. Quite thorough in its coverage of different pain conditions and summarizes the latest clinical information regarding pain treatment."
— *Choice, Association of College and Research Libraries, Jun '98*

"Recommended reference source."
— *Booklist, American Library Association, Mar '98*

■

Pediatric Cancer Sourcebook

Basic Consumer Health Information about Leukemias, Brain Tumors, Sarcomas, Lymphomas, and Other Cancers in Infants, Children, and Adolescents, Including Descriptions of Cancers, Treatments, and Coping Strategies

Along with Suggestions for Parents, Caregivers, and Concerned Relatives, a Glossary of Cancer Terms, and Resource Listings

Edited by Edward J. Prucha. 587 pages. 1999. 978-0-7808-0245-2.

"An excellent source of information. Recommended for public, hospital, and health science libraries with consumer health collections."
— *E-Streams, Jun '00*

"Recommended reference source."
— *Booklist, American Library Association, Feb '00*

"A valuable addition to all libraries specializing in health services and many public libraries."
— *American Reference Books Annual, 2000*

SEE ALSO *Childhood Diseases & Disorders Sourcebook, Healthy Children Sourcebook*

■

Physical & Mental Issues in Aging Sourcebook

Basic Consumer Health Information on Physical and Mental Disorders Associated with the Aging Process, Including Concerns about Cardiovascular Disease, Pulmonary Disease, Oral Health, Digestive Disorders, Musculoskeletal and Skin Disorders, Metabolic Changes, Sexual and Reproductive Issues, and Changes in Vision, Hearing, and Other Senses

Along with Data about Longevity and Causes of Death, Information on Acute and Chronic Pain, Descriptions of Mental Concerns, a Glossary of Terms, and Resource Listings for Additional Help

Edited by Jenifer Swanson. 660 pages. 1999. 978-0-7808-0233-9.

"This is a treasure of health information for the layperson."
— *Choice Health Sciences Supplement, Association of College & Research Libraries, May '00*

"Recommended for public libraries."
— *American Reference Books Annual, 2000*

"Recommended reference source."
— *Booklist, American Library Association, Oct '99*

SEE ALSO *Healthy Aging Sourcebook*

■

Podiatry Sourcebook, 2nd Edition

Basic Consumer Health Information about Disorders, Diseases, Deformities, and Injuries that Affect the Foot and Ankle, Including Sprains, Corns, Calluses, Bunions, Plantar Warts, Plantar Fasciitis, Neuromas, Clubfoot, Flat Feet, Achilles Tendonitis, and Much More

Along with Information about Selecting a Foot Care Specialist, Foot Fitness, Shoes and Socks, Diagnostic Tests and Corrective Procedures, Financial Assistance for Corrective Devices, a Glossary of Related Terms, and a Directory of Resources for Additional Help and Information

Edited by Ivy L. Alexander. 543 pages. 2007. 978-0-7808-0944-4.

"Recommended reference source."
— Booklist, American Library Association, Feb '02

"There is a lot of information presented here on a topic that is usually only covered sparingly in most larger comprehensive medical encyclopedias."
— American Reference Books Annual, 2002

Pregnancy & Birth Sourcebook, 2nd Edition

Basic Consumer Health Information about Conception and Pregnancy, Including Facts about Fertility, Infertility, Pregnancy Symptoms and Complications, Fetal Growth and Development, Labor, Delivery, and the Postpartum Period, as Well as Information about Maintaining Health and Wellness during Pregnancy and Caring for a Newborn

Along with Information about Public Health Assistance for Low-Income Pregnant Women, a Glossary, and Directories of Agencies and Organizations Providing Help and Support

Edited by Amy L. Sutton. 626 pages. 2004. 978-0-7808-0672-6.

"Will appeal to public and school reference collections strong in medicine and women's health. . . . Deserves a spot on any medical reference shelf."
— The Bookwatch, Jul '04

"A well-organized handbook. Recommended."
— Choice, Association of College & Research Libraries, Apr '98

"Recommended reference source."
— Booklist, American Library Association, Mar '98

"Recommended for public libraries."
— American Reference Books Annual, 1998

SEE ALSO Breastfeeding Sourcebook, Congenital Disorders Sourcebook, Family Planning Sourcebook

Prostate & Urological Disorders Sourcebook

Basic Consumer Health Information about Urogenital and Sexual Disorders in Men, Including Prostate and Other Andrological Cancers, Prostatitis, Benign Prostatic Hyperplasia, Testicular and Penile Trauma, Cryptorchidism, Peyronie Disease, Erectile Dysfunction, and Male Factor Infertility, and Facts about Commonly Used Tests and Procedures, Such as Prostatectomy, Vasectomy, Vasectomy Reversal, Penile Implants, and Semen Analysis

Along with a Glossary of Andrological Terms and a Directory of Resources for Additional Information

Edited by Karen Bellenir. 631 pages. 2005. 978-0-7808-0797-6.

Prostate Cancer Sourcebook

Basic Consumer Health Information about Prostate Cancer, Including Information about the Associated Risk Factors, Detection, Diagnosis, and Treatment of Prostate Cancer

Along with Information on Non-Malignant Prostate Conditions, and Featuring a Section Listing Support and Treatment Centers and a Glossary of Related Terms

Edited by Dawn D. Matthews. 358 pages. 2001. 978-0-7808-0324-4.

"Recommended reference source."
— Booklist, American Library Association, Jan '02

"A valuable resource for health care consumers seeking information on the subject. . . . All text is written in a clear, easy-to-understand language that avoids technical jargon. Any library that collects consumer health resources would strengthen their collection with the addition of the Prostate Cancer Sourcebook."
— American Reference Books Annual, 2002

SEE ALSO Men's Health Concerns Sourcebook

Reconstructive & Cosmetic Surgery Sourcebook

Basic Consumer Health Information on Cosmetic and Reconstructive Plastic Surgery, Including Statistical Information about Different Surgical Procedures, Things to Consider Prior to Surgery, Plastic Surgery Techniques and Tools, Emotional and Psychological Considerations, and Procedure-Specific Information

Along with a Glossary of Terms and a Listing of Resources for Additional Help and Information

Edited by M. Lisa Weatherford. 374 pages. 2001. 978-0-7808-0214-8.

"An excellent reference that addresses cosmetic and medically necessary reconstructive surgeries. . . . The style of the prose is calm and reassuring, discussing the many positive outcomes now available due to advances in surgical techniques."
— American Reference Books Annual, 2002

"Recommended for health science libraries that are open to the public, as well as hospital libraries that are open to the patients. This book is a good resource for the consumer interested in plastic surgery."
— E-Streams, Dec '01

"Recommended reference source."
— Booklist, American Library Association, Jul '01

Rehabilitation Sourcebook

Basic Consumer Health Information about Rehabilitation for People Recovering from Heart Surgery, Spinal Cord Injury, Stroke, Orthopedic Impairments, Amputation, Pulmonary Impairments, Traumatic Injury, and More, Including Physical Therapy, Occupational Therapy, Speech/Language Therapy, Massage Therapy, Dance Therapy, Art Therapy, and Recreational Therapy

Along with Information on Assistive and Adaptive Devices, a Glossary, and Resources for Additional Help and Information

Edited by Dawn D. Matthews. 531 pages. 1999. 978-0-7808-0236-0.

"This is an excellent resource for public library reference and health collections."
— American Reference Books Annual, 2001

"Recommended reference source."
— Booklist, American Library Association, May '00

Respiratory Diseases & Disorders Sourcebook

Basic Information about Respiratory Diseases and Disorders, Including Asthma, Cystic Fibrosis, Pneumonia, the Common Cold, Influenza, and Others, Featuring Facts about the Respiratory System, Statistical and Demographic Data, Treatments, Self-Help Management Suggestions, and Current Research Initiatives

Edited by Allan R. Cook and Peter D. Dresser. 771 pages. 1995. 978-0-7808-0037-3.

"Designed for the layperson and for patients and their families coping with respiratory illness. . . . an extensive array of information on diagnosis, treatment, management, and prevention of respiratory illnesses for the general reader." — Choice, Association of College & Research Libraries, Jun '96

"A highly recommended text for all collections. It is a comforting reminder of the power of knowledge that good books carry between their covers."
— Academic Library Book Review, Spring '96

"A comprehensive collection of authoritative information presented in a nontechnical, humanitarian style for patients, families, and caregivers."
— Association of Operating Room Nurses, Sep/Oct '95

SEE ALSO Lung Disorders Sourcebook

Sexually Transmitted Diseases Sourcebook, 3rd Edition

Basic Consumer Health Information about Chlamydial Infections, Gonorrhea, Hepatitis, Herpes, HIV/AIDS, Human Papillomavirus, Pubic Lice, Scabies, Syphilis, Trichomoniasis, Vaginal Infections, and Other Sexually Transmitted Diseases, Including Facts about Risk Factors, Symptoms, Diagnosis, Treatment, and the Prevention of Sexually Transmitted Infections

Along with Updates on Current Research Initiatives, a Glossary of Related Terms, and Resources for Additional Help and Information

Edited by Amy L. Sutton. 629 pages. 2006. 978-0-7808-0824-9.

"Recommended for consumer health collections in public libraries, and secondary school and community college libraries."
— American Reference Books Annual, 2002

"Every school and public library should have a copy of this comprehensive and user-friendly reference book."
— Choice, Association of College & Research Libraries, Sep '01

"This is a highly recommended book. This is an especially important book for all school and public libraries."
— AIDS Book Review Journal, Jul-Aug '01

"Recommended reference source."
— Booklist, American Library Association, Apr '01

Sleep Disorders Sourcebook, 2nd Edition

Basic Consumer Health Information about Sleep and Sleep Disorders, Including Insomnia, Sleep Apnea, Restless Legs Syndrome, Narcolepsy, Parasomnias, and Other Health Problems That Affect Sleep, Plus Facts about Diagnostic Procedures, Treatment Strategies, Sleep Medications, and Tips for Improving Sleep Quality

Along with a Glossary of Related Terms and Resources for Additional Help and Information

Edited by Amy L. Sutton. 567 pages. 2005. 978-0-7808-0743-3.

"This book will be useful for just about everybody, especially the 40 million Americans with sleep disorders."
— American Reference Books Annual, 2006

"Recommended for public libraries and libraries supporting health care professionals." — E-Streams, Sep '05

". . . key medical library acquisition."
— The Bookwatch, Jun '05

Smoking Concerns Sourcebook

Basic Consumer Health Information about Nicotine Addiction and Smoking Cessation, Featuring Facts about the Health Effects of Tobacco Use, Including Lung and Other Cancers, Heart Disease, Stroke, and Respiratory Disorders, Such as Emphysema and Chronic Bronchitis

Along with Information about Smoking Prevention Programs, Suggestions for Achieving and Maintaining a Smoke-Free Lifestyle, Statistics about Tobacco Use, Reports on Current Research Initiatives, a Glossary of Related Terms, and Directories of Resources for Additional Help and Information

Edited by Karen Bellenir. 621 pages. 2004. 978-0-7808-0323-7.

"Provides everything needed for the student or general reader seeking practical details on the effects of tobacco use." — The Bookwatch, Mar '05

"Public libraries and consumer health care libraries will find this work useful."
— American Reference Books Annual, 2005

Sports Injuries Sourcebook, 3rd Edition

Basic Consumer Health Information about Sprains and Strains, Fractures, Growth Plate Injuries, Overtraining Injuries, and Injuries to the Head, Face, Shoulders, Elbows, Hands, Spinal Column, Knees, Ankles, and Feet, and with Facts about Heat-Related Illness, Steroids and Sport Supplements, Protective Equipment, Diagnostic Procedures, Treatment Options, and Rehabilitation

Along with a Glossary of Related Terms and a Directory of Resources for Additional Help and Information

Edited by Sandra J. Judd. 651 pages. 2007. 978-0-7808-0949-9.

"This is an excellent reference for consumers and it is recommended for public, community college, and undergraduate libraries."
— *American Reference Books Annual, 2003*

"Recommended reference source."
— *Booklist, American Library Association, Feb '03*

■

Stress-Related Disorders Sourcebook

Basic Consumer Health Information about Stress and Stress-Related Disorders, Including Stress Origins and Signals, Environmental Stress at Work and Home, Mental and Emotional Stress Associated with Depression, Post-Traumatic Stress Disorder, Panic Disorder, Suicide, and the Physical Effects of Stress on the Cardiovascular, Immune, and Nervous Systems

Along with Stress Management Techniques, a Glossary, and a Listing of Additional Resources

Edited by Joyce Brennfleck Shannon. 610 pages. 2002. 978-0-7808-0560-6.

"Well written for a general readership, the *Stress-Related Disorders Sourcebook* is a useful addition to the health reference literature."
— *American Reference Books Annual, 2003*

"I am impressed by the amount of information. It offers a thorough overview of the causes and consequences of stress for the layperson. . . . A well-done and thorough reference guide for professionals and nonprofessionals alike." — *Doody's Review Service, Dec '02*

■

Stroke Sourcebook

Basic Consumer Health Information about Stroke, Including Ischemic, Hemorrhagic, Transient Ischemic Attack (TIA), and Pediatric Stroke, Stroke Triggers and Risks, Diagnostic Tests, Treatments, and Rehabilitation Information

Along with Stroke Prevention Guidelines, Legal and Financial Information, a Glossary, and a Directory of Additional Resources

Edited by Joyce Brennfleck Shannon. 606 pages. 2003. 978-0-7808-0630-6.

"This volume is highly recommended and should be in every medical, hospital, and public library."
— *American Reference Books Annual, 2004*

"Highly recommended for the amount and variety of topics and information covered." — *Choice, Nov '03*

■

Surgery Sourcebook

Basic Consumer Health Information about Inpatient and Outpatient Surgeries, Including Cardiac, Vascular, Orthopedic, Ocular, Reconstructive, Cosmetic, Gynecologic, and Ear, Nose, and Throat Procedures and More

Along with Information about Operating Room Policies and Instruments, Laser Surgery Techniques, Hospital Errors, Statistical Data, a Glossary, and Listings of Sources for Further Help and Information

Edited by Annemarie S. Muth and Karen Bellenir. 596 pages. 2002. 978-0-7808-0380-0.

"Large public libraries and medical libraries would benefit from this material in their reference collections."
— *American Reference Books Annual, 2004*

"Invaluable reference for public and school library collections alike." — *Library Bookwatch, Apr '03*

■

Thyroid Disorders Sourcebook

Basic Consumer Health Information about Disorders of the Thyroid and Parathyroid Glands, Including Hypothyroidism, Hyperthyroidism, Graves Disease, Hashimoto Thyroiditis, Thyroid Cancer, and Parathyroid Disorders, Featuring Facts about Symptoms, Risk Factors, Tests, and Treatments

Along with Information about the Effects of Thyroid Imbalance on Other Body Systems, Environmental Factors That Affect the Thyroid Gland, a Glossary, and a Directory of Additional Resources

Edited by Joyce Brennfleck Shannon. 599 pages. 2005. 978-0-7808-0745-7.

"Recommended for consumer health collections."
— *American Reference Books Annual, 2006*

"Highly recommended pick for basic consumer health reference holdings at all levels."
— *The Bookwatch, Aug '05*

■

Transplantation Sourcebook

Basic Consumer Health Information about Organ and Tissue Transplantation, Including Physical and Financial Preparations, Procedures and Issues Relating to Specific Solid Organ and Tissue Transplants, Rehabilitation, Pediatric Transplant Information, the Future of Transplantation, and Organ and Tissue Donation

Along with a Glossary and Listings of Additional Resources

Edited by Joyce Brennfleck Shannon. 628 pages. 2002. 978-0-7808-0322-0.

639

"Along with these advances [in transplantation technology] have come a number of daunting questions for potential transplant patients, their families, and their health care providers. This reference text is the best single tool to address many of these questions. . . . It will be a much-needed addition to the reference collections in health care, academic, and large public libraries."
— *American Reference Books Annual, 2003*

"Recommended for libraries with an interest in offering consumer health information."   — *E-Streams, Jul '02*

"This is a unique and valuable resource for patients facing transplantation and their families."
— *Doody's Review Service, Jun '02*

■

Traveler's Health Sourcebook

Basic Consumer Health Information for Travelers, Including Physical and Medical Preparations, Transportation Health and Safety, Essential Information about Food and Water, Sun Exposure, Insect and Snake Bites, Camping and Wilderness Medicine, and Travel with Physical or Medical Disabilities

Along with International Travel Tips, Vaccination Recommendations, Geographical Health Issues, Disease Risks, a Glossary, and a Listing of Additional Resources

Edited by Joyce Brennfleck Shannon. 613 pages. 2000. 978-0-7808-0384-8.

"Recommended reference source."
–*Booklist, American Library Association, Feb '01*

"This book is recommended for any public library, any travel collection, and especially any collection for the physically disabled."
— *American Reference Books Annual, 2001*

SEE ALSO *Worldwide Health Sourcebook*

■

Urinary Tract & Kidney Diseases & Disorders Sourcebook, 2nd Edition

Basic Consumer Health Information about the Urinary System, Including the Bladder, Urethra, Ureters, and Kidneys, with Facts about Urinary Tract Infections, Incontinence, Congenital Disorders, Kidney Stones, Cancers of the Urinary Tract and Kidneys, Kidney Failure, Dialysis, and Kidney Transplantation

Along with Statistical and Demographic Information, Reports on Current Research in Kidney and Urologic Health, a Summary of Commonly Used Diagnostic Tests, a Glossary of Related Terms, and a Directory of Resources for Additional Help and Information

Edited by Ivy L. Alexander. 649 pages. 2005. 978-0-7808-0750-1.

"A good choice for a consumer health information library or for a medical library needing information to refer to their patients."
— *American Reference Books Annual, 2006*

Vegetarian Sourcebook

Basic Consumer Health Information about Vegetarian Diets, Lifestyle, and Philosophy, Including Definitions of Vegetarianism and Veganism, Tips about Adopting Vegetarianism, Creating a Vegetarian Pantry, and Meeting Nutritional Needs of Vegetarians, with Facts Regarding Vegetarianism's Effect on Pregnant and Lactating Women, Children, Athletes, and Senior Citizens

Along with a Glossary of Commonly Used Vegetarian Terms and Resources for Additional Help and Information

Edited by Chad T. Kimball. 360 pages. 2002. 978-0-7808-0439-5.

"Organizes into one concise volume the answers to the most common questions concerning vegetarian diets and lifestyles. This title is recommended for public and secondary school libraries."   — *E-Streams, Apr '03*

"Invaluable reference for public and school library collections alike."   — *Library Bookwatch, Apr '03*

"The articles in this volume are easy to read and come from authoritative sources. The book does not necessarily support the vegetarian diet but instead provides the pros and cons of this important decision. The Vegetarian Sourcebook is recommended for public libraries and consumer health libraries."
— *American Reference Books Annual, 2003*

SEE ALSO *Diet & Nutrition Sourcebook*

■

Women's Health Concerns Sourcebook, 2nd Edition

Basic Consumer Health Information about the Medical and Mental Concerns of Women, Including Maintaining Health and Wellness, Gynecological Concerns, Breast Health, Sexuality and Reproductive Issues, Menopause, Cancer in Women, Leading Causes of Death and Disability among Women, Physical Concerns of Special Significance to Women, and Women's Mental and Emotional Health

Along with a Glossary of Related Terms and Directories of Resources for Additional Help and Information

Edited by Amy L. Sutton. 746 pages. 2004. 978-0-7808-0673-3.

"This is a useful reference book, which makes the reader knowledgeable about several issues that concern women's health. It is recommended for public libraries and home library collections."   — *E-Streams, May '05*

"A useful addition to public and consumer health library collections."
— *American Reference Books Annual, 2005*

"A highly recommended title."
— *The Bookwatch, May '04*

"Handy compilation. There is an impressive range of diseases, devices, disorders, procedures, and other physical and emotional issues covered . . . well organized, illustrated, and indexed."   — *Choice, Association of College & Research Libraries, Jan '98*

640

SEE ALSO *Breast Cancer Sourcebook, Cancer Sourcebook for Women, Healthy Heart Sourcebook for Women, Osteoporosis Sourcebook*

■

Workplace Health & Safety Sourcebook

Basic Consumer Health Information about Workplace Health and Safety, Including the Effect of Workplace Hazards on the Lungs, Skin, Heart, Ears, Eyes, Brain, Reproductive Organs, Musculoskeletal System, and Other Organs and Body Parts

Along with Information about Occupational Cancer, Personal Protective Equipment, Toxic and Hazardous Chemicals, Child Labor, Stress, and Workplace Violence

Edited by Chad T. Kimball. 626 pages. 2000. 978-0-7808-0231-5.

"As a reference for the general public, this would be useful in any library." — *E-Streams, Jun '01*

"Provides helpful information for primary care physicians and other caregivers interested in occupational medicine. . . . General readers; professionals."
— *Choice, Association of College & Research Libraries, May '01*

"Recommended reference source."
— *Booklist, American Library Association, Feb '01*

"Highly recommended." — *The Bookwatch, Jan '01*

■

Worldwide Health Sourcebook

Basic Information about Global Health Issues, Including Malnutrition, Reproductive Health, Disease Dispersion and Prevention, Emerging Diseases, Risky Health Behaviors, and the Leading Causes of Death

Along with Global Health Concerns for Children, Women, and the Elderly, Mental Health Issues, Research and Technology Advancements, and Economic, Environmental, and Political Health Implications, a Glossary, and a Resource Listing for Additional Help and Information

Edited by Joyce Brennfleck Shannon. 614 pages. 2001. 978-0-7808-0330-5.

"Named an Outstanding Academic Title."
— *Choice, Association of College & Research Libraries, Jan '02*

"Yet another handy but also unique compilation in the extensive *Health Reference Series*, this is a useful work because many of the international publications reprinted or excerpted are not readily available. Highly recommended." — *Choice, Association of College & Research Libraries, Nov '01*

"Recommended reference source."
— *Booklist, American Library Association, Oct '01*

SEE ALSO *Traveler's Health Sourcebook*

Teen Health Series
Helping Young Adults Understand, Manage, and Avoid Serious Illness

List price $65 per volume. **School and library price $58 per volume.**

Alcohol Information for Teens
Health Tips about Alcohol and Alcoholism

Including Facts about Underage Drinking, Preventing Teen Alcohol Use, Alcohol's Effects on the Brain and the Body, Alcohol Abuse Treatment, Help for Children of Alcoholics, and More

Edited by Joyce Brennfleck Shannon. 370 pages. 2005. 978-0-7808-0741-9.

"Boxed facts and tips add visual interest to the well-researched and clearly written text."
— *Curriculum Connection, Apr '06*

Allergy Information for Teens
Health Tips about Allergic Reactions Such as Anaphylaxis, Respiratory Problems, and Rashes

Including Facts about Identifying and Managing Allergies to Food, Pollen, Mold, Animals, Chemicals, Drugs, and Other Substances

Edited by Karen Bellenir. 410 pages. 2006. 978-0-7808-0799-0.

Asthma Information for Teens
Health Tips about Managing Asthma and Related Concerns

Including Facts about Asthma Causes, Triggers, Symptoms, Diagnosis, and Treatment

Edited by Karen Bellenir. 386 pages. 2005. 978-0-7808-0770-9.

"Highly recommended for medical libraries, public school libraries, and public libraries."
— *American Reference Books Annual, 2006*

"It is so clearly written and well organized that even hesitant readers will be able to find the facts they need, whether for reports or personal information. . . . A succinct but complete resource."
— *School Library Journal, Sep '05*

Body Information for Teens
Health Tips about Maintaining Well-Being for a Lifetime

Including Facts about the Development and Functioning of the Body's Systems, Organs, and Structures and the Health Impact of Lifestyle Choices

Edited by Sandra Augustyn Lawton. 458 pages. 2007. 978-0-7808-0443-2.

Cancer Information for Teens
Health Tips about Cancer Awareness, Prevention, Diagnosis, and Treatment

Including Facts about Frequently Occurring Cancers, Cancer Risk Factors, and Coping Strategies for Teens Fighting Cancer or Dealing with Cancer in Friends or Family Members

Edited by Wilma R. Caldwell. 428 pages. 2004. 978-0-7808-0678-8.

"Recommended for school libraries, or consumer libraries that see a lot of use by teens."
— *E-Streams, May '05*

"A valuable educational tool."
— *American Reference Books Annual, 2005*

"Young adults and their parents alike will find this new addition to the *Teen Health Series* an important reference to cancer in teens."
— *Children's Bookwatch, Feb '05*

Complementary and Alternative Medicine Information for Teens
Health Tips about Non-Traditional and Non-Western Medical Practices

Including Information about Acupuncture, Chiropractic Medicine, Dietary and Herbal Supplements, Hypnosis, Massage Therapy, Prayer and Spirituality, Reflexology, Yoga, and More

Edited by Sandra Augustyn Lawton. 405 pages. 2006. 978-0-7808-0966-6.

Diabetes Information for Teens
Health Tips about Managing Diabetes and Preventing Related Complications

Including Information about Insulin, Glucose Control, Healthy Eating, Physical Activity, and Learning to Live with Diabetes

Edited by Sandra Augustyn Lawton. 410 pages. 2006. 978-0-7808-0811-9.

Diet Information for Teens, 2nd Edition

Health Tips about Diet and Nutrition

Including Facts about Dietary Guidelines, Food Groups, Nutrients, Healthy Meals, Snacks, Weight Control, Medical Concerns Related to Diet, and More

Edited by Karen Bellenir. 432 pages. 2006. 978-0-7808-0820-1.

"Full of helpful insights and facts throughout the book. ... An excellent resource to be placed in public libraries or even in personal collections."
— *American Reference Books Annual, 2002*

"Recommended for middle and high school libraries and media centers as well as academic libraries that educate future teachers of teenagers. It is also a suitable addition to health science libraries that serve patrons who are interested in teen health promotion and education."
— *E-Streams, Oct '01*

"This comprehensive book would be beneficial to collections that need information about nutrition, dietary guidelines, meal planning, and weight control. ... This reference is so easy to use that its purchase is recommended."
— *The Book Report, Sep-Oct '01*

"This book is written in an easy to understand format describing issues that many teens face every day, and then provides thoughtful explanations so that teens can make informed decisions. This is an interesting book that provides important facts and information for today's teens."
— *Doody's Health Sciences Book Review Journal, Jul-Aug '01*

"A comprehensive compendium of diet and nutrition. The information is presented in a straightforward, plain-spoken manner. This title will be useful to those working on reports on a variety of topics, as well as to general readers concerned about their dietary health."
— *School Library Journal, Jun '01*

Drug Information for Teens, 2nd Edition

Health Tips about the Physical and Mental Effects of Substance Abuse

Including Information about Marijuana, Inhalants, Club Drugs, Stimulants, Hallucinogens, Opiates, Prescription and Over-the-Counter Drugs, Herbal Products, Tobacco, Alcohol, and More

Edited by Sandra Augustyn Lawton. 468 pages. 2006. 978-0-7808-0862-1.

"A clearly written resource for general readers and researchers alike."
— *School Library Journal*

"This book is well-balanced. ... a must for public and school libraries."
— *VOYA: Voice of Youth Advocates, Dec '03*

"The chapters are quick to make a connection to their teenage reading audience. The prose is straightforward and the book lends itself to spot reading. It should be useful both for practical information and for research, and it is suitable for public and school libraries."
— *American Reference Books Annual, 2003*

"Recommended reference source."
— *Booklist, American Library Association, Feb '03*

"This is an excellent resource for teens and their parents. Education about drugs and substances is key to discouraging teen drug abuse and this book provides this much needed information in a way that is interesting and factual."
— *Doody's Review Service, Dec '02*

Eating Disorders Information for Teens

Health Tips about Anorexia, Bulimia, Binge Eating, and Other Eating Disorders

Including Information on the Causes, Prevention, and Treatment of Eating Disorders, and Such Other Issues as Maintaining Healthy Eating and Exercise Habits

Edited by Sandra Augustyn Lawton. 337 pages. 2005. 978-0-7808-0783-9.

"An excellent resource for teens and those who work with them."
— *VOYA: Voice of Youth Advocates, Apr '06*

"A welcome addition to high school and undergraduate libraries." — *American Reference Books Annual, 2006*

"This book covers the topic in a lucid manner but delves deeper into every aspect of an eating disorder. A solid addition for any nonfiction or reference collection."
— *School Library Journal, Dec '05*

Fitness Information for Teens

Health Tips about Exercise, Physical Well-Being, and Health Maintenance

Including Facts about Aerobic and Anaerobic Conditioning, Stretching, Body Shape and Body Image, Sports Training, Nutrition, and Activities for Non-Athletes

Edited by Karen Bellenir. 425 pages. 2004. 978-0-7808-0679-5.

"Another excellent offering from Omnigraphics in their *Teen Health Series*. ... This book will be a great addition to any public, junior high, senior high, or secondary school library."
— *American Reference Books Annual, 2005*

Learning Disabilities Information for Teens

Health Tips about Academic Skills Disorders and Other Disabilities That Affect Learning

Including Information about Common Signs of Learning Disabilities, School Issues, Learning to Live with a Learning Disability, and Other Related Issues

Edited by Sandra Augustyn Lawton. 337 pages. 2005. 978-0-7808-0796-9.

"This book provides a wealth of information for any reader interested in the signs, causes, and consequences

of learning disabilities, as well as related legal rights and educational interventions. . . . Public and academic libraries should want this title for both students and general readers."
— *American Reference Books Annual, 2006*

Mental Health Information for Teens, 2nd Edition
Health Tips about Mental Wellness and Mental Illness

Including Facts about Mental and Emotional Health, Depression and Other Mood Disorders, Anxiety Disorders, Behavior Disorders, Self-Injury, Psychosis, Schizophrenia, and More

Edited by Karen Bellenir. 400 pages. 2006. 978-0-7808-0863-8.

"In both language and approach, this user-friendly entry in the *Teen Health Series* is on target for teens needing information on mental health concerns."
— *Booklist, American Library Association, Jan '02*

"Readers will find the material accessible and informative, with the shaded notes, facts, and embedded glossary insets adding appropriately to the already interesting and succinct presentation."
— *School Library Journal, Jan '02*

"This title is highly recommended for any library that serves adolescents and parents/caregivers of adolescents."
— *E-Streams, Jan '02*

"Recommended for high school libraries and young adult collections in public libraries. Both health professionals and teenagers will find this book useful."
— *American Reference Books Annual, 2002*

"This is a nice book written to enlighten the society, primarily teenagers, about common teen mental health issues. It is highly recommended to teachers and parents as well as adolescents."
— *Doody's Review Service, Dec '01*

Sexual Health Information for Teens
Health Tips about Sexual Development, Human Reproduction, and Sexually Transmitted Diseases

Including Facts about Puberty, Reproductive Health, Chlamydia, Human Papillomavirus, Pelvic Inflammatory Disease, Herpes, AIDS, Contraception, Pregnancy, and More

Edited by Deborah A. Stanley. 391 pages. 2003. 978-0-7808-0445-6.

"This work should be included in all high school libraries and many larger public libraries. . . . highly recommended."
— *American Reference Books Annual, 2004*

"*Sexual Health* approaches its subject with appropriate seriousness and offers easily accessible advice and information."
— *School Library Journal, Feb '04*

Skin Health Information for Teens
Health Tips about Dermatological Concerns and Skin Cancer Risks

Including Facts about Acne, Warts, Hives, and Other Conditions and Lifestyle Choices, Such as Tanning, Tattooing, and Piercing, That Affect the Skin, Nails, Scalp, and Hair

Edited by Robert Aquinas McNally. 429 pages. 2003. 978-0-7808-0446-3.

"This volume, as with others in the series, will be a useful addition to school and public library collections."
— *American Reference Books Annual, 2004*

"There is no doubt that this reference tool is valuable."
— *VOYA: Voice of Youth Advocates, Feb '04*

"This volume serves as a one-stop source and should be a necessity for any health collection."
— *Library Media Connection*

Sports Injuries Information for Teens
Health Tips about Sports Injuries and Injury Protection

Including Facts about Specific Injuries, Emergency Treatment, Rehabilitation, Sports Safety, Competition Stress, Fitness, Sports Nutrition, Steroid Risks, and More

Edited by Joyce Brennfleck Shannon. 405 pages. 2003. 978-0-7808-0447-0.

"This work will be useful in the young adult collections of public libraries as well as high school libraries."
— *American Reference Books Annual, 2004*

Suicide Information for Teens
Health Tips about Suicide Causes and Prevention

Including Facts about Depression, Risk Factors, Getting Help, Survivor Support, and More

Edited by Joyce Brennfleck Shannon. 368 pages. 2005. 978-0-7808-0737-2.

Tobacco Information for Teens
Health Tips about the Hazards of Using Cigarettes, Smokeless Tobacco, and Other Nicotine Products

Including Facts about Nicotine Addiction, Immediate and Long-Term Health Effects of Tobacco Use, Related Cancers, Smoking Cessation, Tobacco Use Prevention, and Tobacco Use Statistics

Edited by Karen Bellenir. 440 pages. 2007. 978-0-7808-0976-5.